Foundations for Health, Science and Sport in Aotearoa New Zealand

Hauora Māori and Environment MAOH501

Health and Environment HEAL504

Lifespan Development and Communication HEAL507

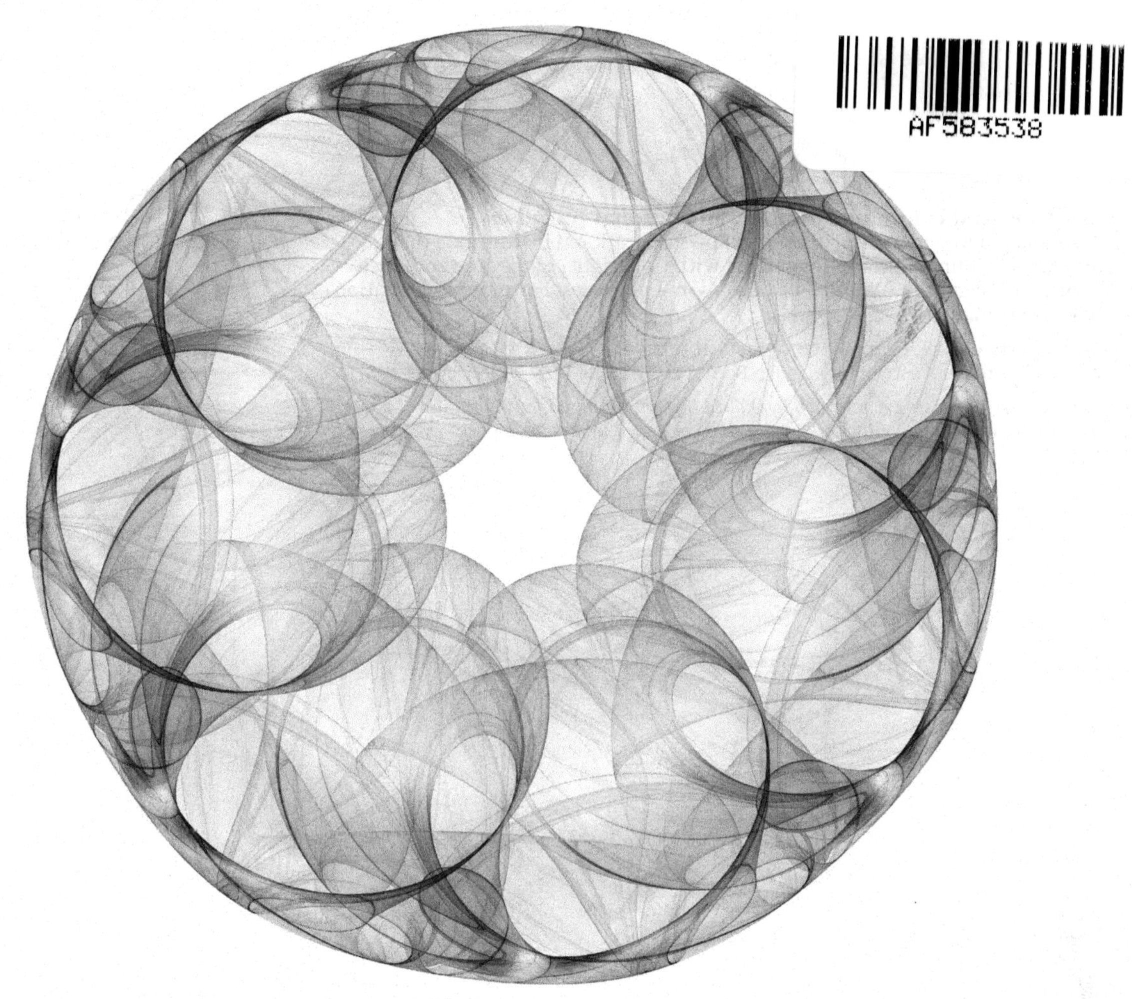

OXFORD

OXFORD
UNIVERSITY PRESS

Oxford University Press is a department of the University of Oxford.

It furthers the University's objective of excellence in research, scholarship, and education by publishing worldwide. Oxford is a registered trademark of Oxford University Press in the UK and in certain other countries.

Published in Australia by
Oxford University Press
Level 8, 737 Bourke Street, Docklands, Victoria 3008, Australia.

First published 2020(D)

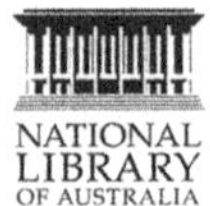

A catalogue record for this book is available from the National Library of Australia

ISBN 9780190326364

Typeset by Kerry Cooke, eggplant communications
Printed and bound in Australia by Ligare Book Printers Pty Ltd

About This Publication

The following Oxford University Press textbooks have been used in this publication:

- Shaw, S., White, L.W., and Deed, B. 2013, *Health, Wellbeing and Environment in Aotearoa New Zealand*, Oxford University Press, Melbourne.
- Shaw, S., Haxell, A., and Weblemoe, T. 2012, *Communication across the Lifespan*, Oxford University Press, Melbourne.
- Durie, M. 2001, *Mauri Ora: The Dynamics of Māori Health*, Oxford University Press, Melbourne.
- Belgrave, M., Kawharu, M., and Williams, D., 2011, *Waitangi Revisited: Perspectives on the Treaty of Waitangi*, Oxford University Press, Melbourne.
- Durie M. 2011, *Whaiora: Māori Health Development 2nd edition*, Oxford University Press, Melbourne.

Pagination, running headers and footers, and cross-references

The pages from the source books have not been altered, except as follows:

- The first page of each chapter/reading gives the reading number for this custom publication, rather than the chapter number from the original publication.
- A shaded strip along the bottom of each page gives information specific to this publication—the page number for this publication, the topic number and name, the reading number and name, and the name/s of the author/s of the reading.

The running headers come from the original publications and contain the page numbers from the original publications. Any cross-references within the chapters refer to the text of the original publications.

Contents

READING 1

A Māori Worldview

ROBERT HOGG

CHAPTER OVERVIEW

This chapter covers the following topics:

- Tīmatanga kōrero (Introduction)
- Tautuhitia te kupu Māori (Defining the word Māori)
- Toi i te āhua o Te Āo Māori whakaaro (Describing a Māori worldview)
- Ētahi mātāpono whakamiramira (Some important principles)
- Toi i te āhua o te ahurea (Describing culture)
- Toi i te āhua o nga āhuatanga Māori (Describing Māori cultural constructs)
- Te kōrero ōrokotīmatanga (The Māori creation story)
- Āhuatanga Māori (Māori cultural constructs)
- Te Āo Hurihuri (The changing world)
- Kupu Whakatepe (Conclusions)

KEY TERMS

Āhuatanga Māori
Aroha
Colonisation
Haka
Iwi
Kaitiakitanga
Karakia
Kaumātua
Kaupapa Māori
Kawa
Kotahitanga
Mana
Mana Atua
Mana Tangata
Mana Whenua
Manaaki
Māori
Marae
Mauri
Mihimihi
Pono
Tā moko

(cont.)

Taonga tuku iho	Te Tiriti o Waitangi
Tapu	Tika
Te Āo Hurihuri	Tikanga
Te Āo Māori	Tino rangatiratanga
Te Āo Māori whakaaro	Waiata
Te Āo Mārama	Whakairo
Te Kōhanga Reo	Whakapapa
Te Kōrero Ōrokotīmatanga	Whakawhānaungatanga
Te Kura Kaupapa	Whānau
Te reo Māori	Whare
Te reo Rangatira	Wharenui

This chapter aims to unpack 'a' **Te Āo Māori whakaaro** (Māori worldview). So to begin this process, it is essential to start with a **mihimihi** (a speech of greeting):

Tēnei au, tēnei au	*Here I am, here I am*
Tēnei au te hōkai nei i taku tapuwae	*Here are my footprints moving swiftly*
Ko te hōkai nuku	*Swiftly over the earth*
Ko te hōkai rangi	*Swiftly through the heavens*
Ko te hōkai ō tō tupuna, ā Tānenuiārangi	*Like the swift movements of your ancestor, Tānenuiārangi*
I pikitia ai ki te Rangi tūhāhā	*Who climbed to the heavens*
Ki Tihi i Manono	*To the summit of Manono*
I rokohina atu rā, ko Io-Matua-Kore anake	*There he found, Io-the-Parentless-one alone*
I riro iho ai	*[Tāne] the one that brought back down*
Ngā kete o te wānanga	*The baskets of knowledge*
Ko te kete Tuauri	*The basket called Tuauri*
Ko te kete Tuatea	*The basket called Tuatea*
Ko te kete Aronui	*The basket called Aronui*
Ka tiritiria, ka poupoua, ki ā Papatūānuku	*To be planted, upright, in Mother Earth*
Ka puta te ira tangata	*Then came forth the life principle of Māori*
Ki te whaiāo, ki Te Āo Mārama	*Into the dawn, into the world of life and light*
Tihei Mauri Ora!	*I sneeze, there is life!*
Ko Mataatua te waka	*Mataatua is the ancestral canoe*
Ko Putauaki te maunga	*Putauaki is the ancestral mountain*

Ko Rangitaiki te awa	*Rangitaiki is the ancestral river*
Ko Ngāti Awa te iwi	*Ngāti Awa is the tribe*
Ko Te Pahipoto te hapū	*Te Pahipoto is the sub-tribe*
Ko Robert Hogg tōku ingoa	*My name is Robert Hogg*
E kore au e ngaro	*I will not be lost*
He kākano i ruia mai i Rangiātea	*I am a seed sown from Rangiātea*
Tuatahi, ngā mihi ki a Io-Matua-Kore	*Firstly, acknowledgements to Io-Matua-Kore*
Tuarua, kei te mihi ki a Ranginui e tu iho nei	*Secondly, acknowledgements to the Sky father above*
Me te whāea e tākato mai ra, a Papatūānuku	*And to the Earth mother that lies below*
Tēnā kōrua, tēnā kōrua, tēnā kōrua	*Greetings to you both*
Nga maharatanga ki ngā tini mate	*We remember the many dead*
Kua wheturangitia	*That shine like stars*
Nō reira, hāere, hāere, hāere atu rā	*Farewell, farewell, go forth*
Hāere ki Hawaiki, ki *Hawaiki nui*	Depart to Hawaiki, to the *great Hawaiki*
Ki *Hawaiki roa*, ki *Hawaiki* pāmamāo	*To the long Hawaiki, to the distant Hawaiki*
Hāere ki te kāinga tūturu	*Go to the true resting place*
I waihotia mō te tangata	*Reserved for Māori*
Āpiti hono tātai hono	*The lines are joined*
Te hunga mate ki te hunga mate	*The dead to the dead*
Āpiti hono tātai hono	*The lines are joined*
Te hunga ora ki te hunga ora	*The living to the living*
Kei te mihi ki a koutou, ngā rangatira mo āpōpō	*Greetings to you, the future leaders*
Kia ū ki te tohu o tēnei whakataukī	*Take heed of the advice of this proverb*
Whāia te iti kahurangi	*Pursue that which is precious*
ki te tuohu koe, me he maunga teitei	*But if you should fail, let it be to a lofty mountain*
Ināianei, me huri ahau ki nga hau e wha	*At present, I turn to the four winds*
Tēnā koutou, tēnā koutou, tēnā koutou katoa.	*Greetings, greetings, greetings to all.*

Mihimihi is an important **Māori** practice (O'Connor & MacFarlane, 2002) that allows Māori, among many other things, the ability to express a sense of belonging and identity (Barlow, 1991). To recite one's pepeha (maxim) is to affiliate to the tribal strata of waka (ancestral canoe), maunga (ancestral mountain), awa (ancestral river), **iwi** (tribe), hapū (sub-tribe) and **whānau** (family) (Papakura, 1986). The narration of pepeha is essential, as it provides an opportunity for individuals not only to connect physically kanohi ki te kanohi (face to face), but also spiritually wairua ki te wairua (spirit to spirit), through a shared **whakapapa** (genealogy). In effect, mihimihi formally acknowledges the cosmos and everything within it, past, present and future, and finally sets the context. It is then essential and appropriate for me as the kaituhi (author) to have opened this chapter with a mihimihi. I did this by starting with a tauparapara (incantation), which depicts one of the many exploits of Tānenuiārangi or Tāne (God of the forest and all that dwell therein), who ascended to the uppermost heaven, Manono, where he received the baskets of knowledge from Io-Matua-Kore. Equipped with this knowledge, Tāne returned to Earth and created Māori.

It is through this very adventure that Tāne is attributed as being the progenitor of Māori. At some stage during a mihimihi (usually towards the beginning), the kaikōrero (speaker) will say the words 'Tihei Mauri Ora', which when translated means 'I sneeze, there is life'. The significance of this phrase is likened to the first sneeze that a newborn baby makes as he or she takes his or her very first breath, symbolising an arrival to **Te Āo Mārama** (the world of life and light). During a mihimihi, the kaikōrero uses this phrase to announce that he is about to speak, as he is present with life. When introducing oneself, it is uncommon for Māori to begin with the family name, as we would not exist without the voyaging encounters of our tūpuna (ancestors). So my pepeha begins by citing my Polynesian lineage to the ancestral canoe Mataatua, which transported my tūpuna to Aotearoa (New Zealand) from Hawaiiki (the ancestral home of Māori). I further reference to the ancestral mountain Putauaki, a majestic and proud entity that provides shelter, food and protection for its people; the awa, Rangitaiki that provides water, food and land access for its people; and finally the people who form my iwi, Ngāti Awa, and hapū, Te Pahipoto. I mention my name last to acknowledge that my immediate whānau is the smallest political unit within the wider Māori social grouping (Papuni & Bartlett, 2006). I then finish my pepeha with the whakataukī (proverb) 'e kore au e ngaro, he kākano i ruia mai i Rangiātea', which when translated means 'I will not be lost, I am a seed sown from Rangiātea'.

As mentioned previously, it was Tāne that acquired ngā kete o te wānanga (the baskets of knowledge), which in turn were the catalysts for the creation of Māori. However, the tauparapara does not indicate 'where' in Manono the baskets were retrieved. It is thought that each basket was suspended in a **whare** (building) called Rangiātea. Many Māori believe that Rangiātea was the very first whare wānanga (higher place of learning) for Māori. I make special reference to this whakataukī, as it begins to unpack Māori ontology and epistemology through whakapapa, and the attainment of knowledge, for it is whakapapa that ensures a sense of identity, belonging and safety.

I continue by paying homage to Io-Matua-Kore, Ranginui (sky father) and Papatūānuku (Earth mother), as an acknowledgment of our whakapapa connection to the spiritual realm. I then remember those loved ones that have passed on, and have returned to the ancestral home of Māori, Hawaiki. I then acknowledge you, the leaders of tomorrow and through the words of the whakataukī, I encourage you to strive for excellence in everything you attempt, and if you are unsuccessful, let it be to a challenge that is unconquerable. I then finish by making reference to the four winds, which is acknowledging North, East, South and West by welcoming one and all. So, welcome, welcome, welcome.

TĪMATANGA KŌRERO (INTRODUCTION)

The purpose of this chapter is to unpack the complexities of 'a' Te Āo Māori whakaaro. To begin, the term 'Māori' will be defined to outline the social hierarchical structure of Māori, and to position the author. Next, the key principles that describe 'a' Te Āo Māori whakaaro will be discussed, followed by an explanation of some important principles, that in part aim to provide a deeper and richer understanding of some important Māori concepts. The term 'culture' will then be defined to contextualise the Māori cultural constructs that aim to describe and define 'a' Te Āo Māori whakaaro. The Māori creation story has been included as a platform to discuss the meaning of the cultural constructs whakapapa, whānau and **whakawhānaungatanga** that begin to describe and define Māori identity. Finally, the author will attempt to weave together the literature and his own personal narratives, in an effort to provide a personalised understanding of 'a' Te Āo Māori whakaaro.

TAUTUHITIA TE KUPU MĀORI (DEFINING THE WORD MĀORI)

It is now timely to define the word 'Māori'. I'd like to start by considering the words of the Tuhoe academic, the late John Rangihau, who stated that:

> I have a faint suspicion that Māori is a term coined by the Pākehā to bring tribes together. Because if you cannot divide and rule, then for tribal people all you can do is unite and rule. Because then they lose everything by losing their own tribal histories and traditions that give them identity (Rangihau, 1975).

Although the fundamental message underpinning this statement is one of power and control, it illuminates two critically important points. First, Māori ontology and epistemology are founded on tribal affiliations, each with their own unique observable artefacts, values and basic underlying assumptions. Second, it would be highly remiss of me to espouse that the way by which 'I' view the world is representative of 'all' Māori. My intention here is simply to share 'a' Te Āo Māori whakaaro, and not to infer that the views expressed are 'the' Te Āo Māori whakaaro.

TOI I TE ĀHUA O TE ĀO MĀORI WHAKAARO (DESCRIBING A MĀORI WORLDVIEW)

Worldviews reflect the different modes for understanding the social world, and can thus influence the approach to and development of theory (Goia & Pitrie, 1990). Within the literature, there are copious Western names for a 'worldview', resulting in the equivalent number of definitions for the same construct (Koltko-Rivera, 2004). Yet in the literature, little can be found to describe a Te Āo Māori whakaaro. Fortunately, after an extensive search of the literature, I offer the following definition. Te Āo Māori whakaaro encapsulates the interconnectedness between **Mana Atua** (spiritual authority), **Mana Whenua** (physical authority) and **Mana Tangata** (human authority), which form the basis of Māori ontology and epistemology. The key principles of a Te Āo Māori whakaaro are Te Āo Mārama (the world of life and light) and **Te Āo Hurihuri** (the changing world). Te Āo Mārama refers to knowledge development as a dynamic process in which an individual interacts within a cosmos, which is defined by his or her own belief structure. Te Āo Hurihuri recognises that the world at one level is always changing, while at another, holds strong to given universal constructs (Wolfgramm, 2008). So it is my intention to use Te Āo Mārama and Te Āo Hurihuri as the frameworks when formulating a thesis of 'a' Te Āo Māori whakaaro.

ĒTAHI MĀTĀPONO WHAKAMIRAMIRA (SOME IMPORTANT PRINCIPLES)

It is important to describe the intimate interconnections between some important principles, these being, **kawa**, **tikanga**, **tapu**, **mauri**, kaitiaki, **tika**, **pono**, **aroha**, **mana** and rahui. To understand kawa (protocols) and tikanga (customs), one must have a deep understanding and appreciation of one's own belief structure. Kawa and tikanga describes a Māori way of 'being' and 'behaving', which may be in contrast to the dominant discourse, and therefore may challenge some societal protocols that are typically accepted as being normal. Kawa deliberately specifies boundaries, especially when encountering episodes of sacredness confronting sacredness. Tapu (sacredness) has a myriad of complexities, which are determined by the context with which it is used. Tapu is the spiritual essence of all things, which derives from mauri (the life principle of all creation). Tapu refers to both personal and communal potentiality for power, growth and enhancement. Understood in the correct context, tapu aims to keep all creation safe by maintaining a sense of cosmological equilibrium, which constantly directs us back to the Supreme Being, that is, Io-Matua-Kore. Therefore, tapu is a sacred state or condition that places an object, animate or inanimate, under the protection and patronage of the Gods. Tapu demands humankind to be the kaitiaki (guardians, stewards) of life by creating and maintaining relationships through the actualisation of tika (that which is right, legal, proper, fair and just), pono (being faithful, honest and sincere to what is tika) and aroha (having concern, compassion and love), for all things. Tapu is increased when all manner of actions, delivered or expressed, are done so in a positive and caring way. As tapu is increased, mana (prestige, personal authority and power to achieve goals) is also increased, as the energy manifested from having tapu is honoured and promoted.

A further extension of tapu is rahui (restrictions, prohibitions, setting boundaries and limits, potentiality for power if tapu is intact, and safety). Rahui puts tapu into action by recognising and acknowledging that an event is about to take place, or that an event has already happened. Rahui acknowledges Mana Atua, Mana Whenua and Mana Tangata by ensuring that dignity and worth of all things, celestial or mortal, are respected, treasured and not belittled. Tapu diminished by acts of violation or discrimination is mana diminished, and consequently restricts the potential for personal authority and the power to achieve. Tapu is about holding and honouring the many journeys of life as we grow and develop from fertility to death. Protection of tapu often requires the implementation of rahui, to ensure that clear boundaries, limits and restraints are implemented to maintain relationships of respect and safety. Finally, to abuse tapu is to violate whakapapa (R. Davis, personal communication, 2 March 2012).

TOI I TE ĀHUA O TE AHUREA (DESCRIBING CULTURE)

At this stage of the journey I'd like to define the term 'culture', as an understanding of this concept will help to contextualise the discussion of Māori cultural constructs that aim, in part, to describe and define my construction of 'a' Te Āo Māori whakaaro.

Sociologists maintain that culture is a critical component of any functioning society (Denison & Mishra, 1995). Keesing (1974) describes culture as the systematic social transmission of behaviours that serve to relate human communities to their ecological surroundings. Furthermore, Smircich (1983) argues that culture is a set of factors that a group produces as an adaptive or regulatory mechanism that connects an individual to his or her environment, resulting in people grouping together within a social structure. Strauss and Quinn (1997) make reference to the 'paradox of culture', which is concerned with centripetal forces, such as beliefs, values, processes and goals; and centrifugal forces, such as demographic strata, economic position and political status that influence social life. Ogbonna and Harris (2000) continue by stating that a group's culture must not only be strong, it must also have unique qualities that cannot be imitated. Finally, Schein (1990) proposes that a culture can be identified by three distinguishable and fundamental criteria, which are: (1) observable artefacts; (2) values; and (3) basic underlying assumptions. At a very simplistic level, a group's culture is manifested through 'what is done, how it is done and who is involved in doing it' (Tierney, 1988, p. 3).

TOI I TE ĀHUA O NGA ĀHUATANGA MĀORI (DESCRIBING MĀORI CULTURAL CONSTRUCTS)

So what are the distinctive features that identify the Māori 'culture'? Or more specifically, what are the beliefs, values, behaviours, assumptions, factors, processes and observable artefacts that identify Māori? To begin to answer these questions, I'd like to start with **Te Kōrero Ōrokotīmatanga** (the Māori creation story). This is a symbolic narrative that presents an account of how the cosmos was created, and how we as Māori (the human element) were fashioned. The Māori creation story has several versions, each with its own diverging nuances, some subtle, while others are more obvious. However, key themes and characters tend to frequent most versions, thereby maintaining a sense of homogeneity between the varying accounts. Remember, Te Āo Mārama challenges us to evaluate the cosmos, and then determine what is important and what is real. Te kōrero ōrokotīmatanga is the genesis of my belief structure; therefore it dictates in part how I negotiate this world of life and light.

TE KŌRERO ŌROKOTĪMATANGA (THE MĀORI CREATION STORY)

In the very beginning there was Io-Matua-Kore, the Supreme Being, the one who is above all Gods, the one who emerged from Te Kore (the nothingness, an energy) (Robinson, 2005). From Te Kore came Te Pō (darkness, the night), which represented a time where Papatūānuku was formed. From Te Pō came Te Āo Mārama, symbolising a time where Papatūānuku and Ranginui came into being. The procreation of Ranginui and Papatūānuku gave birth to nine sons, who are referred to as ira atua (life as possessed by the Gods).

According to Shirres (1997), each sibling is primarily responsible for commanding physical domains within the natural world where all tapu, mana and mauri began. The siblings include Tānenuiārangi or Tāne (God of the forest and all that dwell therein), Tāwhirimātea (God of the wind and storms), Tangaroa (God of the sea, rivers, lakes and all that live within), Tūmatauenga (God of war), Rongo (God of peace), Rūaumoko (God of earthquakes and volcanoes), Rongo mā Tāne (God of kumara and all cultivated foods), Haumia-tiketike (God of wild food) and Whiro (God of evil). As time passed, the sons became frustrated with living in darkness, and after much discussion it was Tāne that eventually separated his parents to allow light. Not long after, Tāne and his brothers went in search of a mortal female to derive ira tangata (human element) (Mead, 2003). The Gods all recognised that it was impossible to obtain ira tangata exclusively from ira atua (Walker, 1990). After much searching of the natural world, the first female was created, Hine-ahuone, who, according to Marsden and Henare (1992), was 'formed and shaped out of the red clay of Onekura—of mother earth' (p. 13). It was Tāne who exhaled his hā (breath of life, essence) of mauri into Hine-ahuone's mouth and nostrils (Walker, 1990). Tāne then 'cohabited with Hine-ahuone' (Walker, 1990, p. 14) and produced Hine-titama. It is through Tāne cohabiting with Hine-titama that ira tangata was formed.

I acknowledge that this is a very simplistic version of the creation story. Nevertheless, it identifies two key concepts. Te kōrero ōrokotīmatanga highlights the intimate connection that ira tangata has with ira atua. It is for this very reason that almost every tikanga that Māori execute has an accompanying **karakia** (incantation, acknowledgment) that seeks to recognise and pay homage to ira atua. Examples include giving thanks to Tāne, Rongo mā Tāne and Haumia-tiketike before eating; and invoking protection from Tāne and Tangaroa before entering into each of their respective domains. Additionally, the exercise of **kaitiakitanga** (guardianship) by Māori over the natural world and everything within it further recognises our connection and obligation to supporting the Gods in their role to command the physical domains, but more importantly, it signifies our commitment (as ira tangata) to protect our primordial mother, Papatūānuku.

In summary, Te kōrero ōrokotīmatanga proposes that all Māori descend from the same common origin (Hine-titama), whose father/partner is a God (Tāne) and a mother (Hine-ahuone) who was formed from the bosom of mother-earth (Papatūānuku). And so I believe that my toto (blood) and therefore my genetic makeup connects me to the spiritual world through Tāne, nature through Papatūānuku, and all Māori through Hine-titama. This is why the root of my belief structure is centred in Mana Atua, Mana Whenua and Mana Tangata.

ĀHUATANGA MĀORI (MĀORI CULTURAL CONSTRUCTS)

There are several cultural constructs that could be used to identify and explain the beliefs, values, behaviours, assumptions, factors, processes and observable artefacts that identify Māori. Āhutanga Māori refers to the cultural constructs that identify Māori. Under the auspices of Te Āo Mārama, I have chosen to discuss whakapapa, whānau and whakawhānaungatanga as the cultural constructs that form my worldview. It is important to note that these cultural constructs are but a mere representation of Māori identity.

Āhutanga Māori—Whakapapa

For Māori, whakapapa is the creation story of all living things from the Gods to us in the present day, and is one of the most prized constructs of knowledge to Māori (Barlow, 1991). Whakapapa establishes our own whakapapa and how we are connected to others by way of ngā kōrero tuku iho (history, stories of the past, traditions) (Bishop, 1998). Hemara (2000) emphasises that 'whakapapa distinguishes Māori from any other race, nationality, or community' (p. 33). Māori may exist in the present, but our tūpuna are forever beside us (Hook et al., 2007). Walker (1990) contends that Māori are people who walk backwards into the future. This reference signifies the importance of seeking guidance from one's ancestors as a means to develop future generations (Paki, 2007). Knowing one's place, connections, obligations and history helps to develop a sense of pride and belonging through acknowledging and understanding that very history (Papuni & Bartlett, 2006). Exploring whakapapa identifies the important connections between both the spiritual and physical realms, and consequently the creation of human beings. Whakapapa represents the interconnections to self, other and nature, and reflects the complex systems that are intertwined from a common origin. It is for this reason that, regardless of each individual's tribal strata, all Māori are connected to the same spiritual beginning, that is, Io-Matua-Kore. Unfortunately, there are many Māori who do not know their whakapapa (Walker, 1989) or have a person through whom whakapapa connections can be maintained and sought (Nikora, 1995). Although this situation is unfortunate, Timoti Karetu offers a slightly different perspective by stating that Māori identity is not dictated by blood quantum; rather it is determined by the upbringing one has had in observing all the rites of passage in a Māori way (Karetu, 1990).

Āhutanga Māori—Whānau

According to Durie (1994), the whānau arena was the place where initial teaching and socialising occurred, which was inevitably based on kinship to the hapū and iwi. A single whānau unit often consisted of three to four generations (Papakura, 1986). This allowed for tuakana-teina (older–younger) relationships to manifest, where the older and more experienced generation(s) would mentor the younger generation(s) to ensure, among many other features, an accurate and meaningful sense of one's identity (Turner & Helms, 1983). The whānau environment encouraged a sense of collective affiliation, maintenance of collaborative relationships, reciprocal obligatory roles and responsibilities and the importance of **kotahitanga** (uniting people as one) (Moeke-Pickering, 1996). Individuals who were considered to have special talents were nurtured and developed by **kaumātua** (an elderly man or elderly woman), who are regarded as repositories of hōhonu (deep) knowledge and wisdom. The attitude was to develop the individual to benefit the wider whānau (Hook, 2007). Whānau provided a place where meaningfulness and belongingness to the tribal strata's could be nurtured, and subsequently formed a pathway for the establishment and sustenance of Māori identity (Moeke-Pickering, 1996). A whakataukī that is relevant here is 'he waka eke noa' (a canoe that we are all in, with no exception). Essentially, whānau creates and promotes a sense of collective oneness, the notion that we are all moving together in the same direction by the same rhythm.

Āhutanga Māori—Whakawhānaungatanga

In traditional Māori settings, learning was conducted within a structure of whakawhānaungatanga (Ka'ai, 1990). Whakawhānaungatanga is critical because it underpins all Māori understandings of human development and learning through a sense of belonging to and relating to others within a context of collective identity and shared responsibility (Macfarlane et al., 2008). Furthermore, Russell Bishop argues that whakawhānaungatanga has a significant impact on the sharing of power and control within the whānau, iwi and hapū (Bishop, 1996). Whakawhānaungatanga presents multiple opportunities for kanohi ki te kanohi, which in turn provides multiple possibilities for wairua ki te wairua through the hongi (Māori greeting, by pressing noses and foreheads) process. While the act of hongi is physical in nature, it is the inhaling of the 'hā' that truly unites ira tangata by connecting us back to Tāne, and therefore back to ira atua. Kia kite a kanohi (a face that is seen) is a demonstration of tautoko (support), by being present at an event both physically and spiritually. Kanohi ki te kanohi continues to strengthen associations by connecting individual's waka, maunga, awa, iwi and hapū. Whakawhānaungatanga elaborates on those imperative interactions and connections that link all involved within a given paradigm. Whakawhānaungatanga is about whakapapa. A whakataukī that is relevant here is 'ko au ko te whānau, ko te whānau ko au' ('I am the family; the family is me'). To explain the meaning of this whakataukī, I draw on the concept of empathy. Empathy can be described as 'the ability to comprehend another's feelings and to re-experience them oneself' (Salovey & Mayer, 1990, p. 194). In order for me to develop whānaungatanga (right relationships), I must first understand my own emotions, and then comprehend the emotions of others. If I am the family, I will understand the family. Whakawhānaungatanga presents multiple opportunities to begin to craft and forge relationships, even those that may be delicate or fragile.

TE ĀO HURIHURI (THE CHANGING WORLD)

The principle of Te Āo Hurihuri challenges Māori to carefully negotiate this ever-changing world, while simultaneously holding strong to those **āhuatanga Māori** that give us identity. In this context, Māori should then strive to perform credibly in a Te Āo Pākehā (the world of a New Zealander of European descent) and **Te Āo Māori**. This may be difficult for some Māori, as these worlds (Pākehā and Māori) can be considered as competing archetypes, because of the opposing nature of individualism and collectivism (Hook, 2006). Ratima and Grant (2007) state that the Pākehā notion of individuality is based on autonomy and self-interest. At this point, I must declare that I often work autonomously in pursuit of perfection. What motivates me to strive to reach such heights is the understanding that everything I do is for a collective, for my whānau, especially my tamariki (children). As whakapapa contends, children are **taonga tuku iho** (treasures from the ancestors). On a daily basis, my wife and I try to create a whānau environment that is underpinned by **manaaki** (take care of, look out for) and aroha, much of which has been learnt through our own lived experiences, both good and bad.

The word manaaki can be divided into two words, 'mana' and 'aki'. As we are aware, the word 'mana' can be defined as power, while 'aki' can be defined as 'to encourage'. So, to manaaki is to 'encourage power'. Should we not manaaki, if in a position to do so? It is sometimes difficult for me to demonstrate manaaki in a surrounding that is forged and driven by individualism. The ideology that achievement is only attained as an individual pursuit is perplexing to me. Here I quote the whakataukı, 'Ehara taku toa i te toa takitahi, engari he takimano, nō ōku tūpuna' ('My strength comes not from one, but from thousands, from my ancestors'). Although whakapapa is very definitive and localised to Māori, all things (animate and inanimate) have genealogy, and therefore have tapu and mana. It is for this very reason that I believe we, as ira tangata, should demonstrate manaaki and aroha in all aspects of our life, through the execution of whakawhānaungatanga.

There are many artefacts that identify the Māori culture, such as **wharenui** (traditional meeting house), **whakairo** (carvings), **tā moko** (Māori tattoo designs), **waiata** (songs) and **haka** (ceremonial performance); however, it is **te reo rangatira** (the Māori language, the language of chiefs) that truly differentiates Māori from any other race. There is a whakataukī that states 'ko te reo te tāhuhu o tēnei whare' ('the language is the ridgepole of this house').

I selected this whakataukī to express the importance of the Māori language, the ridgepole of Māori identity, a feature that is unequivocally unique to Māori. Being able to converse in **te reo Māori** allows one, among many other things, the ability to engage in ngā kōrero tuku iho. A survey on the health of the Māori language in 2001 indicated that approximately 29 000 (9 per cent) of Māori adults were very fluent in te reo Māori. However, many of the very fluent Māori speakers are over the age of 50 (He korero mo te reo Māori, 2009), which invites the question, 'Are we (as Māori) at risk of losing the most important artefact that defines us, as our elders pass on'?' I quote the kīwaha (colloquialism): 'Tōku reo, tōku ohooho' ('My language is my awakening'). Māori are becoming more urbanised, which has led (in many instances) to us prioritising the attainment of material possessions over learning te reo rangatira. A consequence of urbanisation is that a number of Māori do not organise themselves primarily around their iwi, hapū and whānau (Moeke-Pickering, 1996), which significantly reduces the opportunity to speak the language and engage in hui (gatherings). The challenge for Māori is to create communities within the cities that allow Māori to practise those tikanga and āhuatanga Māori that inevitably define us.

Last but not least, as a Māori, I cannot ignore the effect of the processes of **colonisation,** capitalism and assimilation, which have rapidly reduced the primacy of those āhuatanga Māori that are meaningful to Māori (Ministerial Advisory Committee for the Department of Social Welfare, 1988; McKinley et al., 1992). The complexity of de-fragmenting the ideals of the Pākehā culture is to unpack 'patriarchy, racism and ethnocentrisms' and to encourage the 'empowerment of intercultural diplomacy' (Battiste et al., 2002, p. 84). When reflecting on Te Āo Hurihuri, one has no choice but to consider the impact of the current socioeconomic lifestyle characteristics, changing demographic patterns and political realities that now influence the modern Māori sense of identity (Durie et al., 1995). A quote by Manuhuia Bennett in the 1970s concluded that modern Māori will prioritise non-neutral things (such as a car, TV or house) over the things that are happening within their **Marae** (meeting area for whānau or iwi) and/or papa kāinga (original home) (Bennett, 1979). The end result for most Māori has been one of disillusionment, disengagement and disbelief. This is aptly exemplified by Smith (2000), who states that Māori occupy some of the worst categories of social statistics (lower average incomes, a greater prevalence towards life-threatening diseases and a higher level of educational underachievement) in comparison to non-Māori. Although Te Āo Hurihuri urges Māori to cautiously traverse this changing world, it is my contention that the ecological framework of Aotearoa significantly jeopardises Māori ontology and epistemology.

One solution to this dilemma is **Kaupapa Māori** (Māori ideology) theory, a term that grew in the 1970s and 1980s out of Māori aspirations, political consciousness (Bishop, 1999) and **Te Tiriti o Waitangi** (the Treaty of Waitangi) as assurances for the revitalisation of the Māori culture, and therefore Māori identity. Kaupapa Māori theory emphasises co-construction, empowerment and the critical importance of cultural recognition by ensuring the continued existence of Māori identity with the right to reclaim autonomy over one's life (Smith, 2004). The cultural constructs of whānau, whakapapa and whakawhānaungatanga (as discussed previously), among other cultural preferences, form the foundations of Kaupapa Māori theory. Kaupapa Māori theory is an intervention tool for **tino rangatiratanga** (self-determination) that aims to legitimise and validate being, acting and living as Māori (Bishop & Glynn, 1999), and is part of a wider movement by Māori to create new power relationships that recognise Māori as equal Treaty partners in Aotearoa. As Fitzsimons and Smith (2000) explain, 'Kaupapa Māori has the capacity to address Māori social, economic, and educational crises, through which is central to Kaupapa Māori knowledge, pedagogy, discipline, and curriculum' (p. 35). Kaupapa Māori theory is a very powerful tool for transformation to a positive ideological shift for Māori (Paki, 2007), and can be seen as the deconstruction of those hegemonies that have disempowered Māori from controlling and defining their own knowledge within the context of unequal power relations (McNicholas & Barrett, 2005).

Smith (2004) presents three concepts for change with a Kaupapa Māori paradigm. These are conscientisation, resistance and praxis. Conscientisation is a process that involves identifying the various levels of oppression that have marginalised and continue to affect Māori. It is this stage where sorting and transforming existing frameworks occur. The second concept, resistance, aims to transform existing systems by consciously and collectively committing to changing oppressive systems by employing new culturally dynamic strategies and interventions that ensure cultural survival. The third and final concept is praxis. Praxis is inclusive of action and reflection by connecting components within the transformative spectrum.

Although there are a number of Māori-medium initiatives that have grown since the 1980s to address tino rangatiratanga, the greatest success can be seen in the education sector. Enterprises such as **Te Kōhanga Reo** (early childhood centres), **Te Kura Kaupapa** (primary schools), Whare Kura (primary, middle and high school combined) and Whare Wānanga (tribal tertiary institutions) have generated much success. In these settings, Kaupapa Māori theory is embraced in all aspects of the Kura (school) ethos (Fraser, 2004). Central to all of these Māori-medium initiatives is the concept of taonga tuku iho.

Metaphorically, taonga tuku iho refers to the tapu and mana of each person, especially the child. Bishop (2003) suggests that the images and practices created within these Māori-medium settings can be utilised to address power relationships in mainstream education, rather than continuing to propagate the existing deficit discourse.

KUPU WHAKATEPE (CONCLUSIONS)

Te Āo Māori whakaaro is both a set of philosophical beliefs and a set of social practices. Taken together, these form Māori ontology; that is, 'what is real for Māori', which in turn has shaped a Te Āo Māori whakaaro epistemology; that is, 'to live according to tikanga Māori', that which is tika (Henry & Pene, 2001). I have found evidence in the literature that a Te Āo Māori whakaaro is shaped by our assumptions of what is 'real' and what is 'true', which in turn has shaped the way that I view and therefore navigate this world. To be Māori is to be communal through earning apprenticeships by participating in the learning of kawa and tikanga that are part of being of a particular iwi and/or hapū. The intertwined connection between tikanga and tribal strata continue to fundamentally underpin how Māori are identified and conceptualised today. A strong sense of Māori identity is rooted in our connection to Mana Atua, Mana Whēnua and Mana Tangata, which allows tapu and mana to be nurtured, eventually manifesting as a deep-seeded respect for all things. The breadth of Māori cultural literacy is unknown, but te wā (time) informs us to be patient and to allow individuals to explore Te Āo Marama and Te Āo Hurihuri in a time and space that is right for them. I believe that sound whānau leadership is the key to sustaining Māori identity. The existence of a Pākehā ecology has played a significant role in the dilution of Māori identity. Yet, others will argue that this 'perceived loss' has ignited a sense of passion and desire among Māori to defend, protect and assert our identity.

Now that I am nearly at the end of this journey, I have come to the realisation that 'a' Te Āo Māori whakaaro is not actually singular, as evidenced by the many authors that have contributed to this body of work. Ngā mihi nui ki a koutou (acknowledgments to you all). Finally, I am proud to be Māori, I am privileged to learn my culture and I am excited for my children who will grow up appreciating 'a' Te Āo Māori whakaaro. I have enjoyed using whakataukī to express thoughts and ideas; there is much to learn from these beautiful words of wisdom. So with that said, I conclude with the following whakataukī by Waereti Tait-Rolleston (as cited in Moeke-Pickering, 1996), 'E taku mō kai, he wā poto noa koe i waenganui i te wā kua hipa, ki te wā kei te tu mai' ('You are but a speck in the moment of time, situated between two eternities, past and future. Make use of that time so that you may use this moment wisely and for the benefit of your people').

CRITICAL QUESTIONS

Cultural lens

- **What** is meant by the term dominant discourse?
- **Where** do we find support to implement change?

Social lens

- **Is** there room for ethnic-specific health pathways?
- **What** effect do the current social structures have on whānau?
- **Where** does social change begin?
- **Who** is responsible for the existing social structures?

Gender lens

- **Is** status confused with role?

Political lens

- **Do** strategic policy documents lose sight of the finer details?
- **What** position would Tāngata whenua have if there were no Treaty of Waitangi?

Moral lens

- **Can** diverse understandings of right and wrong operate in harmony?
- **Can** a tikanga framework operate within a mainstream environment?

Media lens

- **Why** is it that negative social norms typically dominate the media?

REFERENCES

Barlow, C. (1991). *Tikanga Whakaaro: Key Concepts in Maori Culture*. Auckland: Oxford University Press.

Battiste, M., Bell, L. & Findlay, M. (2002). Decolonizing education in Canadian universities: an interdisciplinary, international, indigenous research project. *Canadian Journal of Native Education*, *26*, 82–95.

Bennett, M. (1979). *He Matapuna*. Wellington: New Zealand Planning Council.

Bishop, R. (1996). *Whakawhānaungatanga: Collaborative Research Stories*. Palmerston North: Dunmore Press.

Bishop, R. (1998). Freeing ourselves from neo-colonial domination in research: a Maori approach to creating knowledge. *International Journal of Qualitative Studies in Education*, *11*(2), 199–219. doi:10.1080/095183998236674.

Bishop, R. (1999). Kaupapa Maori research: an indigenous approach to creating knowledge. In L. Nikora & N. Robertson (eds), *Maori Psychology: Research and Practice* (1–6). Hamilton: Department of Psychology, University of Waikato.

Bishop, R. (2003). Changing power relations in education: Kaupapa Māori messages for 'mainstream' education in Aotearoa/New Zealand. *Comparative Education*, *39*(2), 221–238.

Bishop, R. & Glynn, T. (1999). *Culture Counts: Changing Power Relation in Education.* Palmerston North: Dunmore Press.

Denison, D. & Mishra, A. (1995). Toward a theory of organizational culture and effectiveness. *Organization Science*, *6*(2), 204–223.

Durie, M.H. (1994). Whanau/families and healthy development. Paper presented at Fifth Annual Conference, New Zealand College of Clinical Psychologists. Hamilton: Massey University, Department of Maori Studies.

Durie, M.H., Black, T.E., Christensen, I.S., Durie, A.E., Taiapa, U.K., Potaka, U.K.J. & Fitzgerald, E. (1995). *Te hoe nuku roa Framework: A Maori Identity Measure.* Wellington: Association of Social Science Researchers.

Fitzsimons, P. & Smith, G. (2000). Philosophy and indigenous cultural transformation. *Educational Philosophy and Theory*, *32(1)*, 25–41.

Fraser, D. (2004). Secular schools, spirituality and Maori values. *Journal of Moral Education*, *33*(1), 95–97.

Goia, D. & Pitrie, E. (1990). Multi-paradigm perspectives on theory building. *Academy of Management Review*, *15*(4), 584–602.

He korero mo te reo Māori (2009). *Q3. How Many People Speak Maori?* <http://www.maorilanguage.info/>.

Hemara, W. (2000). *Maori Pedagogies: A View from the Literature.* Wellington: New Zealand Council for Educational Research.

Henry, E. & Pene, H. (2001). *Kaupapa Maori: Locating Ontology, Epistemology and Methodology in the Academy.* London: Sage Publications.

Hook, G.R. (2006). A future for Māori education: Part I: The dissociation of culture and education. *MAI Review*, *1*, 1–14.

Hook, G.R. (2007). A future for Māori education: Part II: The reintegration of culture and education. *MAI Review*, *1*, 1–17.

Hook, G.R., Waaka, T. & Raumati, L.P. (2007). Mentoring Māori within a Pākehā framework. *MAI Review*, *3*(1).

Ka'ai, T. (1990). *Te Hiringa Taketake: Mai i Te Kōhanga Reo ki te Kura: Māori Pedagogy: Te Kōhanga Reo and the Transition to School.* Auckland: Department of Education, University of Auckland.

Karetu, T. (1990). The clue to identity. *New Zealand Geographic*, *5*, 112.

Keesing, R. (1974). Theories of culture. *Annual Reviews*, 3, 73–97.

Koltko-Rivera, M.E. (2004). The psychology of worldviews. *Review of General Psychology*, *8*(1), 3–58. doi:10.1037/1089-2680.8.1.3.

Macfarlane, A.H., Glynn, T., Grace, W., Penetito, W. & Bateman, S. (2008). Indigenous epistemology in a national curriculum framework? *Ethnicities*, *8*(1), 102–127. doi:10.1177/1468796807087021.

McKinley, E., Waiti, P.M. & Bell, B. (1992). Language, culture and science education. *International Journal of Science Education*, *14*(5), 579–595.

McNicholas, P. & Barrett, M. (2005). Answering the emancipatory call: an emerging research approach 'on the margins' of accounting. *Critical Perspectives on Accounting*, *16*, 391–414. doi:10.1016/S1045-2354(03)00098-4.

Marsden, M. & Henare, T.A. (1992). *Kaitiakitanga: A Definitive Introduction to the Holistic World View of the Māori.* Wellington: Ministry for the Environment.

Mead, M.M. (2003). *Tikanga Māori: Living by Māori Values.* Wellington: Huia Publications.

Ministerial Advisory Committee for the Department of Social Welfare (1988). *Puao-te-Ata-Tu: Daybreak. The Report of the Ministerial Advisory Committee of a Maori Perspective for the Department of Social Welfare.* Wellington: Department of Social Welfare.

Moeke-Pickering, T. (1996). *Maori Identity within Whanau: A Review of Literature.* Hamilton: University of Waikato.

Morrison, A. (1999). *Space for Maori in Tertiary Institutions: Exploring Two Sites at the University of Auckland.* Auckland: University of Auckland.

Nikora, L.W. (1995). Race, culture and ethnicity: organisation of Maori social groups. In L.W. Nikora & T.M. Moeke-Pickering (eds), *Maori Development and Psychology* (pp. 20–24). Hamilton: Waikato University.

O'Connor, M. & MacFarlane, A. (2002). New Zealand Maori stories and symbols: family value lessons for Western counsellors. *International Journal for the Advancement of Counselling, 24,* 223–237.

Ogbonna, E. & Harris, L. (2000). Leadership style, organizational culture and performance: empirical evidence from UK companies. *International Journal of Human Resource Management, 11*(4), 766–788. doi:10.1080/09585190050075114.

Paki, V.A. (2007). Kimihia, Rangahaua Nga Tikanga Heke Iho. He Taonga Huahua e Riro Mai: Exploring Whakapapa as a tool towards a Kaupapa Maori assesment framework in early childhood education. Unpublished Masters thesis. Hamilton: University of Waikato.

Papakura, M. (1986). *Makereti: The Old Time Maori.* Auckland: New Women's Press.

Papuni, H.T. & Bartlett, K.R. (2006). Maori and Pakeha perspectives of adult learning in Aotearoa/New Zealand workplaces. *Advances in Developing Human Resources, 8*(3), 400–407.

Rangihau, J. (1975). Being Maori. In M. King (ed.), *Te Ao Hurihuri: The World Moves On: Aspects of Maoritanga.* Auckland: Hicks Smith.

Ratima, M. & Grant, B. (2007). Thinking about difference across and within mentoring. *MAI Review, 3.*

Robinson, S.T. (2005). *Tohunga: The revival: Ancient Knowledge for the Modern Era.* Auckland: Reed Publishing.

Salovey, P. & Mayer, J.D. (1990). Emotional intelligence. *Imagination, Cognition and Personality, 9*(3), 185–211.

Schein, E. (1990). Organizational culture. *American Psychologist, 45*(2), 109–119.

Shirres, M. (1997). *Te Tangata: The Human Person.* Auckland: Accent Publications.

Smircich, L. (1983). Concepts of culture and organizational analysis. *Administrative Science Quarterly, 28*(3), 339–358.

Smith, G.H. (2000). Maori education: revolution and transformative action. *Canadian Journal of Native Education, 24*(1), 57–72.

Smith, G.H. (2004). Mai te Maramatanga, ki te Putanga Mai o te Tehuritanga: from conscientization to transformation. *Journal of the College of Education/University of Hawai'i at Manoa, 37*(1).

Strauss, C. & Quinn, N. (1997). *A Cognitive Theory of Cultural Meaning.* Cambridge: Cambridge University Press.

Tierney, W. (1988). Organizational culture in higher education: defining the essentials. *Journal of Higher Education*, *59*(1), 2–21.

Turner, J.S. & Helms, D.B. (1983). *Lifespan Development*. New York: Holt, Rinehart and Winston.

Walker, R. (1989). *Maori Identity*. Wellington: Government Printer.

Walker, R. (1990). *Ka Whawhai Tonu Matou: Struggle without End*. Auckland: Penguin.

Wolfgramm, R. (2008). Creativity and institutional innovation in intercultural research. *MAI Review*, *3*(6).

WEBSITES

<http://www.maorilanguage.info/>

Maori language website.

<http://history-nz.org/maori9.html>

New Zealand history and Maori legends.

TE KAWENATA Ō WAITANGI

THE APPLICATION OF THE TREATY OF WAITANGI TO HEALTH

In 1985, the Standing Committee on Māori Health recommended that the Treaty of Waitangi be regarded as a foundation for good health.[1] The parent body, the New Zealand Board of Health, immediately responded in a positive way and itself recommended that 'All legislation relating to health should include recognition of the Treaty of Waitangi'.[2] It was a bold step but not one entirely understood nor fully endorsed by Government. Having barely had time to come to grips with the Waitangi Tribunal's sweeping revisions of New Zealand's history and substantiated criticisms of a century or so of unfair legislation, Government was now being pressured to examine social policy areas from a Treaty perspective. Māori claims on the property rights of physical resources such as land and fisheries, based on the Treaty of Waitangi, were beginning to receive long overdue attention, but health, education, welfare, and housing had received virtually no consideration at all, and their relevance to the Treaty of Waitangi remained largely unexplored.[3]

Probably no direct connection between Māori health and the Treaty of Waitangi had been entertained this century although, as already described in Chapter Three, motivation for the Treaty stemmed in part from health concerns as long ago as 1837. Busby, the British Resident in New Zealand since 1832, was convinced that, because disease and death prevailed to the extent that they did, the Māori population could disappear entirely. He urged the Colonial Office to take action, maintaining that without Crown intervention Māori would continue to be vulnerable to the 'evils' of *ad hoc* British settlement. His influence, along with pressures from the missionaries through the Church Missionary Society, played a significant part in convincing the British Government that positive intervention was essential. Although Busby had favoured a 'protecting state' rather than an annexation of sovereignty, the Treaty of Waitangi was the proposed solution.[4] They were armed with Lord Normanby's 'Instructions', which among other things noted the deleterious health consequences of colonization, and the need for protection against 'any Contracts which they might be the ignorant and unintentional authors of injuries to themselves. You will not for example, purchase from them any Territory the retention of which by them would be essential, or highly conducive, to their own comfort, safety or subsistence. The acquisition of Land by the Crown for the future Settlement of British Subjects must be confined to such districts as the Natives can alienate without distress or serious inconvenience to themselves'.[5]

Normanby's 'Instructions' linked economic and social objectives and promoted policies of positive protection, a burden on the Crown to ensure that Māori were not unfairly marginalized by British settlement and that their well-being was ensured. Similarly, the report of the Aborigines Committee to Parliament in 1837 had recommended that the executive (rather than Parliament) should adopt a distinct policy towards indigenous peoples with prohibition of alcohol sales and social and political sensitivity. Treaties with indigenous chiefs were also advocated.[6]

TREATY TEXTS

The 1840 Treaty of Waitangi was the outcome. Phrased in broad, non-specific terms, the Preamble to the Treaty contained the objectives (based to some extent on Normanby's 'Instructions'), while the three articles provided for a transfer of sovereignty (Article One), a continuation of existing property rights (Article Two), and citizenship rights (Article Three). Of the two texts, English and Māori, the English version was more expansive in Article One and the Māori version broader in its interpretation of Article Two provisions.

Much depended on the translation of the word 'sovereignty', but Henry Williams, the Church of England missionary asked by Hobson to translate the English text, chose to avoid the obvious Māori equivalents (mana, rangatiratanga). He preferred instead a transliteration of governorship, kāwanatanga, which did not convey any sense of a transfer of sovereignty, rather a lesser notion of administrative authority.[7] This was surprising in view of the fact that Williams had used different words when he translated the 1835 Declaration of Independence; then he described Māori sovereignty as 'te Kingitanga, te mana'.[8] The wording in the Treaty was more consistent with Busby's idea of a Protectorate than a formal annexation of absolute power. Whatever else, however, Article One did provide for the Crown to establish a government.

Of more interest to a discussion on Māori health is Article Two. While the English version amounted to a confirmation of existing property rights, and a guarantee that they would not be unjustly alienated, the Māori version went wider to incorporate social and cultural guarantees. By equating 'full exclusive and undisturbed possession' with 'tino rangatiratanga' the effect was to recognize the authority of chiefs, generally. Moreover, the translation of 'other properties' (by implication the English version meant physical properties) as 'taonga katoa' further extended the meaning to include cultural as well as material properties.[9] The Waitangi Tribunal agreed that the Māori version was broader, concluding that Māori language was a taonga and admonishing the Crown for failing to protect it 'as required by article 2 of the Treaty'.[10]

At health hui held in the 1980s and 1990s, Māori often claimed that health could be described as a taonga and therefore entitled to protection under the Treaty. Government acknowledged that view but did not agree with it. 'The claim that the protection of the health of Māori has (through Article 2) a special claim on New Zealanders as a whole, over and above the responsibility of the Crown to secure the health of all citizens is, however, not one the Government accepts'.[11]

Article Three of the Treaty of Waitangi, however, has more obvious and direct implications for health. Prior to 1840, Māori as individuals had no claims on a Government. If anything, individual rights were subsidiary to those of the tribe, the survival of the group taking precedence. The Treaty changed that. By promising 'all the Rights and Privileges of British subjects', Māori individuals acquired new citizenship rights. While in 1840 those may not have been as extensive as they are today, they at least included the right to a fair trial and the right to carry a British passport. But the undertaking also implied that there would be no serious gaps between Māori and other New Zealanders, and that, if necessary, the Crown would exercise 'royal protection' in order to meet its new obligations. Thus Article Three was as much about equity as citizenship. Its significance for health is particularly evident in light of continuing disparities in standards of health between Māori and non-Māori.

While the three articles contain the essence of the provisions, it is useful to consider the Preamble in order to understand the Treaty's original purposes. Protection of Māori well-being was obviously contemplated. Her Majesty Victoria, Queen of the United Kingdom, regarded 'the Native Chiefs and Tribes of New Zealand' with royal favour and was 'anxious to protect their just Rights and Property and to secure to them the enjoyment of Peace and Good Order …'. As well, 'a settled form of Civil Government' was proposed 'with a view to avert the evil consequences which must result from the absence of the necessary Laws and Institutions, alike to the native population and to Her subjects …'. Taken together with Normanby's 'Instructions' and Busby's 1837 dispatch, it becomes apparent that the Treaty of Waitangi was concerned with much more than the protection of physical resources; human protection was also intended.

Table 14 lists the provisions of the Treaty of Waitangi derived from both the English and Māori versions.

Table 14: Treaty of Waitangi provisions

	Article One	*Article Two*	*Article Three*
English Text	Crown sovereignty	Tribal property rights	Royal protection and citizenship rights
Māori Text	Crown authority to govern	Tribal authority over cultural, social, and economic resources	Royal protection and citizenship rights
Twentieth-century Implications	Parliament's right and authority to govern	Tribal right to exercise tino rangatiratanga	Māori individuals' right to expect a fair share of society's benefits

TREATY PRINCIPLES

The two versions of the Treaty did not say the same thing and created quite different expectations. Māori believed that greater recognition of Māori authority was promised, and Government insisted that a full and complete transfer of sovereignty had occurred. Some compromise can be reached by attending to the Treaty's principles rather than relying totally on the actual texts. To some extent this approach can overcome the criticisms that time has rendered the Treaty obsolete and that it was insufficiently detailed to allow firm rules to be laid down. Certainly, the Treaty of Waitangi Act 1975 required the newly established Waitangi Tribunal to take into account the principles of the Treaty and gave it statutory authority to decide what the principles were. Māori, placing greater emphasis on the actual words of the Treaty, have never been entirely comfortable with a focus on principles, sometimes because the definition of principles has been left to the Crown, acting on its own. Nonetheless, such an approach has enabled the issues to be debated and contemporary Treaty applications to be determined.

The terms of reference for the Royal Commission on Social Policy described the principles of the Treaty of Waitangi as one of the foundations of New Zealand society and economy, and the Commission took them into account in its work, concluding that the Treaty was relevant to all social and economic policies and relevant to the future as much as the past.[12] 'The Commission believes that the Treaty is always speaking and that it has relevance to all economic and social policies. Not only must the past be reviewed in light of its principles, but the Treaty's promise must also be seen as fundamental to those principles which will underline social wellbeing in years to come.'[13]

Rejecting a Treasury conclusion that the Treaty was 'silent, as in respect of employment, incomes, and economic development',[14] the Royal Commission view was that the Treaty's relevance could not be excluded from the range of Government policies. Even before then, a number of Government departments, including those in social policy areas, had accepted that Treaty principles were important. A report, *Puao-te-ata-tu*, from a Ministerial Advisory Committee[15] had rather forced the Department of Social Welfare to reconsider its structures, programmes, and processes as they related to Māori. The Department later submitted to the Royal Commission that 'all State agencies will have to come to terms with their responsibilities under the Treaty of Waitangi'.[16]

Earlier still, in 1986, the fourth Labour Government Cabinet had taken what seemed to be a decisive stand on Treaty issues by agreeing that all future legislation should be examined to determine any implications for the Treaty of Waitangi and that departments should consult with Māori on significant matters as well as assessing financial and resource implications arising from Treaty considerations.[17] One of the first departments to respond was the Department of Health. A circular memorandum for hospital boards and area health boards, authored by the Director-General of Health, Dr George Salmond, recommended that the Treaty of Waitangi be integrated into health services. He firmly stated the Department's views: 'For the Department of Health, the Treaty has special significance. Concepts of health are firmly based in Māori culture (which according to the Treaty, has a right to official recognition and protection) and Māori people have a right to appropriate services—funded through our health system. The Department accepts this view which is in accord with the WHO principles set out in the Alma Alta Declaration of 1978 on Primary Health Care'.[18]

There was, however, a gap between recognition of the importance of the Treaty to social policy and health, and actual implementation of Treaty-based policies and programmes. For one thing, the principles of the Treaty as they might apply to social policy areas had not been defined; legal decisions had concerned principles relating to physical resources such as land.[19] The only Waitangi Tribunal report relevant to cultural matters was about Māori language.[20] In 1988, however, the Royal Commission on Social Policy recommended three principles relevant both to social policy and the Treaty of Waitangi: partnership, participation, and protection.[21]

Partnership

The first of these, partnership, had also been proposed by the Bicultural Commission of the Anglican Church,[22] the Waitangi Tribunal, and the Court of Appeal. Partnership is strongest when it refers to an agreement between Iwi or hapū and the Crown, although it is sometimes used with limited justification to describe a working relationship between Māori and government agencies. It was the theme of *Tirohanga Rangapū: Partnership Perspectives*, a discussion document promoted by the Hon Koro Wetere, Minister of Māori Affairs, in 1988 and intended to reshape the relationship between Māori and the Crown. 'The Government will be working to develop mechanisms that provide for practical partnership within the state sector. Practical partnership will be achieved through consultation with iwi and government agencies over policies of concern to the iwi.'[23]

However, although partnership implies an association of equals, in fact it more often refers to a reassignment of government authority to a tribal group within deliberately constrained guidelines. At least in the eyes of the Crown, it is not a licence to take constitutional liberties. Not all tribes are happy with that understanding and have declined to engage in so-called partnerships with the Government. But many have eagerly entered into partnerships with the Department of Health, area health boards, and, more recently, regional health authorities, maintaining that the real significance lies in the underlying constitutional symbolism whereby the two partners to the Treaty work together to realize mutually acceptable goals.

Because New Zealand does not have a written constitution, however, and has never explicitly defined the constitutional position of Māori, partnerships may be forced to function within ill-defined parameters, relying on good faith and agreed-upon goals more than formal conventions or clearly demarcated lines of authority. In an attempt to formalize the partnership process, several Iwi in the Bay of Plenty established a confederation, Te Whānau Poutirirangiora ā Papa, to explore, on behalf of Māori, a relationship with the Bay of Plenty Area Health Board.[24] They opted for a parallel partnership plan in which the united tribes and the Board shared in decision-making, policy development, and service provision for Māori client groups.[25]After lengthy discussion the partnership proceeded with mutual enthusiasm and was seen as a model for other areas.[26] But before its contribution to Māori health could be assessed, the health reforms had led to a dismantling of the area health board system.

Determined to maintain the initiative, Te Whānau Poutirirangiora then pursued a similar arrangement with the Midland Regional Health Authority, though this time it was as a co-purchaser rather than a provider of health services.

Participation

Participation, a second principle recommended by the Royal Commission on Social Policy, refers to Māori involvement in a particular activity or sector. The basis for Māori participation in health has been inconsistent in the past (as discussed in Chapter Four). With an increasing reliance on health professionals, Māori participation has been marginalized. A survey undertaken in 1987 showed that in some disciplines, such as clinical psychology, there were only one or two Māori, and no clinical psychology programmes included any substantial Māori perspective.[27] Social work participation rates were higher, around 7 per cent, and both of the university training programmes had significant Māori input. However, only 0.7 per cent of the medical workforce was Māori. Even by 1991 fewer than 1 per cent of medical practitioners and only 2 per cent of registered nurses were Māori, and, despite a range of Māori health initiatives, Māori are underrepresented in policy development and service provision.[28] At the same time, a passive consumer position has been replaced by a determination to take an active leadership role in defining health needs and then arranging (if not providing) health services. 'The last decade has seen a health revolution occur in New Zealand. A revolution led by Māori people who have questioned the definition of health and the definition of health professional, who participates in and benefits from health planning, decision making, and the delivery of health services. This has led to a range of Māori initiated, Government funded health projects that have contributed to the greater participation of Māori in the health sector. For example, Marae based health centres, and iwi based health service delivery contracts with health sector agencies.'[29]

Recognizing the importance of Māori participation at policy making levels, and conscious that local body elections seldom returned Māori candidates, the Hon Helen Clark, who was Minister of Health in 1989, appointed Māori members to all area health boards. She was using powers given to the Minister under a 1989 amendment to the Area Health Boards Act. Although she had taken advice on suitable appointees, in some situations it was never clear whether the newly appointed Māori members had a mandate from Māori people or whether they were simply Māori members who could bring their own Māori perspective. The difference was to become an increasingly important one as Māori sought to participate in national and local affairs on their own terms without depending on party political patronage.

Concerned that area health boards would fail to distinguish between having a Māori board member and active Māori participation in health services, the Ministerial Advisory Committee on Māori Health produced a set of policy guidelines.[30] Two models were recommended for boards to consider. The first, a partnership model, allowed for Iwi, separately or collectively, to interact with a board in determining health policy, at least in respect of Māori. The second model proposed a standing committee, consistent with section 28 of the Area Health Boards Act, which would be representative of Māori within the region and able to provide the board with policies for Māori health. The Committee's three recommendations were: that Māori health policies at a board level should be guided by representative Māori opinion; that dialogue should be established between boards and Iwi for the advancement of their respective health plans; and that

Māori community committees should be established to address specific health goals and targets. Generally, boards found the guidelines useful.

From 1991, appointments to Crown research institutes, regional health authorities, and Crown health enterprises were made after consultation with Māori, but in the end the selections were determined at ministerial levels. When appointments to the Treaty of Waitangi Fisheries Commission were being considered at a national meeting of Māori leaders held at Parliament, the National Māori Congress agreed that the Minister of Māori Affairs had the constitutional authority to make the appointments, but urged him to allow Māori to make the selections.[31] The distinction, important in Māori eyes, would have overcome the uncertainties concerning the mandate held by Māori appointees to public bodies.

Protection

A third Treaty principle, protection, refers to the State's policies and programmes to guarantee Māori the same 'rights and privileges' as other New Zealanders. It includes proactive measures to promote health and prevent illness. The Waitangi Tribunal has emphasized the principle of active protection, describing it as an obligation on the Crown to remedy past mistakes through measures which will give Māori opportunities to take full advantage of the benefits of contemporary society. In deciding on the Ngāti Pāoa claim, and having made the observation that the Crown had allowed Ngāti Pāoa to become virtually landless, Chief Judge Durie concluded, 'It seems then a reasonable expectation today, and in keeping with the spirit of the Treaty, that the Crown should not resile from any opportunity it may have to provide at least a part of those endowments that it ought to have guaranteed, and to ensure, that proper policies to that end are maintained'.[32] Rather than simply allowing Māori to take their chances alongside other groups, the principle of active protection requires the Government to intervene positively, not because Māori deserve better health than anyone else, but because they are entitled to no less a standard of health than that of their neighbours. At the risk of paternalism, the Crown's Treaty undertaking is to safeguard Māori interests to the extent that Māori themselves can enjoy similar health outcomes to other New Zealanders.

THE CROWN TREATY PRINCIPLES

The fourth Labour Government came into office in 1984 with a greater commitment to the Treaty of Waitangi than any previous Government: 'The Government had the Treaty as a centrepiece of its Māori policy'.[33] Not only did it begin to appear in legislation, but it was also included in the terms of reference of the Royal Commission on Social Policy and had been intended to feature prominently in the proposed Bill of Rights. However, enthusiasm for the Treaty changed after 1987 when the Courts found in favour of the New Zealand Māori Council (in relation to the State Owned Enterprises Act 1986), several tribes (in connection with the fisheries quota management system in 1987), and the Tainui Māori Trust Board (in respect of a transfer of the Huntly coal mines to Coalcorp in 1989).

Whether the Government had anticipated the extent and force of Māori legal endeavours is not clear, but it soon became apparent to them that they were ill-prepared to take on Māori in Court. Consequently a Treaty of Waitangi Policy Unit was established in the Department of Justice in 1989, primarily to act as a focus for Crown Treaty activities but also to coordinate the increasingly large number of departments involved in Treaty claims and to negotiate with Iwi on behalf of the Crown.[34] Having been quite prepared to act on behalf of Māori interests, the Government now faced the prospect of having to defend itself against Māori claims and to define its own Treaty stance. In short, it needed to reclaim the Treaty as a political rather than a legal issue, and the Prime Minister, the Rt Hon Geoffrey Palmer said so: 'It must be made clear that the roles of Parliament, the Government and the courts are understood and certain. It must be made clear that the Government will make the final decisions on treaty issues'.[35]

The Crown principles for action on the Treaty of Waitangi emerged as one indicator of the Government's resolve to assert itself.[36] Unlike the earlier principles defined by the Waitangi Tribunal, Court of Appeal, and Royal Commission on Social Policy, the Crown principles were to guide Crown action. They were not principles of the Treaty itself, though were derived from it,[37] neither were they intended for Māori and the State alike. Significantly they did not include partnership nor did they suggest an extension into social policy areas. Instead the focus was on government departments being prepared and able to handle themselves when negotiating with Māori. The five Crown principles were: the kāwanatanga principle—the principle of government; the rangatiratanga principle—the principle of self-management; the principle of equality; the principle of cooperation; the principle of redress.

Māori reaction to the principles was less than enthusiastic. The rules, it seemed, had changed. Just as Māori were gaining confidence in the courts and the Waitangi Tribunal, Government was attempting to bypass them, favouring instead a system which was under its own control. It had the same ring as the 1852 Constitution Act when fundamental changes to the Māori–Crown relationship were instituted without consultation. Up until then, Māori had regarded the Colonial Office, if not the British Parliament, as a more objective arbiter between tribal and settler interests, but with the establishment of a settler Government in New Zealand in 1854 the rules and the refereeing were conducted by one party only. So in 1989 it appeared that the Government was seeking ways to avoid involving the more neutral third parties such as the courts and the Waitangi Tribunal.

Of particular concern was the so-called rangatiratanga principle which had been presented in terms of management rather than mana, and, though acknowledging physical and cultural properties, failed to mention a possible role for Iwi in social arenas, including health. That presumably could be accommodated under the principle of equality, provided the law was able to recognize Māori interests and the Māori position. In any event a change of Government in 1990 left the Crown principles suspended. Though never formally discounted by the National Government, neither were they endorsed.

A summary of the relevant principles of the Treaty of Waitangi is contained in Table 15.

Table 15: Principles of the Treaty of Waitangi

	Waitangi Tribunal	*Court of Appeal*	*Royal Commission on Social Policy*	*Crown Principles for Action on Treaty Issues*
Main Principles	Partnership Tribal rangatiratanga Active protection Mutual benefit Consultation	Honour Good faith Reasonable actions Partnership	Partnership Participation Protection	Kāwanatanga Rangatiratanga Equality Cooperation Redress
Application	Claims to the Tribunal	State Owned Enterprises Act 1986	Social policies	Government departments and Treaty negotiators

LEGISLATION

The resolution of Treaty grievances is enabled under certain legislation: the Treaty of Waitangi Act 1975, the Treaty of Waitangi (State Enterprises) Act 1988, the Crown Forest Assets Act 1989, and the Treaty of Waitangi (Fisheries Claim) Settlement Act 1992. Apart from these, legislation also exists to give effect to the Treaty in a variety of situations.

However, even though it has been used to aid the interpretation of the law generally, the Treaty of Waitangi has been enforceable only when it has been incorporated into legislation. In deciding on the landmark New Zealand Māori Council State Owned Enterprises case,[38] for example, the Court of Appeal would not have been able to comment so positively on the Treaty of Waitangi[39] if section

9 of the State Owned Enterprises Act 1986 had not been worded the way that it was.[40] The two outstanding instances when the Treaty was used to assist in defining the law occurred in *Huakina Development Trust* and the radio frequencies case. In the former, Justice Chilwell in 1987 considered that the Treaty was so much part of the 'fabric of society' that he used it to assist in the definition of the public interest when considering the Water and Soil Conservation Act 1967. He subsequently found in favour of the Huakina Development Trust which had brought an action against the Waikato Valley Authority. Similarly, Heron J granted an injunction preventing the allocation of radio frequencies on the grounds that the disposal of the resource could affect Treaty rights. While the Radio Communications Act 1989 contained no reference to the Treaty, nonetheless the judge felt that Māori had reasonably expected the Treaty to form part of the background against which the Act should apply.[41]

There are a significant though not abundant number of Acts which contain a reference to the principles of the Treaty of Waitangi: the Treaty of Waitangi Act 1975, the Environment Act 1986, the State Owned Enterprises Act 1986,* the Conservation Act 1987, the Crown Minerals Act 1991,* the Foreshore and Seabed Endowment Revesting Act 1991, the Harbour Boards Dry Land Endowment Revesting Act 1991, the Resource Management Act 1991, the Crown Research Institutes Act 1992.[42]

There are other Acts which refer to Māori interests but fall short of specifying the Treaty of Waitangi as an obligation on the Crown. These other Acts include: the Law Commission Act 1985, the Education Act 1989, the Broadcasting Act 1989, the Mental Health (Compulsory Assessment and Treatment) Act 1992, and the Health and Disability Services Act 1993. Each of them requires that some aspect of the Māori situation be taken into account. In the case of the Mental Health Act, section 5, reinforced by section 65, requires that any Court or Tribunal who exercises powers under the Act must have respect for a patient's cultural and ethnic identity, language, and religious or ethical beliefs. They must also show proper recognition of the importance to the patient's well-being of family ties, as well as whānau, hapū, and Iwi links. Further, section 6 requires an interpreter to be made available 'wherever practicable' if the first or preferred language of the patient is Māori (or any other language). Winston Maniapoto considered that these provisions would make it virtually impossible for a non-Māori psychiatrist to assess a Māori-speaking patient adequately. However, the Director of Mental Health, Dr Janice Wilson, replied that under the Act it would be sufficient to have an interpreter and, even then, only if practicable.

In the Health and Disability Services Act 1993, section 8 refers to the ability of the Minister to give to a purchaser written notice of the Crown's social and other objectives. These objectives may be in relation to a number of matters including (in subclause (e)) 'the special needs of Māori and other particular communities or people for those services'. These legislative provisions are summarized in Table 16.

Table 16: The Treaty of Waitangi, legislation, and Māori interests

Resolution of Claims under the Treaty of Waitangi	*Legislation to Secure Rights Protected by the Treaty of Waitangi*	*Provisions Relating to the Principles of the Treaty of Waitangi*	*Provisions Relating to Māori Interests or the Māori Perspective*
Treaty of Waitangi Act 1975 Treaty of Waitangi (State Enterprises) Act 1988 Crown Forest Assets Act 1989 Treaty of Waitangi (Fisheries Claims) Settlement Act 1992	Māori Language Act 1987 Te Ture Whenua Māori Act 1993	Environment Act 1986 State Owned Enterprises Act 1986 Conservation Act 1987 Crown Minerals Act 1991 Foreshore and Seabed Endowment Revesting Act 1991 Harbour Boards Dry Land Endowment Revesting Act 1991 Resource Management Act 1991 Crown Research Institutes Act 1992	Law Commission Act 1985 Education Act 1989 Broadcasting Act 1989 Mental Health Act 1992 Health and Disability Services Act 1993

There are two points to be made concerning the Treaty in legislation. First, there is no reference to the Treaty in any social policy legislation. Where express Treaty reference is made, it is in relationship to physical resources such as the environment, land, or the sea. Second, a recognition of Māori interests in social policy legislation appears to arise from a concern about cultural values or disparities in Māori/non-Māori standards rather than from any sense of a Treaty-based obligation or rights quite apart from equity issues. The implication of this is that, although the Government can accept the relevance of the Treaty to tribal property (as provided for in Article Two), it has not yet been able to accept the full implications of the Māori version of the same article with its broad definition of taonga and its promise of tino rangatiratanga.

In this regard the Health and Disability Services Act 1993 was a disappointment to Māori. Its predecessor, the Area Health Boards Act 1983, contained no express reference to Māori interests and, despite Māori submissions urging the Minister to include a Treaty clause in the 1993 Act, it was omitted. On more than one occasion during the Hon Simon Upton's public relation tours to explain the health reforms, he was asked about the place of the Treaty in the proposed legislation. His reply was that New Zealand had not yet agreed on the significance of the Treaty to social policy areas and, in any case, section 8(e) of the new Bill would 'meet the health needs of Māori and help address the improvement of their health status'.[43] Māori were less convinced. They felt that the 153-year debate on the Treaty of Waitangi had established the applicability of the Treaty across all sectors and for the future as well as the past. Nor did they feel that the main issue was simply one of reducing disparities in health (or education or income levels or housing).

Considerable interest in the Health and Disability Services Act 1993 also focused on any provisions for the disposal of surplus health land. Ever since the State Owned Enterprises case, the Government had been aware of intense Māori interest in surplus Crown properties and the need to have a transparent process in place before disposal. In addition, special arrangements had often been made between tribes and community leaders for the endowment of hospitals with land. Members of the Ngāti Whakaue tribe, for example, had been promised free hospital care in recognition of the land they gifted for a hospital at Rotorua.

Anticipating significant disposal of assets, the Minister agreed that the new health authorities should utilize a surplus land protection mechanism which would protect Māori interests.[44] Section 42(1)(a) of the Health and Disability Services Act 1993 advised accordingly. Eventually, though not before the Act was passed, a mechanism was developed. Known as the consultative clearance process, it required that a schedule of surplus lands be published at least a month before sale. Hapū or Iwi who could demonstrate a substantive interest would be able to lodge their claims with the Department of Survey and Land Information as a prelude to negotiations. Until negotiations were complete the land would be placed in a land bank and could not be sold without ministerial approval. Surplus lands were divided into three categories: category A sites comprised wāhi tapu (sacred sites) or burial grounds; category B sites were lands of special importance to Iwi (such as mountains or streams) which were already the subject of a claim; and category C lands were those which might be useful in the settlement of valid claims against the Crown.[45]

While a Treaty clause in legislation affords maximum protection in terms of claims against the Crown, it is not the sole basis for a claim. For the purposes of the Treaty of Waitangi Act 1975 it is sufficient to demonstrate that a Crown policy or practice has amounted to a breach of the Treaty, even if appropriate legislation is not available to support the case. Some Māori groups, concerned about poor standards of Māori health in comparison with other New Zealanders, have threatened to take a claim to the Waitangi Tribunal, fully realizing the difficulties in proving Crown negligence rather than individual or family carelessness.[46] Moreover, it would not be an easy task to untangle the multi-causal factors which underlie illness or disease. Unsatisfactory social conditions might be more relevant than inadequate hospital care or delays in gaining access to treatment.

While the Waitangi Tribunal has not been asked to inquire into a claim based on a failure of the Crown to safeguard Māori health, it has reported on a claim concerning Māori rights to hospital resources. The Domett Avenue claim was made in respect of a property which was being used as a centre for Māori health education and cultural training by Te Taou Reweti Charitable Trust. The Auckland Area Health Board proposed to sell the property which was now considered surplus to Board requirements. The Māori claimants, not wishing to leave the building, raised with the Tribunal their understanding that a condition of the Ngāti Whātua land sales in Auckland was to be special health services for Māori. Land sale deeds contained a proviso by which 10 per cent of the resale price was to be returned to Ngāti Whātua in cash or services, for '. . . the construction of hospitals in which persons of our own race may be tended, for the payment of medical attendance for us . . .'.[47]

In other words, the claimants' case was based on the assumption that Ngāti Whātua were entitled to special provisions, above and beyond those for all citizens. Before the Tribunal report was issued the land was sold but the funds from the sale were to be held in a Board trust fund, pending a successful claim or agreement with local Iwi. The Tribunal recommended that the future disposal of surplus area health board properties should be consistent with a general policy (to be developed after consultation with Māori) and that consideration should be given as to whether any particular arrangements should be made to fund Māori health needs.

This last recommendation took into account the undertakings made in various parts of the country that Māori land sales would be accompanied by special provisions for education and health. Māori had provided an economic base for hospitals in a variety of ways. Sometimes land was compulsorily taken for a hospital site but without compensation; in other cases land was gifted but on an understanding that Māori needs would not be overlooked; and, as in the Ngāti Whātua case, sometimes there was an agreement that land sales would be linked to special provisions for Māori.

By 1992, over 150 years after its signing, the Treaty of Waitangi had been accepted by the Minister of Health as the 'founding document of New Zealand'.[48] Though the acceptance did not go as far as Māori would have liked, and did not include any mention of the Treaty in the new health legislation, nonetheless it represented a significant move towards a more logical appreciation of health as a combination of social, cultural, economic, and political factors. Māori health now stood some chance of being considered within a context that was meaningful both in terms of New Zealand's historical development and the contemporary aspirations of Māori people.

True, a large gap existed between acceptance of the Treaty and the translation of its aims into performance indicators, output measures, staff profiles, and, above all, actual health gains for Māori. Two ideological movements eventually helped to shape the pathway. The first was biculturalism and its radical realignment of New Zealand's approaches to health; the second was the health reforms, a move towards greater accountability for the expenditure of public funds, and a refocusing of health priorities towards earlier forms of intervention, quality care, and a reduction of unacceptable disparities.

ENDNOTES

1 New Zealand Board of Health, (1987), *Annual Report of the New Zealand Board of Health 1986–87*, New Zealand Board of Health, Wellington.

2 New Zealand Board of Health, (1988), *Priorities for the New Zealand Health Services*, New Zealand Board of Health, Wellington.

3 M. H. Durie, (1989), 'The Treaty of Waitangi: Perspectives for Social Policy', in I. H. Kawharu (ed.), *Waitangi: Māori and Pākehā Perspectives of the Treaty of Waitangi*, Oxford University Press, Auckland, p. 298.

4 P. Adams, (1977), *Fatal Necessity: British Intervention in New Zealand 1830–1847*, Oxford University Press, Auckland, p. 88.

5 Lord Normanby's 'Instructions' are contained in: Waitangi Tribunal, (1987), *Orakei Report*, Department of Justice, Wellington.

6 Adams, *op cit.*, p. 92.

7 Bruce Biggs, (1989), 'Humpty Dumpty and the Treaty of Waitangi', in Kawharu, *op cit.*, pp. 305–6.

8 R. M. Ross, (1972), 'Te Tiriti o Waitangi: Texts and Translations', *New Zealand Journal of History* 6 (2): 139–42.

9 Biggs, *op cit.*, pp. 307–8.

10 Waitangi Tribunal, (1986), *Te Reo Māori Report*, Department of Justice, Wellington.

11 Te Wāhanga Hauora Māori (1992), *Whaia te Ora mō te Iwi: Strive for the Good Health of the People*, Department of Health, Wellington, p. 23.

12 Royal Commission on Social Policy, (1988), *The April Report*, II, Royal Commission on Social Policy, Wellington, pp. 26–151.

13 Ibid., p. 80.

14 Treasury, (1987), *Government Management: Brief to the Incoming Government, vol. 1*, Treasury, Wellington, p. 348.

15 Ministerial Advisory Committee on a Māori Perspective for the Department of Social Welfare, (1986), *Puao-te-ata-tu*, Department of Social Welfare, Wellington.

16 Department of Social Welfare, (1987), *Submission to the Royal Commission on Social Policy*, Department of Social Welfare, Wellington.

17 Geoffrey Palmer, (1992), *New Zealand's Constitution in Crisis: Reforming Our Political System*, John McIndoe, Dunedin, pp. 82–3.
18 Department of Health, (1986), *Circular Memorandum No. 1986/70*, Department of Health, Wellington.
19 The 1987 landmark Court of Appeal case, concerning the State Owned Enterprises Act 1986, was about the transfer of physical assets, principally land and forests. The Court emphasizes the principles of partnership, good faith, and honour.
20 Waitangi Tribunal, (1985), *op cit.*
21 Royal Commission on Social Policy, *op cit.*, vol II, pp. 47–69.
22 Bicultural Commission, (1986), *Te Ripoata a te Komihana mo te Kaupapa Tikanga Rua mo te Tiriti o Waitangi: The Report of the Bicultural Commission of the Anglican Church on the Treaty of Waitangi*, Church of the Province of New Zealand.
23 Department of Māori Affairs, (1988), *Te Urupare Rangapū: Partnership Response*, Department of Māori Affairs, Wellington, p. 12.
24 The Iwi were Ngāti Ranginui, Ngāi Te Rangi, Ngāti Pukenga, Waitaha, Tapuika, Ngāti Pikiao, Ngāti Rangiwehi, Ngāti Whakaue, Tuhourangi, Ngāti Rangitihi, Tuwharetoa ki Kawerau, Ngāti Awa, Tuhoe, Whakatōhea, Ngāi Tai, Te Whānau ā Apanui.
25 Pia Callaghan, (1990), *Te Whānau Poutirirangiora ā Papa*, a discussion paper prepared for the Bay of Plenty Area Health Board.
26 Ministerial Advisory Committee on Māori Health, (1990), *He Ara Tohutohu Mō Nga Hauora ā Rohe: Guidelines for Area Health Boards*, Department of Health, Wellington.
27 M. W. Abbott and M. Durie, (1987), 'A Whiter Shade of Pale: Taha Māori and Professional Psychology Training', *New Zealand Journal of Psychology* 16: 58–71.
28 D. Ropiha, (1993), *Whakarawa mai te Hau Maori: Increasing the Participation of Maori in the Health Workforce*, Health Research and Analytical Services, Internal Report, Department of Health, Wellington.
29 Te Wāhanga Hauora Māori, *op cit.*, p. 20.
30 Ministerial Advisory Committee on Māori Health, (1990), *op cit.*
31 M. H. Durie, (1993), *Submission to the Minister of Māori Affairs on the Appointment of Commissioners to the Treaty of Waitangi Fisheries Commission*, National Māori Congress, Wellington.
32 Waitangi Tribunal, (1987), *Report on the Waiheke Claim*, Tribunals Division, Department of Justice, Wellington.
33 Palmer, *op cit.*, p. 82.
34 Alex Frame, (1990), 'A State Servant Looks at the Treaty', *New Zealand Universities Law Review* 14 (1): 82–96.
35 Geoffrey Palmer, (1990), 'Treaty of Waitangi Issues Demand Clarity, Certainty', *New Zealand Herald*, 2 January 1990.
36 Department of Justice, (1989), *Principles for Crown Action on the Treaty of Waitangi*, Department of Justice, Wellington.

37 W. Renwick, (1990), *The Treaty Now*, GP Books, Wellington, pp. 128–30.

38 Court of Appeal, (1987), *The Treaty of Waitangi in the Court of Appeal: The Full Judgements of the Court in the New Zealand Maori Council's case*, CA 54/87, Department of Justice, Wellington.

39 K. Keith, (1990), 'The Treaty of Waitangi in the Courts', *New Zealand Universities Law Review* 14 (1): 37–61.

40 Section 9 of the State Owned Enterprises Act reads, 'Nothing in this Act shall permit the Crown to act in a manner which is inconsistent with the principles of the Treaty of Waitangi'.

41 P. McHugh, (1991), *The Māori Magna Carta: New Zealand Law and the Treaty of Waitangi*, Oxford University Press, Auckland, pp. 270–9.

42 A (*) denotes where Treaty principles have been accorded priority.

43 Te Wāhanga Hauora Māori, *op cit.*, p. 23.

44 Ibid., pp. 22–3.

45 Hon Douglas Graham, Minister of Justice (1993), circular letter to Iwi authorities.

46 In 1987 there was debate at a national hui about taking a claim to the Waitangi Tribunal on the basis that health was a taonga and that the Crown had failed to protect it. See *Gisborne Herald*, 8 July 1987.

47 Waitangi Tribunal, (1991), *The Auckland Hospital Endowments Claim*, Department of Justice, Wellington.

48 Hon Simon Upton, Minister of Health, (1992), in Te Wāhanga Hauora Māori, *op cit.*, p. 23.

READING 3

Hauora Tāngata

Māori Health Status

No single measure can give an accurate indication of the state of Māori health. Because health encompasses at least the dimensions of wairua, hinengaro, tinana, and whānau, the indices normally used are limited and tend to reflect only one dimension and, even then, focus on sickness and illness rather than the wider view of health. Furthermore, an assessment of contemporary Māori health status requires more precise definition of the terms 'Māori' and 'health'. In the past neither have been described in a consistent manner, so that accurate comparisons of past and present, or Māori and non-Māori, have been hindered by differing understandings and definitions.

Much depends on the way in which statistics are collected and then used. Questionable political motivation has sometimes led to biased and unethical practices and to the application of ethnic statistical data for dubious purposes. For instance, a 'race alien' classification was developed to discourage Asian migration to New Zealand and the classification of some Māori as 'half castes living as Europeans' was designed to speed up Māori integration into a homogenous society.[1] Yet, in spite of those problems and others, ethnic statistics have been useful in allowing some assessment of Māori health status both for comparative purposes and for future health planning.

DEFINING MĀORI

The definition of a Māori has taken several courses. Prior to 1840, Māori regarded themselves as 'normal' and other races were seen as different, the term Pākehā being used for Europeans.[2] Subcategories, based on nationality and ethnicity, were also used to distinguish different types of Pākehā: Wiwi for the French, Kotimana for Scots, Ingarihi for the English. Tauiwi was also used, though in a less specific sense, to describe settlers from other countries, no matter what their ethnic background.[3] After the Treaty of Waitangi, however, and particularly from 1860 when the declining Māori population had become a minority, euro-centric views of race came to dominate. It was Māori who were regarded as different.

Māori were either full-blooded or half-caste. Quite apart from the inaccuracy of Māori statistics, the distinction between half-castes living as Māori and half-castes living as Europeans introduced a further source of error and confused the rationale for recording half-castes anyway. Half-castes living as Europeans were not considered Māori even though the basis for classification then was biological rather than cultural. By 1926 that distinction had gone and a Māori was defined as a person with half or more Māori blood. A Māori who had less than 50 per cent Māori blood was considered European. The result was that, even after the registration of births and deaths became compulsory for Māori in 1913,[4] cultural self-identification was so strong that the 'full Maori' category was grossly over-enumerated.[5] The Maori Affairs Act 1953 defined a Māori as 'a person belonging to the aboriginal race of New Zealand, including a half-caste and a person intermediate between half-caste and a person of pure descent from that race'.[6]

Biological inheritance as the sole determinant of ethnicity was replaced by the concept of cultural identification in the 1974 Māori Affairs Amendment Act. Sponsored by Hon Matiu Rata, the Act described a Māori as 'a person of the Māori race of New Zealand; and includes any descendent of such a person'. The broader approach no longer required an estimation of racial percentages. In fact, though said to be more accurate, such a percentage system had become a grossly inaccurate method, many describing themselves as 'full' Māori simply to register disapproval at having to calculate their identity. It also contained overtones of colonial assumptions about racial superiority. After the new definition was introduced the Crown Law Office considered that a Māori was either a person of pure Māori blood or a person of less than pure blood who elected to be considered as a Māori for the purpose of the Electoral Act 1975.

In the 1986 census, self-identification was the method used to determine ethnic identity (by then the term 'race' had all but been dropped because of its discriminatory associations) and by 1991 the process had been further refined. Questions 7, 8, and 9 in the 1991 census related to Māori identity. Question 7 contained nine choices, respondents being asked to indicate which ethnic group or groups they belonged to. New Zealand Māori was one option. Question 8 asked if there were any Māori ancestry and, if so, in question 9, what were the main and other tribal affiliations (a total of three could be mentioned).

The 1991 census was significant in two respects. First, it enquired into tribal affiliation, largely in response to pressure from central government who needed the information for the implementation of the Rūnanga Iwi Act 1990. The Act provided for Iwi development and the redistribution of resources to Iwi according to population.[7] Second, the 1991 census distinguished between people who were descended from a Māori and those who opted to identify as Māori. There was a significant difference. 434,847 New Zealand residents specified that they belonged to the Māori ethnic group (12.9 per cent) while 511,278 persons claimed Māori ancestry (15.1 per cent).[8] In addition, 110,000 people indicated that they belonged to another ethnic group as well as Māori. Some doubt therefore arose as to how many Māori there actually were: 511,278 or 434,847 or (excluding those who had more than one ethnic identity) 321,000? If the larger figure were used for a claim to resources based on population, at least one commentator considered that it would be misleading.[9] Māori on the other hand took heart that the population, however defined, had increased to over half a million and that they were now again able to define their own identity. The 1996 census confirmed continued growth in both descent and ethnic identity: 579,714 reported descent from a Māori while 523,371 identified as ethnic Māori. By now the gap between the two measures was reducing, although the difference remained high enough to pose the same question as it did in 1991. And the distinction between 'sole Māori' and multiple ethnic identities had still to be resolved.

Vital statistics meanwhile remained based on the biological concept of race. Births and deaths required an estimation of the degree of Māori blood, and a Māori child was one who had at least 50 per cent Māori genetic make-up. In hospitals there was no deliberate policy for determining whether patients were half or more Māori. In practice, hospital clerical staff completed most statistical forms and sometimes made up their own minds rather than asking patients or relatives. As a result they tended to under-report Māori.[10] Cultural identity became used more often than the biological method in hospitals but the retention of the word 'race' on the admission form suggested that a biological estimation was intended. Similar difficulties in reporting ethnicity occurred with funeral directors. A study on deaths due to coronary artery disease showed that there was quite serious under-reporting of Māori deaths largely due to funeral directors choosing to leave the ethnicity question blank.[11]

Guesses about ethnicity are highly inaccurate since physical appearance is no longer a reliable indicator, and often members of staff are too embarrassed to ask.[12]

Table 18 summarizes the differences between the two main methods of defining Māori, and highlights the inconsistencies arising from each method in, for example, recording live births. Although there has been a general move towards cultural affiliation and self-identification, there is still considerable variation between government departments and agencies. The obvious variation is between statistics from the Justice Department, with its biological approach, and data from the 1991 census which are based on self-identification. As shown in Table 18, the Justice Department recorded 6946 Māori births in 1991 whereas the census figures were as high as 13,000 for the same year.

Table 18: Statistical definitions of Māori

	Biological Determination	*Ethnic Affiliation*	*Māori Descent*	*Mixed (i.e., unclear)*
Estimation of Race	Parental inheritance Degree of Māori blood	Self-identification	Genealogy used as basis for entitlement to be Māori	Self-identification used in practice but concept of race retained on forms
Basis	Constitutional genetic	Cultural	Whakapapa	Best estimate
Current Usage	Justice Department (births, deaths) Schools Adoptions Foetal and neo-natal deaths	Census enumeration (Q 7) Household labour-force survey Post-secondary education Cancer registration	Census enumeration (Q 8) Iwi registers	Health statistics Psychiatric statistics Some schools
Minimum Requirement	Half-Māori	Choose to identify as Māori	One Māori ancestor	Estimate of Māori descent
Sub-groupings	Full-blooded Half-caste Less than half	Māori identity Māori descent	Māori Iwi Hapū	Māori Belonging to Māori race
Application to Births 1991	6,946	13,000		

MEASURING HEALTH

Three limitations are particularly obvious in assessing Māori health status.

First, for the most part health statistics are about hospital activities. While they are useful, they should not be confused with indicators of health which can be applied outside hospital situations and which relate more directly to people and families in their usual environments. In its first report, the Core Services Committee drew attention to the limited information about community care services (including out-patient services): 'Detailed data on how many services are provided in the community area is also not known, nor are the demographic characteristics of those receiving services or the reasons people use these services'.[13]

Second, consistent with a hospital orientation, health statistics focus on illness and injury. More is known, for example, about hospitalization due to psychiatric illness and disability than about family patterns of emotional stress or reactions due to bereavement. Although some studies have been made on the prevalence of certain conditions within a community, few have focused on health incidents which are relatively minor, though frequent. The Māori Women's Welfare League Rapuora study was an exception; it asked women for their own assessment of their health status and in terms which made sense given their cultural affiliations.[14] Compulsory reporting of some conditions such as communicable diseases is required by law, and a greater emphasis on accountability, as expected in the health reforms, may lead to a more comprehensive data base. In the meantime, health profiles are decidedly sickness profiles.

Third, health indicators are designed for specific purposes. Diagnostic-related groupings are useful for determining in-patient cost categories; the International Classification of Diseases is based on clusters of signs and symptoms as well as knowledge about natural history and is useful for treatment purposes; death rates are useful to compare gross characteristics of various groups; and discharge rates reflect hospital turnover and usage. None of these alone is able to provide a comprehensive or accurate profile of the health of Māori people. Another method, taken by the Ministry of Health in conjunction with the Department of Statistics, is the household survey. *A Picture of Health*, a report about the health of 7000 New Zealanders, emphasized self-assessment of health status, health risks, and utilization of health services.[15] Though less reliable for small populations, and favouring healthy populations (because hospitalized patients were not included), the study provided a useful complement to other reports. It confirmed high smoking rates for Māori, higher Māori attendances at accident and emergency departments, and slightly higher hospital admission rates.

MĀORI HEALTH STATUS REPORTS

Comprehensive Comparisons

Māori health data has usually been presented by way of comparison with non-Māori. An early systematic tabulation of Māori health standards was compiled by R. J. Rose for the Department of Health in 1960. It showed that Māori health standards were 'very low in comparison with the European' and that Māori were 'affected to an even greater degree than the pakeha in many diseases which occur in late middle life or in old age. . . . There has been a misconception common among physicians and health workers that the Māori is comparatively free from these types of disease'.[16] If there were misconceptions, they rapidly vanished as similar themes were repeated in many subsequent reports. The Hunn Report[17] presented an improving but still dismal picture of Māori health. In 1951 a difference of fourteen to seventeen years separated life expectancy between Māori men and women and their European counterparts, respectively. Infant mortality, a sensitive indicator of the health of a population, was better than in earlier decades, but in 1958 Māori rates were almost three times as high as non-Māori. Similarly, as shown in Table 19, age-adjusted death rates were nearly twice as high. Birth rates on the other hand were double those of European.

Māori Standards of Health

The first of three special reports compiled by Eru Pomare, a grandson of the first Māori medical officer, Maui Pomare, was published in 1980.[19] Bringing together data from hospitals sources, it provided an overview of Māori health standards from the years 1955 to 1975 and served to underline the point that, although Māori life expectancy had dramatically improved, major disparities between Māori and non-Māori existed for most disease categories. Unlike earlier reports which had noted the high incidence of infectious diseases, the pattern had changed and the degenerative disorders were more apparent: hypertension, coronary artery disease, diabetes, obesity, hyperuricaemia, and gout. A relationship with lifestyle was demonstrated and over-nutrition, smoking, alcohol, and accidents were highlighted as causative factors.

Pomare's second report examined health statistics between the years 1970 and 1984.[20] In those years the Māori fertility rates suddenly reduced, almost to the same level as non-Māori. From an average of 6.2 births in 1962, by 1985 the average had fallen to 2.2 births. Other changes were also noted. There were improvements in life expectancy (2.8 years for Māori males and 3.5 years for Māori females), a reduction in mortality rates of over 25 per cent, and a reduced average length of stay in hospital (14.3 days down to 7.1 days). The third report, published in 1995 after Pomare's untimely death earlier that year,

Table 19: Māori health status 1950–1959

	Māori	*European*
Life Expectancy (1951)	55 years (female) 54 years (male)	65 years (female) 68 years (male)
Birth Rate (per 1000) (1956)	45	25
Infant Mortality (per 1000) (1958)	54	19
Death Rate (per 1000) (1959)	6.61 (under 20) 13.09 (over 20)	1.92 (under 20) 13.28 (over 20)

Source: Hunn Report, (1961)[18]

commented on the overall improvements in mortality but expressed concern about the continuing rise in psychiatric admissions, higher levels of alcohol and drug abuse, and the often increasing disparities between Māori and non-Māori standards of health. The significance of socio-economic factors, especially unemployment, as one set of determinants of poor health, was discussed, and there was a recommendation for adequate resourcing of Māori health services—a strategy seen as 'likely to alleviate' disparities between Māori and non-Māori.[21]

Māori Health Data

He Kākano, a handbook of data on Māori health prepared by Te Puni Kōkiri,[22] contained comparative statistics across the range of health services. Health risks over the life-cycle were analysed and compared to non-Māori. Risks for Māori were especially high for respiratory disease (hospitalization rate of 2.2 times as great), diabetes (2.1 times), cataracts (1.9 times), kidney disease (1.5 times), circulatory disease (1.5 times), female reproductive system disorders (1.4 times), and complications of pregnancy and childbirth (1.3 times as high as non-Māori). *He Kākano* also included cost data, largely derived from the first report of the Core Service Committee,[23] relating to Māori ill-health. The ten highest total expenditure areas were normal birth, injury/accident, newborn problems, complications of birth, bronchitis and asthma, pneumonia and pleurisy, stroke, heart failure and shock, digestive disorders, and chronic obstructive lung disease.

The Public Health Commission, one of the new health authorities established after the health reforms were announced in 1991, prepared a report on the health status of all New Zealanders, highlighting a range of public health issues.[24] *Our Health, Our Future/Hauora Pakari, Koiora Roa* demonstrated significant disparities between Māori and non-Māori in most areas. Of the lifestyle factors contributing to poor health, socio-economic status, food and nutrition, alcohol, tobacco, and pathological gambling were held to be especially relevant. A higher Māori incidence was described for a variety of conditions, including communicable diseases (such as meningitis and rheumatic fever), ischaemic heart disease (with higher death rates than for non-Māori or rates recorded in Australia, England, Wales, and Scandinavia), asthma and diabetes mellitus, lung cancer (twice the non-Māori rate), deaths from motor vehicle crashes, schizophrenia. Those differences mirrored the gaps in socio-economic circumstances, Māori being substantially less well-off on all counts.[25] On the other hand, Māori had a lower incidence of melanoma, cancer of the bowel, and suicide.[26] Comparative data between Māori and non-Māori, from various sources, are shown in Table 20.

Table 20: Māori/non-Māori health status, 1990/91[1]

	Māori	*Non-Māori*
Life Expectancy (years at birth)	72.9 (female) 68 (male)	79.2 (female) 73.4 (male)
Death Rates (per 100,000 population)	675.5 (female) 850.8 (male)	414.6 (female) 665.2 (male)
Infant Death Rates (per 1000 live births)	18.4	11.4
Total Fertility Rates (average number of children per woman)	2.28	2.10
Hospitalisation rates—Non-Mental Health (per 1000 population)	190.0	138.0
Hospitalisation rates—Mental Health (per 100 population)	850.0	560.0
Average Length of Stay in Hospital[2] (days)	5.20	5.99

1 All rates are adjusted for age

2 The age and diagnostic-related-growth adjusted length of stay in hospital indicates that Māori patients spend less time in hospital than non-Māori, but the discrepancy may reflect differing patterns of hospital use. If lack of effective primary care is a factor in higher Māori admission rates to hospital, it could also account for slightly shorter lengths of stay, i.e., many who could reasonably have been managed through primary care were admitted for brief periods in hospital.

Sources: *Our Health Our Future; He Kākano; Picture of Health; Core Services 1993/94; Department of Statistics*

SPECIFIC HEALTH PROBLEMS

A number of reports have examined specific aspects of Māori health, using comparisons with non-Māori as the baseline. Some of these, outlined in Table 21, are discussed to illustrate the range of health problems which have been identified as significantly different from the non-Māori experience to warrant extra attention.

Mental Illness

Data from psychiatric admissions was the major source of information used by the New Zealand Health Information Service (previously the National Health Statistics Centre) in comparing Māori and non-Māori standards of mental health. Annual reports demonstrated a growing trend for higher Māori psychiatric admission rates, especially in the twenty- to twenty-nine-year-old age group, and

Table 21: Specific Māori health problems

Health Problem	*Particular Concern*	Reports
Mental illness	High psychiatric admission rates	*Mental Health Data* *Tino Rangatiratanga and Māori Mental Health* *Ngā Ia ō te Oranga Hinengaro Māori*
Mental illness	Special patients	*Psychiatric Report*
Psychiatric disability	Psychiatrically disabled	*Atawhaitia*
Hearing impairment	Otitis media in children	*Whakarongo Mai*
Cancer and respiratory diseases	Smoking	*Te Taonga-mai-Tawhiti*
Respiratory disease	Asthma	*He Mate Huango*
Child health	Sudden infant death syndrome	*Hui Hauora Mokopuna*
Women's health	Cervical cancer	*National cervical screening programme*
Infectious diseases	AIDS	*Te Puni Kōkiri*

correspondingly lower admission rates for non-Māori.[27] Māori under-representation in psychiatric hospitals, the rule prior to 1970, had changed to the extent that Māori rates became two or three times higher than non-Māori, even by 1982.[28] Alcohol-related admissions represented the greatest area of increase. Reasons for the reversal were complex and could have included a greater utilization of psychiatric facilities, more accurate ethnic statistics, an actual greater incidence of mental illness, urbanization and its attendant turmoil, inadequate primary health care, and cultural bias, if not frank discrimination.[29] The extent of the problem and the plight of psychiatric patients were further discussed at the first national hui for mental health workers at Wainuiomata Marae in June 1993. Alcohol and drug misuse, inadequate support systems, and ineffective treatment services were held to be responsible.[30]

The *Psychiatric Report*[31] was concerned with patients known to the criminal justice system who had been ordered by the court to receive compulsory treatment. Māori representation among these so-called special patients was disproportionately high: in 1986, although Māori comprised only 10–12 per cent of the population, they accounted for 67 per cent of special patient admissions. Several concerns relating to Māori were outlined, including the absence of taha Māori in the training of health professionals. They led to recommendations for better regional facilities with closer attention to cultural factors in the genesis and management of Māori patients. The report also showed that Māori patients were more likely than non-Māori to be committed for treatment rather than receiving voluntary treatment at an earlier stage of illness.

After yet another report authored by Judge Ken Mason,[32] a Mental Health Commission was established in 1996 to monitor the implementation of the Ministry of Health's strategic mental health plan, *Looking Forward*. The Commission's *Blueprint* document, released in 1997, recommended the provision of kaupapa Māori services and more realistic levels of servicing in all communities. In addition, recommendations were made for a client-centred recovery approach, and a sufficient workforce to deliver high quality services.[33]

Psychiatric Disability

Apart from the *Psychiatric Report*, Ken Mason also undertook another Māori health review.[34] The Māori Trustee, Neville Baker, considered that the Māori Trustee could have a potential role as trustee for ex-psychiatric patients who were living in the community and asked for a report on the matter. Deinstitutionalization had become part of Government health policy and Māori patients appeared to be particularly vulnerable once they left hospital.[35] The review established that Māori were over-represented among the psychiatrically disabled, accounting for 32 per cent of patients in community care in the region served by the Tairawhiti Area Health Board, 30 per cent of intellectually handicapped patients at Tokanui Hospital, 21 per cent of psychiatrically disabled under the care of the Hawke's Bay Area Health Board, and 31 per cent of disabled patients at Lake Alice Hospital, Marton. It was recommended that the Māori Trustee should play a prime role to ensure that the health and welfare of those people was protected. However, the report itself was never accepted as policy.

Hearing Impairment

During 1988 the Hon Koro Wetere, Minister of Māori Affairs, became increasingly perturbed by reports of hearing impairment among Māori. As early as 1965 the problem had been identified but there was little indication that the situation was improving, and, somewhat to the surprise of his colleague the Minister of Health, Wetere decided to commission a review.[36] The report of the review team, *Whakarongo Mai*, concluded that levels of hearing impairment among Māori children were excessively high in Northland, South Auckland, Waikato, the East Coast, and the Bay of Plenty.[37] In a Ruatoki Valley study, one-quarter of all children tested had a hearing loss.[38] Inadequately treated infection of the middle ear (otitis media), with the subsequent development of glue ear, was regarded as the major cause, exacerbated by adverse socio-economic conditions. The consequences of hearing impairment were serious: underachievement in schools, unemployment, offending, and an inability to participate in society. Though not all of the report's recommendations were acted on, reducing hearing loss in children under the age of five became one of the ten health goals in the 1989 New Zealand Health Charter. Higher risks for Māori children were acknowledged.[39] Hearing loss was also one of the six public health goals identified by the Public Health Commission in 1992.

Cancer and Respiratory Diseases

High levels of smoking among Māori, particularly women, became a matter of considerable concern when a causal relationship was shown between smoking, respiratory diseases, including cancer of the lung, and cardio-vascular diseases. Lung cancer rates for Māori are high, being twice the non-Māori rate, and for Māori females they are among the highest in the world. Paparangi Reid and Robert Pouwhare examined the historical and contemporary significance of tobacco-smoking for Māori and provided statistical information on the prevalence and the costs.[40] While there were signs of reduced smoking among Māori men, the reverse appeared to be the case for women, especially young Māori women. They estimated that 600 Māori deaths each year could be attributed to tobacco and that over $163.7 million was spent on tobacco products. More resources for smoke-free campaigns and deliberate efforts to separate children from the direct and indirect effects of smoking were recommended.

Māori youngsters were doubly at risk; not only was there a positive correlation between smoking and socio-economic circumstances, but parental habits were also shown to be important in deciding to commence smoking.[41] By 1993 it was estimated that 46 per cent of Māori aged fifteen years and over were regular smokers compared to the total New Zealand rate of 23 per cent.[42] Māori women rates were even higher—58 per cent being regular smokers and, according to a Plunket Society survey, 69 per cent of Māori women smoked during pregnancy. In October 1993 the Public Health Commission held a consultation hui at the Turangawaewae Marae, Ngaruawahia, to bring together Māori health workers to discuss goals for a nationally focused Māori smoke-free coordination service.[43] Auahi kore, smoke-free, became the slogan and the focus for an active campaign within Māori communities. Sponsorship of events for Māori youth took the message onto sports fields, marae, schools, and cultural festivals, attempting to link high self-esteem, cultural pride, and physical fitness with the absence of tobacco products. Although the results do not yet confirm any serious trend towards major reductions in the prevalence of smoking among Māori,[44] auahi kore has at least gained Māori attention and provided a focus for reviewing practices and assumptions about lifestyle which were all too often taken for granted.

Respiratory Diseases

Alarm at the excessive number of deaths from asthma in Māori people and the large numbers requiring hospital treatment prompted the Minister of Māori Affairs, the Hon Koro Wetere, to launch another health review, this time into asthma. The review team could find no evidence to confirm that asthma was more frequent among Māori, but did conclude that there were significant differences in the way the illness was managed. Hospital admission rates for asthma were twice as high for Māori as for non-Māori and the death rate was higher up until 1987. Inadequate access to appropriate health care, the use of accident and emergency departments as the first line of medical assistance, and asthma education were blamed for the discrepancies.[45] The report's recommendations favoured a national Māori asthma education coordinator, Māori asthma resource people, voluntary workers, and education programmes in Kōhanga Reo.[46]

Child Health

At the Hui Hauora Mokopuna held at Rātana Pā in June 1990, sudden infant death syndrome (SIDS) was identified as a major issue for Māori, death rates under one year of age being twice as high as for non-Māori, and largely attributable to cot deaths.[47] The New Zealand Cot Death Study identified several risk factors which included low birth weight (less than 2,500g), smoking in the baby's environment, sleeping position, and socio-economic status.[48] Māori were disproportionately represented on at least three of those measures. For example, the rate of low birth weight among Māori infants—80 per 1000 live births—is the highest in the OECD countries.[49] Māori SIDS workers met with the Public Health Commission at Tirahau Marae, Auckland, in 1993 to plan further strategies to reduce the problem. While some overall reduction in cot deaths had been achieved (in 1989 the rate was as high as 9.2 per 1000), Māori rates in 1992 were still unacceptably high (6.5 deaths per 1000 live births, compared to less than 2.5 per 1000 for non-Māori).[50] Three significant risk factors for Māori infants were highlighted at the hui: maternal smoking, lower attendance at antenatal clinics, and a failure of national campaigns to reach the Māori population. National and regional coordination for Māori well-child care was recommended together with health promotional programmes designed specially to reach Māori parents.[51] Māori health programmes were given strong endorsement; in the Rotorua area a sharp reduction in SIDS was linked to the time that the Tipu Ora programme had been active.

Women's Health

Increased Māori rates of cervical cancer were noted in 1988 and registration increased by 35 per cent from 1989 to 1990 (though the increase might be a reflection of registration procedures).[52] In any event the incidence rate among Māori females, who have a high international rate, is more than twice that for non-Māori females.[53] Cervical cancer seemed an ideal opportunity to take preventative action since effective and practical screening tests had been devised and, theoretically at least, early intervention could prevent invasive cancer.

The Cartwright Report in 1988 had revealed what many Māori knew only too well: that screening procedures and information about cancer were often geared to meet the needs of doctors rather than consumers.[54] The report rekindled Māori determination to take an active role in cervical screening programmes and the Ministerial Review on the Implementation of a National Cervical Screening Programme concurred.[55] Māori women were not well acquainted with cervical screening, so active Māori participation would require special initiatives including regional Māori coordinators and programmes which guaranteed cultural appropriateness and safety.[56] A single national register became a much debated topic, Māori women often being unconvinced that personal information would be adequately safeguarded. In the debate, screening was nonetheless promoted, and by 1993 knowledge about cervical screening had increased even though reasons for its use were poorly understood.[57]

Infectious Diseases

Early in the 1980s a new disease made its appearance in New Zealand. Once tuberculosis had been brought under control, infectious diseases ceased to be a major cause of death for Māori. However, the emergence of acquired immunodeficiency syndrome (AIDS) presented global health risks on a scale never contemplated in the past. Māori were not to escape. By June 1992, of the 335 notified cases of AIDS, 36 (11 per cent) were Māori. Though not any more frequent among Māori, Māori were seen to be more at risk because of the greater prevalence of associated factors. Needle-sharing among drug users, a higher incidence of sexually transmitted diseases, a lower level of knowledge about AIDS, higher levels of imprisonment, and lower socio-economic status were all warning signs suggesting that a higher Māori incidence might be expected, warranting specific strategies.[58] Māori had already reached a similar conclusion and, under the leadership of Rex Perenara, a small group, Te Roopu Tautoko, was active in increasing awareness within Māori communities. Not infrequently they had to overcome bias and prejudice before their concerns about the risks of AIDS for Māori could be seriously addressed.

PERFORMANCE MONITORING

Life expectancy, mortality rates, hospitalization data, and prevalence rates are incomplete measures of health status and give little indication of quality of care. Increases in the number of Māori health initiatives and health programmes targeted specifically towards Māori created a need for measures which were appropriate in Māori terms. The Department of Health suggested certain principles to guide area health boards in the delivery of services to Māori: respect for individual dignity (culturally safe services), equity of access (adequate resourcing, accessible venues), community involvement (Māori participation), disease prevention and health promotion (rather than an exclusive focus on treatment of illness), effective resource use (including appropriate monitoring and evaluation procedures). Boards were urged to work closely with Māori groups, to reduce disparities between Māori and non-Māori, and to maintain health status data for Māori.[59]

Specific indicators for Māori health against which area health board performance could be measured were recommended by the Department of Health in 1990.[60] An attempt was made to acknowledge the whare tapa whā model of health by employing indicators which would measure wairua, hinengaro, tinana, and whānau. Three measures for taha wairua were suggested: language and cultural awareness, spiritual healers, work-force composition. Boards were asked to indicate such items as the number of staff members attending Māori culture courses, the percentage of doctors and nurses who could conduct a karakia (prayer service), the patterns of interaction with healers, and the percentage of the work-force who were Māori. Cultural sensitivity was to be measured with indicators such as rituals surrounding death in a hospital, delays in returning bodies to relatives, and making the placenta available to families after childbirth. More systematic recording of Māori health initiatives was incorporated into the Maori health performance schedule with particular attention to Māori participation in decision-making and consumer satisfaction.

While the proposed indicators were a major step towards greater accountability and practical recognition of Māori perspectives, they were weighted more to staff development and hospital politics than to actual health gains for Māori. Notwithstanding the good intention and abundant goodwill, the links between-staff being able to conduct karakia or say a few words in Māori and the health of Māori people are tenuous and may not be sufficient to justify the use of scarce health resources.

A Māori health status review, useful for health care funders and providers, has also been developed by the Department of Health.[61] It focuses on six main areas: the population profile, the profile of the region (Iwi, history, food sources, local authorities), lifestyle (smoking, nutrition, alcohol use, drug use, injury, exercise,

Table 22: Goals and themes for a Māori health audit

Goal Category	*Themes*
Māori development	Treaty of Waitangi Empowerment
Gains in Māori health	Government obligations Data and information Active involvement
Māori cultural values and beliefs	Cultural safety Intellectual property rights

Table 23: Māori development themes and indicators

Goal Category	*Theme*	*Indicators*
Māori development	Treaty of Waitangi	The dual-focused framework (DFF)* Kāwanatanga Tino rangatiratanga Ōritetanga Partnership Participation Active protection
	Empowerment	Extent of Māori involvement in programme - planning - delivery - monitoring Opportunity for Māori ownership Māori community involvement Links to positive Māori development

* The dual-focused framework is further discussed in Chapter Ten.

sexuality, leisure, cultural activities), health indicators (life expectancy, mortality, hospitalization, registration, surveys), health service utilization, and health service responsiveness.

As contractual arrangements become more frequent in health activities, it is important that relevant indicators be used so that activities designed to improve Māori health can be monitored and assessed. The Public Health Commission has adopted a model for monitoring providers which allows for flexibility and a Māori development approach while at the same time attempting to measure health gains and cultural sensitivity.[62] The CHI audit model incorporated three goals and several themes, as shown in Table 22.[63]

For each theme a number of indicators were suggested. Tables 23, 24, and 25 contain the themes and indicators for each goal.

Table 24: Themes and indicators to measure gains in Māori health

Goal Category	*Theme*	*Indicators*
Gains in Māori health	Government obligations	Relevance to Government objectives for Māori health Recognized Māori health priority Link to Public Health Commission pilot health goals
	Data and information	Arrangements for obtaining ethnic data Level of accuracy of ethnic data Reasons for seeking ethnic data Method for transfer of technology to Māori
	Active involvement	Level of programme priority for Māori Per cent Māori work-force Numbers of Māori likely to be targeted Circumstances of Māori targeted in the programme

In the CHI model, providers are invited to develop their own set of measurements, subject to Public Health Commission endorsement, for each indicator. The project is then audited according to those measurements.

SOCIO-ECONOMIC INDICATORS

Health status cannot be measured outside the socio-economic realities of Māori experience. There is abundant evidence that health is directly related to general standards of living as determined by employment, education, income levels, housing, and household configurations.[64] Nor is there any evidence of improvement, except perhaps in early childhood education, school retention, and home ownership rates. Large increases in unemployment are considered to be the main factor blocking Māori economic progress.[65] Data from the 1991 census, summarized in Table 26, show that the Māori position was significantly different from other New Zealanders. On that basis alone, disparities in standards of health could be predicted confidently.

Table 25: Themes and indicators relevant to Māori cultural values and beliefs

Goal Category	*Theme*	*Indicators*
Māori cultural values and beliefs	Cultural safety	Consultation with appropriate tangata whenua Identification of areas where cultural factors will be significant Strategy to satisfy cultural needs Involvement of Māori in planning and implementing strategies for cultural safety
	Intellectual property rights	Sources of cultural information acknowledged Permission obtained to use cultural knowledge Cultural material given due respect Efforts made to retain an appropriate context when using cultural information or practices

AN OVERVIEW OF MAORI HEALTH STATUS

Because there is no single measure of Māori health status, a comprehensive picture is dependent on data from several sources. Correlations between socio-economic, cultural, mortality, and morbidity data are needed in order to assess the vitality, the mauri, of Māori individuals and family. There is no single Māori reality and a statistical Māori may differ markedly from another Māori in terms of lifestyle, cultural affiliations, and degree of health. Most studies have been sectoral and cross-sectional; they have been oriented to a particular sector such as health or education or employment and have presumed that Māori is a definable measure. In statistical terms it might be, but the cultural parameters, at least as they apply to diverse situations for contemporary Māori, have yet to be analysed.[66]

While conventional health measures such as life expectancy, death rates, fertility rates, and hospitalization rates give some indication of Māori health, they are imperfect measures and fail to capture Māori vitality or mauri. Nor, for that matter, do the range of socio-economic indices. More correctly they are statements about the ways in which Māori differ from non-Māori and imply that Māori should aspire to similar standards as other New Zealanders. It might make good sense but it fails to answer the question about Māori aspirations and perspectives. At best, health and socio-economic measures suggest that Māori and non-Māori positions are converging but significant differences abound.

Table 26: Māori socio-economic standing, 1991 census data

Sector	*Māori Position*	*Comment*
Labour	23.8% male unemployment 24.7% female unemployment 36.7% of Māori aged between 15 and 24 years were unemployed	37,050 Māori were unemployed and seeking work Māori are over-represented in manual, unskilled occupational groups
Income levels	Income less than $20,000 received by over 75% of Māori Over 85% of Māori females received less than $20,000	Annual median income for Māori aged over 15 years was $11,001 One-parent families had a median annual income of $14,525 compared with $35,050 for two-parent families
Education	66.8% of Māori women over 15 years had no educational qualification 63.6% of Māori men over 15 years had no educational qualification	13,500 children attend 719 Kōhanga Reo 4221 children attend Māori medium classes at primary or secondary school levels
Housing	Fewer than 50% of Māori adults own their own home (cf. 75% non-Māori) Two-thirds of Māori are living in overcrowded homes	Overcrowding and substandard housing is linked to infectious diseases, respiratory problems, and mental health problems
Households	14.4% of the Māori population live in sole parent situations (36,000 families)	Whānau isolation is a significant health risk

Sources: Department of Statistics, *New Zealand Māori Population and Dwellings*; Analysis and Monitoring Group, Public Health Commission, *Our Health Our Future*; Te Puni Kōkiri, *He Kākano: A Handbook of Māori Health Data*.

Conventional indicators and measurements are weighted towards illness and dysfunction rather than health and equilibrium. Moreover, they can easily be interpreted as representing personal failure rather than system failure and lend themselves to aggravating a sense of discouragement and alienation. What remains to be determined are the characteristics which underlie Māori capacities for adaptability, resurgence, and positive development. Health status should be about those very qualities. The Decade of Māori Development, prescribed at the 1984 Hui Taumata, sought to emphasize them and, in the process, to balance negative descriptions with priorities for positive Māori futures.

ENDNOTES

1 Review Committee, (1988), *Report of the Review Committee on Ethnic Statistics 1988*, Department of Statistics, Wellington, pp. 47–9.

2 The word 'māori' was used to mean normal or usual.

3 'Tauiwi' was used by the Royal Commission on Social Policy when referring to New Zealanders who were not Māori. It did not exclude non-Europeans as the term Pākehā might have.

4 The Births and Deaths Registration Amendment Act 1912 came into force in 1913.

5 D. I. Poole, (1977), *The Maori Population of New Zealand 1769–1971*, Auckland University Press and Oxford University Press, Auckland, p. 241.

6 J. Metge, (1976), *The Maoris of New Zealand: Rautahi*, (2nd edn), Routledge and Kegan Paul, London, p. 41.

7 As it happened, the Rūnanga Iwi Act was repealed in 1991 after a change of Government.

8 Department of Statistics, (1993), *1991 Census of Population and Dwellings: Iwi Population and Dwellings*, Department of Statistics, Wellington.

9 J. Gould, (1991), 'The Gene Pool and Self Determination', *The Dominion*, 20 November 1991.

10 P. G. Brown, (1983), *An Investigation of Official Ethnic Statistics*, Occasional Paper No. 5, Department of Statistics, Wellington.

11 P. Graham, R. Jackson, R. Beaglehole, and G. de Boer, (1989), 'The Validity of Māori Mortality Statistics', *New Zealand Medical Journal* 102: 124–6.

12 R. Kilgour and V. Keefe, (1992), *Kia Piki te Ora*, Department of Health, Wellington, p. 54.

13 Core Services Committee, (1992), *Core Services 1993/94, First Report of the National Advisory Committee on Core Health and Disability Support Services to the Minister of Health*, Wellington, p. 8.

14 E. Murchie, (1984), *Rapuora: Health and Māori Women*, Māori Women's Welfare League, Wellington.

15 Statistics New Zealand and Ministry of Health, (1993), *A Picture of Health*, Department of Statistics and Ministry of Health, Wellington.

16 R. J. Rose, (1960), *Māori—European Standard of Health*, Special Report No. 1, Department of Health, Wellington.

17 J. K. Hunn, (1961), *Report on Department of Māori Affairs, Appendix to the Journals of the House of Representatives, 1960*, Wellington.

18 Ibid., pp. 19–22.

19 E. W. Pomare, (1980), *Maori Standards of Health: A Study of the 20-year Period 1955–75*, Special Report Series No. 7, Medical Research Council of New Zealand, Auckland.

20 E. Pomare and G. M. de Boer, (1988), *Hauora: Maori Standards of Health—A Study*

of the Years 1970–1984, Special Report Series 78, Medical Research Council and Department of Health, Wellington.

21 E. Pomare, V. Keefe-Ormsby, C. Ormsby, N. Pearce, P. Reid, B. Robson, N. Wātene-Haydon, (1995), *Hauora Māori Standards of Health III—A Study of the Years 1970–1991*, Te Rōpu Rangahau Hauora a Eru Pomare, Wellington School of Medicine, Wellington.

22 Te Puni Kōkiri, (1993), *He Kākano: A Handbook of Māori Health Data*, Ministry of Māori Development, Wellington.

23 Core Services Committee, *op cit.*

24 Analysis and Monitoring Group, (1993), *Our Health, Our Future/Hauora Pakari, Koiora Roa: The State of the Public Health in New Zealand 1993*, New Zealand Public Health Commission, Rangapū Hauora Tumatanui, Wellington.

25 Ibid., pp. 55–74.

26 Though the number of deaths due to suicide is not high, it is the second leading cause of death for males and females aged fifteen to twenty-four years, and since 1974 death rates from suicide have increased four times in that age group. Māori rates have increased at a corresponding rate.

27 New Zealand Health Information Service, (1993), *Mental Health Data 1991*, Department of Health, Wellington.

28 National Health Statistics Centre, (1983), *Mental Health Data 1982*, Department of Health, Wellington.

29 M. H. Durie, (1994), 'Māori Psychiatric Admissions: Patterns and Policy Implications', in J. Spicer, A. Trlin, and J. Walton (eds), *Social Dimensions of Health and Illness: New Zealand Perspectives*, Dunmore Press, Palmerston North (1994).

30 L. Dyall and J. Bridgeman, (1993), 'Tino Rangatiratanga and Mental Health', in V. Keefe-Ormsby *et al.* (eds), *Tino Rangatiratanga and Maori Mental Health*, Department of Health, Wellington, p. 21.

31 Committee of Inquiry, (1988), *Psychiatric Report*, report to the Minister of Health, Wellington. All members of this committee were Māori. Chaired by retired Judge Ken Mason, other members included pyschiatrists Dr Henry Bennett and Dr Erihana Ryan. Lorna Dyll was secretary to the Committee.

32 K. Mason, J. Johnston, and J. Crowe, (1996), *Inquiry Under Section 47 of the Health and Disability Services Act 1993 in Respect of Certain Mental Health Services, Report to the Minister of Health Hon. Jenny Shipley*, Ministerial Inquiry, Christchurch.

33 Mental Health Commission, (1997), *Blueprint for Mental Health Services in New Zealand*, Mental Health Commission, Wellington.

34 K. Mason, (1991), *Atawhaitia: The Māori Trustee Report on the Care of Māori under the Protection of Personal and Property Rights Act 1988 and Part X of the Māori Affairs Act 1953*, Māori Trustee, Wellington.

35 M. H. Durie, (1988), 'Social Policy Perspectives', in J. Martin and J. Harper (eds), *Devolution and Accountability*, New Zealand Institute of Public Administration,

Wellington, pp. 37–45.

36 R. G. Phillips-Turner, (1965), *Diseases of the Ear, Nose and Throat in Māori Children*, Special Report Series No. 14, Department of Health, Wellington.

37 M. H. Durie, T. Black, K. Coddington, G. S. Douglas, S. Kay, P. W. Eisdell Moore, E. Tawhiri, and M. H. Te Koha, (1989), *Whakarongo Mai: Māori Hearing Impairment*, a report to the Minister of Māori Affairs, Department of Māori Affairs, Wellington.

38 M. Giles, and P. O'Brien, (1989), 'Otitis Media and Hearing Loss in the Children of the Ruatoki Valley: A Continuing Public Health Problem', *New Zealand Medical Journal* 102: 160–1.

39 Hon H. Clark, Minister of Health, (1989), *New Zealand Health Goals and Targets*, Department of Health, Wellington.

40 P. Reid and R. Pouwhare, (1991), *Te-Taonga-mai-Tawhiti*, Niho Taniwha, Auckland.

41 G. H. Ree, (1986), 'Smoking Habits and Associated Factors in School Children', *New Zealand Medical Journal* 99, 812: 807–9.

42 *The Dominion*, 9 December 1993.

43 M. Glover, (1993), *Smoke-free Māori; Hui Summary Report*, Public Health Commission, Wellington.

44 Ministry of Health, (1997), *Progress on Health Outcome Targets*, Ministry of Health, Wellington, pp. 135–41.

45 J. E. Garrett, J. Mulder, and H. Wong-Toi, (1989), 'Reasons for Racial Differences in A & E Attendance Rates for Asthma', *New Zealand Medical Journal* 102: 121–4.

46 E. Pomare, H. Tutungaehe, I. Ramsden, M. Hight, N. Pearce, and V. Ormsby, (1991), *He Mate Huango: Māori Asthma Review*, report to the Minister of Māori Affairs, Ministerial Asthma Review Team, Wellington.

47 Ministerial Advisory Committee on Māori Health, (1990), *Hui Hauora Mokopuna*, Department of Health, Wellington.

48 'Cot Death Risk Factors', *Health* 40, 14 Summer 1991: 11–12.

49 Analysis and Monitoring Group, *op cit.* pp. 219–21.

50 Ibid., pp. 216–7.

51 Public Health Commission, (1993), 'Healthy Lives', *Newsletter of the Public Health Commission*, 2 August 1993.

52 Pomare and de Boer, *op cit.*

53 Public Health Commission, *op cit.*

54 S. Cartwright, (1988), *The Report of the Cancer Inquiry*, Department of Justice, Auckland.

55 Ministerial Review Committee, (1989), *Report on the Implementation of a National Cervical Screening Programme*, Department of Health, Wellington.

56 K. Ratima, C. Paul, and D. C. G. Skegg, (1993), 'Cervical Smear Histories of Māori Women Developing Invasive Cervical Cancer', *New Zealand Medical Journal* 106, 969: 519–21.

57 K. H. Ratima, M. H. Durie, and M. M. Ratima, (1993), *Cervical Screening in Māori*

Women—Knowledge and Service Factors: A Report prepared for Health Waikato Limited, Te Manawa Hauora, Massey University, Palmerston North.

58 Te Puni Kōkiri, (1992), *Māori and AIDS: Report to the National Council on AIDS*, Ministry of Māori Development, Wellington.

59 Department of Health, (1991), *Service Statement: Hauora Māori—Māori Health*, Department of Health, Wellington.

60 Coopers and Lybrand Associates, (1991), *Performance Monitoring System Improving Direction, Performance and Accountability (Māori Health)*, Department of Health, Wellington.

61 Health Research Services, (1993), *Guidelines for a Review of Māori Health Status: Draft Report*, Department of Health, Wellington.

62 M. H. Durie, (1993), *A Culturally Appropriate Auditing Model: The C.H.I. Audit Model*, Public Health Commission, Wellington.

63 CHI is abbreviated from the initial letters of consolidation (of current initiatives), holistic (approaches to health), and interactive (between purchaser and provider).

64 H. Barwick, (1992), *The Impact of Economic and Social Factors on Health*, a report prepared by the Public Health Association of New Zealand for the Department of Health, Wellington.

65 J. Davey, (1993), *From Birth to Death III*, Institute of Policy Studies, Victoria University of Wellington, Wellington, pp. 206–7.

66 The Department of Māori Studies at Massey University, Palmerston North, commenced a longitudinal study on Māori households in 1993. The study, *Māori Profiles: Te Hoe Nuku Roa*, links socio-economic variables with cultural measures and assesses the impact of Māori policies on households.

READING 4

Tirohanga Māori

Māori Health Perspectives

At the opening of the Hui Whakaoranga, a national Māori health conference held on the Hoani Waititi Marae, Auckland, in 1984, the Hon Ben Couch, Minister of Māori Affairs in the National Government, declared, '. . . there is no such thing as Māori health or Pākehā health; there is only people health'. He went on to ascribe differences in health standards to self-inflicted lifestyle choices, '. . . most people who enjoy good health have earned it. The rules are the same for people of all races; good eating, plenty of sleep and exercise, and moderation in all things'.[1] His views were not atypical of the era but they were out of step with Māori thinking in two respects. First, they ignored Māori experience and the growing body of evidence which linked culture and health; and, second, they disregarded socio-economic status as a significant determinant of good health, quite apart from individual motivation.

Over the succeeding two days the Hui Whakaoranga rejected the notion that cultural factors were irrelevant to health and concluded on quite a different note, recommending that 'health and educational institutions recognise culture as a positive resource' and that 'the feasibility of including Māori spirituality in health education programmes in schools and in tertiary educational institutions be investigated'.[2]

ILLNESS AND TREATMENT

Prior to 1976, professional and academic interest in Māori perspectives on health and sickness tended to confine discussion to particular clinical syndromes which were unique to Māori and of anthropological as much as medical interest. Mākutu and mate Māori, for example, attracted considerable comment from Western-trained psychiatrists, though tended to be reinterpreted as superstitious phenomena and of doubtful diagnostic significance.[3,4] Māori concepts of illness were increasingly reinterpreted by the medical anthropologists in mental and psychic realms, scarcely relevant to the vast majority of human illnesses and hardly applicable to contemporary times. It was left to Māori writers to point out the continuing relevance of culture to illness and treatment, and to provide some balance for the more esoteric ideas which had appeared in the earlier medical and scientific literature.

The process started with an examination of medical practice and hospital procedures to determine the significance of culture to Māori patients in everyday situations. Durie concluded that, although Māori were more often than not Westernized, or at least appeared to be, cultural heritage continued to shape ideas, attitudes, and reactions, particularly at times of illness. 'The concepts of tapu and the perception of illness as an infringement against tapu are central to much of the anxiety and depression which surround the Māori patient while in hospital. Family involvement at times of illness is likewise a very traditional and culturally necessary attitude which must be recognised in the management of the whole patient and not just his impaired organ.'[5]

The relationship between tapu and noa, and explanations of illness based on a postulated breach of tapu, continued to have meaning for Māori and therefore had implications for doctors in the management of Māori patients as well as the care of the deceased as long as they were still in hospital custody. Because early retrieval of a relative's body was critical to uphold the mana of the family and the individual, mourning Māori families were grossly offended if the body were not released within twenty-four hours of death. Post-mortem delays, or simple administrative inefficiencies, could add immeasurably to the grief of an already distressed family.[6]

Tipene-Leach, writing about aspects of the doctor–patient relationship, described a number of sensitivities and behaviours relevant to communication during a clinical examination.[7] For instance, immediately asking patients to reveal their names, without any preliminary remarks, could lead some Māori to feel threatened even before the examination had commenced. Similarly, expecting a Māori patient to engage in direct eye-to-eye contact could be interpreted as an invitation to demonstrate bad manners since looking an older person in the eye was a sign of haughtiness or disrespect. Various parts of the body were also described as having special significance, though not necessarily at a conscious level. Medical or nursing interventions involving the head, sexual organs, hair, and nail clippings, required a measure of caution and a greater degree of circumspection than was customary in busy hospital wards.

The gradual introduction of Māori concepts into medical routines was not entirely welcomed, but nor was it dismissed outright. By the mid-1970s there was some tentative recognition that ethnicity and culture had implications for health. Māori views, though not always understood, were often taken on board at face value, even though they could not be rationalized in medical terms. Moreover, discussions of similarities between tohunga and doctor in the *New Zealand Medical Journal* had generated sympathetic interest.[8] Both, it seemed, were experts in history-taking as a prelude to making a diagnosis; both took extensive family histories (tohunga more than doctor); both employed specific treatment methods; and both recommended periods of rehabilitation. By removing Māori concepts from the realms of the supernatural, and emphasizing their continuing importance even when a patient did not profess to subscribe to them, Western-trained health professionals were more able to appreciate their significance and respect them.

HEALTH AND WELL-BEING

Having shown the relevance of culture to health and sickness, Māori interest then turned to the wider contexts of health and community. For some years it had been acknowledged that there were many dimensions to health. In its 1947 definition, the World Health Organization concluded that health was greatly influenced by social and cultural factors: 'Health is a state of complete physical, mental and social wellbeing and not merely the absence of disease or infirmity'.[9] The definition was a reminder to the world that there was more to health than biological dysfunction and that it went well beyond the province of the health sector. Neither was it the exclusive province of the medically trained doctor or nurse, although they had a particular interest in some aspects of it having made spectacular advances in the treatment of physical illnesses, especially infections, from the 1940s onwards. The problem was, or at least was perceived as being, that medical interest in physical disease greatly outweighed an interest in the person as a whole within a sociological and ecological environment. A cellular focus no longer seemed adequate for understanding the complexities of health even though it had been a useful step in the past.

During the 1970s Māori were beginning to insist that a narrow focus on micro-organisms or even on physical illness created a distorted framework within which to consider health and to plan for the future. Interest moved towards a view of health that made sense to Māori in Māori terms, and outside hospital. As Māori participation in the health debate escalated, a number of Māori perspectives were advanced. All emphasized the value of traditional belief systems to health, though not necessarily at the expense of Western medical practice. Indeed, seldom did debate move towards an exclusively Māori system. Greater balance was the goal.

Several views emerged, but one which subsequently gained wide acceptance as 'the Māori health perspective' was a four-sided health construct, later known as whare tapa whā (a four-sided house).[10] Though often described as a traditional

Māori approach to health, more correctly it was a view of health which accorded with contemporary Māori thinking. Its ready acceptance by Māori was to some extent proof of that. The characteristics of whare tapa whā are shown in Table 12.

Table 12: The whare tapa whā model

	Taha Wairua	*Taha Hinengaro*	*Taha Tinana*	*Taha Whānau*
Focus	Spiritual	Mental	Physical	Extended family
Key Aspects	The capacity for faith and wider communion	The capacity to communicate, to think, and to feel	The capacity for physical growth and development	The capacity to belong, to care, and to share
Themes	Health is related to unseen and unspoken energies	Mind and body are inseparable	Good physical health is necessary for optimal development	Individuals are part of wider social systems

Whare Tapa Whā

Briefly, the whare tapa whā model compared health to the four walls of a house, all four being necessary to ensure strength and symmetry, though each representing a different dimension: taha wairua (the spiritual side), taha hinengaro (thoughts and feelings), taha tinana (the physical side), taha whānau (family). The concept of health as an interaction of wairua, hinengaro, tinana, and whānau was first presented at the Rahui Tane Hostel in Hamilton in August 1982 during a training session for fieldworkers in the Māori Women's Welfare League research project, Rapuora.[11] During the welcome , kaumātua Tupana te Hira had emphasized in Māori the importance of wairua as a starting-point for health. It was a view that many kaumātua shared and which was frequently heard on marae throughout the country. Later that evening, psychiatrist Henry Bennett spoke about mental illness and mental health, while Dr Jim Hodge of the Medical Research Council described some of the common disorders such as kidney failure which affected Māori disproportionately. Dr Mason Durie, also a psychiatrist, drew these themes together, calling them taha wairua, taha hinengaro, taha tinana, and taha whānau and leaving League members with a broadly based view of health which seemed to combine the four basic ingredients for good health. Importantly, a notion of balance between them was also introduced. The model later appeared in the Rapuora report: 'To say that a person is a psychosomatic unity, a personality formed jointly by physical and mental processes, only partly embraces the Māori concept. A study of Māori health must follow more than two strands. Tinana is the physical element of the individual and hinengaro the mental state, but these do not make up the whole. Wairua, the spirit and whanau the wider family, complete the shimmering depths of the health pounamu, the precious touchstone of Māoridom'.[12]

The four-part framework was again presented by Durie at a health hui held at the Palmerston North Hospital in December 1982[13] and further developed for the 10th Young People's Hui held at the Raukawa marae in May 1983.[14] The four dimensions of health were originally portrayed as a set of interacting variables, not dissimilar from a holistic view, nor for that matter from the World Health Organisation 1947 definition but, unlike them, firmly anchored on a spiritual rather than a somatic base.

Taha wairua is generally felt by Māori to be the most essential requirement for health. It implies a capacity to have faith and to be able to understand the links between the human situation and the environment, Without a spiritual awareness and a mauri (spirit or vitality, sometimes called the life-force) an individual cannot be healthy and is more prone to illness or misfortune. A spiritual dimension encompasses religious beliefs and practices but is not synonymous with regular churchgoing or strong adherence to a particular denomination. Belief in God is one reflection of wairua, but it is also evident in relationships with the environment. Land, lakes, mountains, reefs have a spiritual significance, quite apart from economic or agricultural considerations, and all are regularly commemorated in song, tribal history, and formal oratory.[15]A lack of access to tribal lands or territories is regarded by tribal elders as a sure sign of poor health since the natural environment is considered integral to identity and fundamental to a sense of well-being.[16]

Spiritually, the hours immediately following death are particularly significant. As the deceased person's spirit hovers tentatively between the visible world and the world of spirits, mourners themselves are able to feel a spiritual presence and to experience a renewed sense of continuity with their own ancestors, their history, and their future. For that reason a rapid retrieval of a deceased relative from hospital becomes a matter of urgency.

Taha hinengaro is about the expression of thoughts and feelings. In Māori nomenclature, thoughts and feelings derive from the same source, located within the individual. The notion that they are vital to health is a well-recognized concept among Māori. Western authorities have reached similar conclusions though through circuitous routes that have traversed psychological and psychiatric observations, a path that other cultures have not needed in order to finish up at the same point. Māori thinking can be described as holistic. Understanding occurs less by division into smaller and smaller parts, the analytical approach, than by synthesis into wider contextual systems so that any recognition of similarities is based on comparisons at a higher level of organization.

Consistent with this style of thinking, health is viewed as an interrelated phenomenon rather than an intra-personal one. Healthy thinking from a Māori perspective is integrative not analytical; explanations are sought from searching outwards rather than inwards; and poor health is typically regarded as a manifestation of a breakdown in harmony between the individual and the wider environment. There are several words and expressions which bind the individual to the outside world. Whenua, for example, can mean both placenta and the land, rae is either the forehead or a land promontory, iwi refers equally to a bone (kō-iwi) or to a nation of people, while hapū can denote pregnancy and a section of a large tribe. The word for birth is whānau, the same term used to describe a family, and wairua, spirituality, can also be used to refer to an insect, just as kāpō can mean blind or a species of eel. Whakapo is to darken (as in approaching night) and, as well, to grieve, waimate is a hereditary disease but also polluted water, kauae can be the jawbone or a major supporting beam in a building, and tāhuhu refers both to the vertebral column and the ridge pole of a meeting-house.

A further distinctive feature of taha hinengaro is its relevance to both thoughts and feelings. While Western thinking distinguishes between the spoken word and emotions (and generally encourages the word more than the feeling), Māori do not draw such a sharp distinction. Communication, especially face-to-face, depends on more than overt messages. Māori may be more impressed by the unspoken signals conveyed through subtle gesture, eye movement, or bland expression, and in some situations regard words as superfluous, even demeaning. Emotional communication can assume an importance which is as meaningful as an exchange of words and valued just as much. Condolences, for example, are frequently conveyed with tears; infrequently with words. So, when Māori children who are chided by their teachers for showing what they feel, instead of talking about their feelings, they are not only made to feel unworthy (of their feelings) but must also contend with a sense of frustrated expression.

Taha tinana (bodily health) is a more familiar health dimension, though the Māori emphasis is different in that there is the clear separation of tapu and noa. Certain parts of the body, and the head in particular, are regarded as special (tapu), and bodily functions such as sleeping, eating, drinking, and defecating are imbued with their own significance, reflecting various levels of importance and requiring quite different rituals. Food, for example, is a leveller which removes any vestige of sacredness or distance (as between people). Because cleaning the body and eating are polar opposites, separation of food from toileting functions is regarded as necessary to maintain good health, a condition severely tested in hospital wards where all functions are frequently conducted in the same confined space.

Body image may be regarded differently by Māori. Slender body forms are not necessarily prized more than well-rounded shapes, nor does obesity provoke the same sense of disapproval encountered in society generally. Perhaps because of this, anorexia nervosa remains relatively infrequent among Māori girls. By the same token, however, health workers report difficulties in trying to convince Māori patients that they should lose weight. Their efforts might be better spent in appealing to health risks, especially for future generations, rather than to personal vanity.

The fourth dimension of health, taha whānau, acknowledges the relevance of the extended family to health. There are at least two important considerations. The first is that the family is the prime support system for Māori, providing care and nurturance, not only in physical terms but culturally and emotionally. Reported rises in the prevalence of family dysfunction, including signs of abuse, do not lessen the point but underline its significance. Māori still maintain that ill health in an individual is a reflection on the family and may well blame a family for allowing a person to become ill or to die, even when there is no direct causal link. The practice of muru is still observed in some areas. When there is evidence that a lack of quality care by the family has contributed to death, neighbours and more distant relatives may seek retribution by removing family property or personal belongings, especially when the deceased is a community leader. Similarly, in cases of child abuse or neglect the extended family may take it upon themselves to remove the boy or girl from parental custody and take over the caring role. Parental rights often tend to be seen as secondary to the interests of the whānau or even the tribe to ensure that future generations are protected.

A second consideration of taha whānau relates to identity and sense of purpose. The much-lauded state of self-sufficiency or self-realization does not convey a sense of health to Māori. Quite the reverse, since an insistence on being overly independent suggests a defensive attitude, while a failure to turn to the family when the occasion demands is regarded as immaturity, not strength. Interdependence rather than independence is the healthier goal.[17] Sometimes this goal clashes with the European regard for independence in teenagers as 'one of critical developmental tasks of adolescence, . . . a fundamental building block of health'.[18]

Even in modern times a sense of personal identity derives as much if not more from family characteristics than from occupation or place of residence. Interest in family and tribal background rivals personal qualifications or achievements so that credibility, certainly in Māori settings, depends on an individual being able to make the links and demonstrate that there is active whānau and tribal support. On that basis, it has become a common occurrence for family members to accompany job-seeking applicants to an interview. Their role is a dual one: to convince the interview panel that their relative is the best person for the job, but also to ensure that the job itself is suitable and not likely to lead to exploitation, unfulfilled expectations, or disrespect. There have been instances when an applicant has been successful but the family, unhappy about the interview, has counselled against accepting the position. Similarly, there are numerous anecdotal accounts of candidates being passed over because of the family's confronting attitude during the interview.

Underlying the whare tapa whā model is the consistent theme of integration. Individual health is built into a wider system, the boundary between personal and family identity being frequently blurred. Similarly the divisions between temporal and spiritual, thoughts and feelings, mental and physical are not as clear-cut as they are have been in Western thinking since the advent of Cartesian dualism.[19]

Māori interest in redefining health in their own terms and reclaiming a positive role in shaping health services was accelerated when the whare tapa whā model was introduced. It was simple, even simplistic, but that was also its appeal. In addition, it appeared at a time when Māori were debating the general direction which health services were taking. Widespread concern had focused on three issues.

First, Māori were not impressed by the overemphasis on physical aspects of health with its biological constructs and increasing preoccupation with cellular phenomena. Nor for that matter were a number of other New Zealanders. At a national conference to consider the role of the doctor, holistic care was emphasized to balance a perception that many doctors had acquired too narrow a focus, their work often lacking ecological and caring dimensions. 'Because the scientific and technical aspects of practice cannot be separated from human concerns and social skills, particular attitudes are required: the readiness to treat people as equals; empathy; willingness to share information two ways; and a recognition that patients have a responsibility for their own health.'[20]

Second, many Māori felt that their relationship with health professionals, and with the health system generally, had become strained. Rightly or wrongly a feeling of alienation had arisen, not necessarily because of poor access or even inadequate care, but mainly because there was a lack of shared decision-making and limited recognition of Māori views. The more professionals acted as if they knew best, the less tolerant Māori became. Surely, they argued, Māori health belonged to Māori people. Māori health perspectives such as whare tapa whā were welcomed because they provided the necessary framework within which a semblance of ownership over health could be entertained.

Third, despite a century and a half of colonization, Māori remained convinced that good health could not be gauged by simple measures such as weight, blood pressure, or visual acuity. Spiritual and emotional factors, though more difficult to measure, were equally important.

TE WHEKE

There were other Māori health perspectives which gained acceptance in the 1980s. One of these, te wheke (the octopus), was discussed by Pere at the Hui Whakaoranga in 1984. In order to illustrate the main features of health from a Māori family perspective, she compared health to an octopus.[21] Each of the eight tentacles of the octopus symbolized a particular dimension of health while the body and head represented the whole family unit. The intertwining of the tentacles indicated the close relationships between each dimension.

Like te whare tapa whā, the model included wairuatanga (spirituality), taha tinana (the physical side), hinengaro (the mind), and whanaungatanga (the extended family, similar to taha whānau). The other dimensions were: mana ake, the uniqueness of the individual and each family and the positive identity based on those unique qualities; mauri, the life-sustaining principle resident in people and objects, including language; hā a Koro mā a Kui mā, literally the breath of life that comes from forebears and an acknowledgment that good health is closely linked to a positive awareness of ancestors and their role in shaping the family; whatumanawa, the open and healthy expression of emotion, necessary for healthy human development; and waiora, total well-being for the individual and the family, represented in the model by the eyes of the octopus.

NGĀ POU MANA

In 1988 the Royal Commission on Social Policy described another set of values and beliefs—four supports, ngā pou mana—as pre-requisites for health and well-being.[22] As with the other models a set of interacting variables was proposed, the combination leading to individual and group well-being manifest by the retention of mana, cultural integrity, a sound economic base, and a sense of confidence and continuity. This model, unlike the other two, placed greater stress on the external environment and the significance of oral tradition as a stabilizing influence. Though prepared primarily to examine foundations for social policies and social well-being, nonetheless it has relevance for health and has similarities with Durie's three 'institutions of health'—land, language, and family.[23]

The four supports—family (whanaungatanga), cultural heritage (taonga tuku iho), the physical environment (te ao tūroa), and an indisputable land base (turangawaewae)—brought together social, cultural, and economic dimensions in a way which could be readily appreciated by Māori and which demonstrated the links between the three. Particular reference to the environment (te ao tūroa) was perhaps influenced by the Waitangi Tribunal's landmark decisions in respect of claims made by tribes against the Crown and on the basis of pollution of tribal waterways.[24] These claims had all recognized the significance of a clean environment for good health and drew attention to the overlap between physical and cultural pollution. Quite apart from the effects of effluent on seafood and the consequent risks of hepatitis or other alimentary diseases, Māori claimants also described a type of pollution which debased spiritual and cultural values. Disposal of human waste, treated or not, onto potential food sites or into wāhi tapu (historical sites declared tapu) offended Māori just as the depletion of traditional foods through pollution created embarrassment when families were unable to meet customary hospitality obligations when visitors arrived.

Turangawaewae is a pou mana with cultural, social, and economic significance. Not only does it refer to land rights and access to an economic base, it also includes the marae, an institution, perhaps like no other, where Māori customs and tradition, including language, have priority. A measure of Māori identity, and indirectly a health measure, is the level of access, as of right, which an individual has to a marae. Since the marae is the epitome of a collective identity and one of the few remaining opportunities for social relationships to be strengthened in a manner which is mutually supportive, it enables Māori to redress some of the imbalance between individual and group pursuits inevitably created by life in suburbia.

Taonga tuku iho, cultural heritages upon which intellectual and philosophical traditions are based, are also valued by Māori because they suggest a continuity with past wisdom and consolidate a Māori identity. Increasing recognition of language as a taonga (treasure), important for cultural and health reasons, has resulted in extensive revitalization strategies locally and nationally. After considering a claim brought by Ngā Kaiwhakapumau i te Reo (the Wellington Māori Language Board), the Waitangi Tribunal described language as a taonga, categorizing it along with physical resources such as land.[25] The Tribunal report made it very clear that there was a Treaty of Waitangi obligation on the Crown to ensure that Māori language was strengthened before it was lost altogether, and the point was made on several occasions that without language any sense of pride or cultural integrity is seriously undermined.

Cultural heritage, as a basis for well-being if not health, also concerns the ownership of intellectual and cultural property. Cultural erosion has come about not only because of assimilation but also because history, traditions, art forms, healing methods, and poetry have often been appropriated by others and in the process Māori have been denied a guardian or custodial role, or have lost access to their own material altogether.

The Draft Declaration on the Rights of Indigenous Peoples recognizes both the significance of intellectual property to indigenous peoples as well as indigenous forms of health care, based on traditions passed down over the generations.[26]Article 22 of the Draft Declaration states that 'Indigenous peoples have the right to their traditional medicines and health practices, including the right to the protection of vital medicinal plants, animals and materials'. Article 27 is more specific: 'Indigenous peoples have the right to special measures to protect, as intellectual property, their sciences, technologies and cultural manifestations, including genetic resources, seeds, medicines, knowledge of the properties of fauna and flora, oral traditions, literatures, designs and visual performing arts'.

Table 13 summarizes the main features of the three perspectives.

Table 13: Māori health perspectives–three models

	Whare Tapa Whā	*Te Wheke*	*Ngā Pou Mana*
Components	Wairua Hinengaro Tinana Whānau	Wairuatanga Hinengaro Tinana Whanaungatanga Mana ake Mauri Hā a Koro mā a Kui mā Whatumanawa	Whanaungatanga Taonga tuku iho Te ao tūroa Turangawaewae
Features	Spirituality Mental health Physical Family	Spirituality Mental health Physical Family Uniqueness Vitality Cultural heritage Emotions	Family Cultural heritage Environment Land base
Symbolism	A strong house	The octopus	Supporting structures

GAINING PERSPECTIVE

Other Māori health perspectives were advocated on various occasions. Te Roopu Awhina ō Tokanui, a group of Māori health professionals at a psychiatric hospital, became active in promoting Māori health, particularly mental health, and were instrumental in establishing a Māori unit, Whaiora, within Tokanui Hospital. At the Australian Congress of Mental Health Nurses held at Adelaide in 1986, they presented a nine-part framework to guide psychiatric nursing: taha wairua (spirituality), taha whānau (family), taha hinengaro (well-being), taha tinana (physiology), taha whenua (environment), taha tikanga (compliance), Māoritanga (old world), Pākehātanga (new world), taha tangata (self).[27]

All Māori health perspectives had similar themes. Essentially they sought to widen understandings of health, to translate health into terms which were culturally significant, and to balance physical and biological approaches with cultural and sociological views. The Department of Health agreed that, 'Māori people in general believe that their current health status is ultimately linked to their historical, social, cultural, economic, political and environmental circumstances. In order to achieve any improvement in health status, health initiatives must incorporate a holistic definition and approach and be part of a developmental strategy to improve the overall status and wellbeing of a Māori community, tribal or family group. In doing so Māori people would like to define health for themselves; identify their own specific health concerns; . . . take responsibility for their own health; be involved in their own health care'.[28]

The appearance of the Māori health perspectives in the early part of the 1980s was not altogether surprising, given the strong moves towards positive Māori development and a rejection of assimilationist ideals. In education, housing, social welfare, and political representation Māori were intent on injecting a genuine Māori point of view as a prelude to reclaiming some degree of ownership and autonomy over social as well as economic arenas. Health was no exception.

But the perspectives also reflected a more general re-examination of New Zealand's health goals and its health services. Māori often articulated issues which had worried a wide cross-section of New Zealanders but which had not otherwise been able to find expression. The S-Factor for example was a concept used to encompass spirit, spirituality, or even 'something which represents that which defies being placed into the categories of ethics, psychology, medicine, and sociology'.[29] It was seen to be similar to taha wairua, but more relevant to Western than Māori culture, and it was introduced to balance a preoccupation with measurable and quantifiable health outcomes. Once Māori began to talk about spirituality, thoughts, feelings, and family in connection with health, others followed.

However, not everyone was impressed by the Māori health perspectives. To sceptics, they were based on romantic visions of the past, devoid of practical application, and likely to discourage Māori patients from seeking appropriate health care. At a time when scientific and technological advances were enabling organ transplants and new hopes for the disabled, Māori, it seemed, were longing for the quiet life and a return to a world now recognizable only in the history books. Further, because whare tapa whā extended the focus for health well beyond the individual, a sense of futility often developed among health workers. How could a diabetic regain health if the land injustices of the past century were ignored? By taking the debate to the widest possible levels, health programmes ran the risk of being so general and indistinguishable from welfare programmes that they would have no significant impact. Worse, if cultural factors were so important, sometimes it seemed pointless to treat a diabetic unless steps were also taken to provide parallel cultural enrichment; and health workers sometimes felt that they should take the initiative.

Far from improving treatment opportunities, it was argued that the new perspectives would displace clinical priorities and resources with sociological, economic, or political agendas. A further issue concerned the difficulty in measuring concepts as diffuse as taha wairua. While measurements of physical illness and subsequent medical interventions lacked accuracy, they were improving and at least there was some agreement about the desirable indicators. Not so in mental health (taha hinengaro) and even less so in spiritual matters. Was taha wairua of any practical value if it could not be measured? The critics felt not.

Generally, however, Māori health perspectives were consistent with new orientations and global trends: general systems theory, family psychotherapy, the community health movement, health promotion, primary health care, and calls for de-medicalization of the human life cycle. New Zealand was moving in the same direction and, in recommending a national health policy in 1988, the New Zealand Board of Health advocated five principles: holism, empowerment, social and cultural determination, equity of access and devolution, and equitable and effective resource use.[30] The Board had borrowed extensively from Māori views and writings.

By 1990, Māori views on health had made a significant impact on New Zealand health services generally, but more importantly they had given Māori people the necessary confidence, based on their own understandings of health, to challenge the system and reclaim a more active participatory role in society and within the health sector.

ENDNOTES

1 Komiti Whakahaere, (1984), *Hui Whakaoranga: Māori Health Planning Workshop*, Department of Health, Wellington.

2 Ibid.

3 G. Blake-Palmer, (1954), 'Tohungaism and Makutu', *Journal of the Polynesian Society* 63 (2): 147–63.

4 L. K. Gluckman, (1976), *Tangiwai: A Medical History of 19th Century New Zealand* Whitcoulls, Christchurch, pp. 232–60.

5 The psychoanananalyst Carl Jung used the term 'collective unconscious' to describe the continuing influence of cultural beliefs even when they were beyond conscious appreciation.

6 M. H. Durie, (1977), 'Māori Attitudes to Sickness, Doctors and Hospitals', *New Zealand Medical Journal* 86: 483–5.

7 D. Tipene-Leach, (1978), 'Māoris: Their Feelings About the Medical Profession', *Community Forum*, Auckland.

8 Durie, (1977), *op cit.*

9 World Health Organization, (1947), 'Constitution of the World Health Organization', *Chronicles of the World Health Organization* 1: 12.
10 M. H. Durie, (1985), 'A Maori Perspective of Health', *Journal of Social Sciences and Medicine* 20 (5): 483–6.
11 E. Murchie, (1984), *Rapuora: Health and Māori Women*, Māori Women's Welfare League, Wellington, p. 112.
12 Ibid., p. 81.
13 The 1982 Hui Ora was arranged by a Māori health interest group, made up mainly of Māori professional staff from the Palmerston North Hospital. It was attended by representatives of major Māori organizations in the area. The keynote speakers were Drs David Yates, Paratene Ngata, and Mason Durie.
14 W. Winiata, (1984), 'The Raukawa Tribal Planning Experience and Health', in *Hui Whakaoranga, op cit.*
15 D. S. Sinclair, (1975), 'Land: Māori Views and European Response', in M. King (ed.), *Te Ao Hurihuri*, Hicks Smith, Wellington.
16 M. H. Durie, (1979), 'Land and Mental Health', unpublished paper presented at the the RANZCP Conference, Queenstown.
17 M. H. Durie, (1987), 'Implications of Policy and Management Decisions on Maori Health: Contemporary Issues and Responses', *International Journal of Health Planning and Management* 2, Special: 201–13.
18 C. Maskill, (1991), *A Health Profile of New Zealand Adolescents*, Discussion Paper 14, Health Research Services, Department of Health, Wellington.
19 M. H. Durie, (1986), 'Te Taha Hinengaro: An Integrated Approach to Mental Health', *Community Mental Health in New Zealand* 1 (1): 4–11.
20 C. J. Heath (ed.), (1985), *Summary Report—National Conference on the Role of the Doctor in New Zealand: Implications for Medical Education*, University of Otago Medical School, Dunedin, p. 8.
21 R. R. Pere, (1984), 'Te Oranga o te Whānau: The Health of the Family', in *Hui Whakaoranga, op cit.*
22 M. Henare, (1988), 'Nga Tikanga me nga Ritenga o te Ao Māori: Standards and Foundations of Māori Society', in *The April Report*, III, part 1, Royal Commission on Social Policy, Wellington, pp. 24–232.
23 M. H. Durie, (1985), 'Māori Health Institutions', *Community Mental Health in New Zealand* 2 (1) 63–9.
24 W. H. Oliver, (1991), *Claims to the Waitangi Tribunal*, Department of Justice/Daphne Brasell Associates, Wellington. The major claims were brought by Te Ātiawa (the Motunui claim), Ngāti Pikiao (Kaituna River), Ngāti Te Ata (Manukau Harbour), and Ngāti Kahu (Mangonui Inlet).
25 Waitangi Tribunal, (1986), *Te Reo Māori Report*, Department of Justice, Wellington.
26 Working Group on Indigenous Populations, (1993), *Draft Declaration on the Rights of Indigenous Peoples. Report on the Eleventh Session of the United Nations Working Group*

on *Indigenous Populations,* United Nations, Geneva.

27 Te Roopu Awhina ō Tokanui, (1987), 'Cultural Perspectives in Psychiatric Nursing: A Maori Viewpoint', *Nursing Praxis in New Zealand* 2 (3): 3–11.

28 P. Ngata and L. Dyall, (1984), 'Health: A Māori View', *Health* 36: 2.

29 C. Benland, (1988), 'The S-Factor: Taha Wairua', in *The April Report, op cit.*, pp. 450–68.

30 New Zealand Board of Health, (1988), *Priorities for the New Zealand Health Services,* New Zealand Board of Health, Wellington, p. 6.

The Wai 262 Claim: A Claim by Māori to Indigenous Flora and Fauna: *Me o Rātou Taonga Katoa*

MAUI SOLOMON

Background

The Wai 262 claim was filed in 1991 on behalf of six claimant iwi.[1] The claim began as a vision of two kuia, Dell Wihongi and Saana Murray in collaboration with elders from four other iwi. These kaumātua were becoming concerned at the apparent loss of native flora and fauna to overseas interests and the lack of Māori involvement and participation regarding decision making concerning the granting of intellectual property rights over this flora and fauna.[2]

Much has been written and published about the Wai 262 claim both in New Zealand and overseas. Sir Hugh Kawharu, of Ngāti Whatua, an anthropologist, linguist, and tribal elder, had this to say to the Waitangi Tribunal hearing the Wai 262 claim in May 2002:

> *In my opinion the present claim has had no equal in terms of significance to Māori since the Te Reo Māori claim in 1985. Such a statement is not made lightly … . The Te Reo Māori claim was a historic moment in the history of our people, bringing together as it did voices from the four winds, to decry the loss and devaluing of the Māori language. Te reo is the stalwart of culture, the bastion of self-determination. The Tribunal heard evidence at that time from some of the last tohunga of the language—holders of a type of knowledge which could only faithfully be expressed through their own reo … .*
>
> *The Wai 262 claim takes another step forward from that auspicious claim in 1985. It focuses on that simple phrase in the second article of the Māori version of Te Tiriti o Waitangi—Te tino rangatiratanga o o rātou taonga katoa. It talks of a way of life, a world view, a culture, an identity. Denial by the Crown partner of these matters is the cause of historical and contemporary Treaty breaches.*[3]

The Wai 262 claim has also received widespread attention from the international community and indigenous peoples' organisations in particular. The late Darrell Posey, an internationally renowned anthropologist, noted that the Wai 262 claim was one of the most important initiatives by indigenous peoples anywhere in the world to seek recognition and protection of their cultural and intellectual property rights.[4]

What is the claim all about?

The Statement of Claim, which was filed in 1991 with the Waitangi Tribunal and amended in 1997, states as follows:

> *THE CLAIM*
> The claim relates to te tino rangatiratanga of Ngāti Kuri, Te Rarawa, and Ngāti Wai in respect of indigenous flora and fauna me o rātou taonga katoa (and all their treasures) within their respective tribal rohe, including but not limited to te reo, mātauranga, knowledge systems, laws, customs and values, whakairo, wāhi tapu, biodiversity, natural resources, genetics and genetic derivatives, Maori symbols, images, designs, and their use and development and associated indigenous, cultural and customary heritage rights (including intellectual property and property rights) in relation to such taonga. 'Taonga' in this claim refers to all elements of the claimants' estates, material and non-material, tangible and intangible.[5]

The claim has been described in various ways since it was filed with the Tribunal in 1991. It was the 262nd claim to be registered, hence the abridged version 'Wai 262'. It was initially described as a claim to indigenous flora and fauna. It has been called the 'claim to intellectual and cultural property' or the 'mātauranga Māori claim'. The statements of claim of some claimants refer to it as a claim to 'indigenous flora and fauna me o rātou taonga katoa', a reference back to article two of the Treaty. Perhaps it was best encapsulated by Mason Durie when giving evidence on behalf of the claimants in 2002. He described the claim as 'te ao Māori claim'—the claim about the Māori world.

The claim is about ensuring that appropriate recognition, protection, and provision is made for Māori rights in relation to indigenous flora and fauna, their special relationship with that indigenous flora and fauna, and all knowledge and intellectual property rights that flow from that relationship. The claimants assert that these are rights that were guaranteed and protected under article two of both the English and Māori versions of Te Tiriti o Waitangi/Treaty of Waitangi.[6]

Should New Zealanders be concerned about the place of the Treaty in modern-day New Zealand?

There is a common belief among many New Zealanders that Māori wish to turn the clock back and live as they did before Europeans arrived. These attitudes are perhaps understandable in light of the widely held misconceptions about Māori self-determination and the lack of any serious endeavour to educate New Zealanders about the Treaty of Waitangi and its historical and contemporary importance in New Zealand today. In the current political environment, politicians such as the leader of the National Party, Don Brash, are claiming that policies based upon recognition of Treaty rights amount to 'special privileges' and foster 'racial divisiveness'.

The Treaty has received minimal exposure in our education system so that generations of New Zealanders have grown up quite ignorant of its existence or meaning. The media thrive on conflict, so often portray the most negative aspects of Māori and Treaty issues. Little wonder, therefore, that New Zealanders are up in arms when politicians deliberately manipulate poorly informed public opinion for their own political ends.

The current debate over the foreshore and seabed demonstrates the high level of misunderstanding and public animosity that has been generated by misinformation and politicisation of the issues. Māori have sought for the past decade or more to engage with the Crown to discuss the nature and extent of their Treaty interests in the coastal marine area. Having been repeatedly rejected in their entreaties to the Crown, they sought redress through the only avenue available to them: the legal system. Then having had their right to seek redress upheld in the highest court in the land,[7] the government announced that they would legislate to remove those rights and replace them with a set of 'interests' that the Crown would unilaterally determine. The notion of 'one law for all' espoused by Brash does not appear to apply to Māori, whose legal rights can be so easily trampled and extinguished in the interests of appeasing the misinformed views of the majority population.

After undertaking twelve hui around the country and engaging with various Māori groups about their proposals over a period of six months, the Crown proposals for the foreshore and seabed essentially remained unchanged. The Crown simply ignored what Māori had said despite several alternative options being put forward by Māori that could have resulted in a more robust result. Instead Māori have been accused through the media of wanting to 'exclude Pākehā from the beaches', and 'sell off the land to overseas interests' and of advocating 'separatism'. Māori are not only offended by these statements, but also deeply hurt. Their record of kaitiakitanga (equated with caring) and manaakitanga (sharing) of the environment in post-European times is beyond reproach. These factors were pointed out *ad nauseum* to the Crown representatives and to the media but largely fell on deaf ears. Perception, especially when it promotes your own political agenda, is more potent than reality. It is possible for the foreshore and seabed debate to be resolved in a way that enhances the Treaty relationship between the Crown and Māori and the developing sense of nationhood of all New Zealanders. It should not be done to appease the politics of the day but rather with the long term vision of a nation united, not a nation divided. Hopefully, it is not too late.

The Wai 262 claimants and Māori generally are concerned to ensure that their legitimate cultural and property rights are recognised and respected within Aotearoa New Zealand and that their relationship with their natural world is equally recognised and respected. Respect for the Māori world view and their cultural values (in a country and society that is largely Eurocentric in its outlook) is at the very core of the Wai 262 claim. Unfortunately for the claimants, their property rights and cultural values have not been accorded the legal protection and political recognition that was guaranteed to them under the Treaty of Waitangi. It should not be automatically assumed by ordinary New Zealanders that the recognition of these rights and obligations is somehow a denial or erosion of their own heritage or values. Non-Māori New Zealanders will benefit from a greater involvement of Māori in the cultural, social, and economic environment within New Zealand. In many cases Māori claims are synonymous with concerns shared by the majority of New Zealanders. For example, decades before the environmentalist movement gained popularity in New Zealand and the passage of the Resource Management Act in 1991, Māori tribes had been actively involved in claims to the Waitangi Tribunal and through the Planning Tribunal to protect the environment from the adverse consequences of pollution.[8] Māori claims to prevent the wholesale disposal of state-owned assets to foreign interests in the 1980s and 1990s and the more recent upsurge of overseas investors buying vast tracts of New Zealand's coastal and high-country estates has also resonated with many New Zealanders who are equally concerned about New Zealand remaining in New Zealand hands.

What did the Treaty guarantee to Māori?

In interpreting the principles of the Treaty of Waitangi, the Waitangi Tribunal is required to look at both the English and Māori versions. However, the significant majority of chiefs signed the Māori version of the Treaty because that is the language they spoke and it is the version that contained concepts they understood. There has been on-going debate surrounding what Māori were agreeing to give up in exchange for the article two guarantee. The English version records Māori as ceding their sovereignty to Queen Victoria while the Māori version records Māori agreeing to grant to the Queen kāwanatanga (the 'governorship') over their lands. Whatever the the perspective about whether Māori agreed to cede to the Queen in 1840, both the English and Māori versions of the Treaty are quite explicit as to what Māori were getting in return.

The second article of the English version confirmed and guaranteed to the chiefs and tribes and the respective families and individuals thereof 'the full exclusive and undisturbed possession of their lands and estates, forests, fisheries and other properties which they may collectively or individually possess so long as it is their wish and desire to retain the same in their possession'.[9]

Article two of the Māori version guarantees 'te tino rangatiratanga o o rātou wenua o rātou kainga me o rātou taonga katoa'.[10] So, according to the widely accepted translation by Hugh Kawharu, it 'arranges [and] agrees to the Chiefs to the subtribes to people all of New Zealand the unqualified exercise of their chieftainship over their land over their villages and over their treasures all'.[11] It is, therefore, clear that both the English and Māori versions guaranteed to Māori a specific set of property rights and 'other properties' (English version) and taonga katoa (and 'treasures all') (Māori version). In exchange for sovereignty (English version) and kāwanatanga (Māori version), Māori were being guaranteed their full chieftainship over all of their property rights and all other taonga. This is what Māori would have understood when signing the Treaty in 1840.

It is interesting in the context of the debate occurring today notwithstanding these clear and unambiguous words that several political parties would seek to deny the relevance of the Treaty in the assertion and recognition of Māori property rights. Instead, as both the National Party leader, Don Brash, and the ACT party would have it, the Treaty is a blueprint for a 'special privileges', 'racial separatism', and 'racial conflict'. Ironically, both National and ACT are proponents for the recognition and protection of private property rights. It seems the only caveat is that recognition is refused if those property rights are held by Māori. The current Labour government is also guilty of seeking to deny Māori access to the courts to pursue their legitimate claims in relation to the foreshore and seabed despite the highest court in the land ruling to the contrary.[12]

As noted above, Wai 262 concerns claims in relation to both tangible assets (property rights and natural resources) and intangible assets (taonga such as language, designs, traditional knowledge, and cultural practices).

What is mātauranga Māori?

One of the taonga said by the claimants to have been guaranteed to individual rangatira and hapū is their mātauranga Māori, or Māori knowledge. One kaumātua of Ngāti Kahungunu defined mātauranga Māori in these terms:

> *Mātauranga Māori in a traditional context means the knowledge, comprehension or understanding of everything visible or invisible that exists across the universe (i.e.: Aorangi sometimes referred to as Rangi and Papa). This meaning is related to the modern context as Māori research, science and technology principles and practices.*[13]

The Wai 262 claim seeks the protection of mātauranga Māori from inappropriate use and its control by Māori. Included in the protection of knowledge is the knowledge system itself, and its internal mechanism for transmission, dissemination, tuition, and development. The evidence presented to the Tribunal has asserted that such systems existed at the time of the Treaty, but have been seriously eroded and disrespected to the point where the systems and the knowledge itself are at risk. This has been a consistent theme as the Tribunal has travelled from hapū to hapū to hear the testimony of elders. Generally speaking, it was explained that mātauranga Māori had as its basis the notion of whakapapa, leading to the following characteristics:[14]

- the inter-relatedness of all things
- the basis of knowledge being in the natural environment
- the inseparability of the spiritual (tapu) and life force (mauri) from every aspect of knowledge.

In more recent times, there has been a growing recognition of the importance of mātauranga Māori and its relationship and relevance to Western science. As noted by Murray Parsons:

> *If science is the study of the world around us using a hypothetico-deductive process (the scientific method) then this is not exclusive to Western or European-derived cultural traditions but is also found in the cultures of all indigenous peoples. All indigenous peoples have science according to their needs and cultural understandings of their surroundings, the environment. The same thought processes that allowed Polynesians to voyage between the islands of the Pacific and to settle them, also has sent people into space. The term Māori Science has been used to emphasise Māori people too used the scientific method and that it is not the prerogative of Western countries only.*[15]

The significance of mātauranga Māori to sustainability of the environment

While New Zealand has a clean, green, and healthy environmental image internationally, the reality is that the country's biodiversity has been greatly affected by human interactions with the environment. A recent press release by NZ Forest and Bird Society commenting on the proposed changes to the Resource Management Act 1991 noted that:

> *New Zealand's environmental performance is poor. New Zealand holds world records in the number of threatened species, rivers are still being polluted, important wetlands are still being drained and forests are still being cleared. If New Zealand is to achieve sustainable management, a lot will need to be done.*[16]

New Zealanders are becoming more aware of the importance of preserving and enhancing biodiversity. Mātauranga Māori, or Māori knowledge, innovations and practices, have a key role to play in the future conservation and sustainable use of New Zealand's biological diversity. A practical example of this is the current management of Whakaki Lake in the Hawkes Bay. This is a Māori-owned lake, comprising the biggest wetland on the whole of the east coast of the North Island and as such is of very high ecological value. For many years the lake had been managed by the predecessor to the Hawkes Bay Regional Council, which had focused on turning the wetland into productive farmland. The result was that a formerly pristine area was turned into a salty marsh of much lower ecological value. Following years of negotiations, the local iwi were granted management over their lake. As a result of reinstating traditional management techniques and knowledge, the lake is once again thriving as is evident from the re-growth in the tuna (eel) populations in the lake.[17]

Robert McGowan, who has worked with Māori for the past thirty years in helping to preserve the knowledge and practices of mātauranga Māori in New Zealand, says that it is:

More important—because it is not given much emphasis in my experience—of preserving that living relationship of those who have the knowledge with the environment. That's what gives life to the knowledge—upholding the mauri. At the end of the day it is not about compiling data, it is about upholding the mauri, ensuring that it continues to live and thrive and bestow its gift of wholeness, health, integrity. That is so much more difficult when Māori are largely alienated from the land, either by loss of ownership or loss of access...[18]

Over millennia of inhabiting the shores of Aotearoa, Māori have built up a large storehouse of knowledge about their natural world. Māori consider themselves to be an intrinsic part of the natural world rather than apart from it. Everything in the natural world of the Māori can be explained in terms of whakapapa or genealogy.

In the beginning was te kore or total darkness. There was no life, only potential. Papatūanuku, the earth mother and Ranginui, the sky father were locked together in an embrace that stifled all growth. Their children, desperate for light, devised a plan to forcibly separate their parents. This job fell on the shoulders (literally) of one of the children, Tāne Mahuta, god of the forests. Binding to his mother below, he pushed upwards with his legs with all his strength and pushed his father apart from the earth.

Into the light created between Papatūanuku and Ranginui sprang the raging winds of Tāwhirimatea (god of the winds), the swirling seas of Tangaroa (god of the sea) and all his progeny, the towering forests of Tāne Mahuta and all his progeny, and the varieties of cultivated and uncultivated crops. Tāne Mahuta fashioned the first human, Hine-ahu-one from the clay of his mother.

Tangata whenua literally means 'people of the land'. The Moriori people of Rekohu (Chatham Islands) claim to have sprung from the earth ('no ro whenua ake'). Legends tell of different waka or canoes arriving on Rekohu and Aotearoa from Hawaiki in various migrations from about 900 AD. They named every landmark, stream, rock, mountain, and other natural features in the landscape, including the flora and fauna they found there. Māori regard themselves as one with their natural world.

During a period of 1000 years occupation, the ancestors of the Māori developed complex rituals and protocols for regulating behaviour between themselves and their environment. This may best be described as a relationship of reciprocity and respect between themselves and the world that sustained them both physically and spiritually. Concepts such as mauri, tapu, kaitiaki, and rāhui (prohibitions imposed over the taking of resources), evolved as mechanisms of sustaining humankind's relationships with their natural world.

There were rights and obligations in relation to the taking of resources for human sustenance. So before a tree was taken from the domain of Tāne, karakia must be said and permission sought from the deity of the forest for the taking of one of his children. Karakia were said before fishing expeditions and the first catch of the day was gifted to Tangaroa as an expression of thanks and gratitude. Creatures of the sea and the landscape were imbued with special powers to guard over the people and the resources. So on Rekohu the most important gods of the sea were the Great White Sharks, which are still found in abundance in the waters around Rekohu.[19] To Moriori these creatures were kaitiaki or guardians of the oceans. Traditional knowledge passed down tells of these kaitiaki guiding fishermen to the safety of harbour if they were in trouble at sea. Moriori fishermen rather than fearing these creatures imbued them with great mana and consequently learned to live in harmony with them. As a people who relied so heavily on the sea for their survival, it is not difficult to see why Moriori held the lord of the oceans in such high regard and developed a relationship of respect and reciprocity. This is in stark contrast to the manner in which most people regard the Great Whites today where fear is the predominant factor.

Ngāti Kurī, one of the claimant tribes in the Wai 262 claim, has traditionally harvested the native kūaka bird (godwit) for many centuries. The kūaka migrates between New Zealand and Siberia on its long annual journey north. The kūaka is now a protected bird under New Zealand law and it is illegal for Māori to take it for food. However, Ngāti Kurī has a long-standing relationship with this bird, and for them the kūaka is equally important as a source of spiritual nourishment as it is for kai or food. An elder of Ngāti Kurī once described how when she was very ill, what she craved for most was the taste of the kūaka, which she claimed was food for her spirit and that she maintained helped restore her to good health.[20]

Ngāti Kurī has long been involved in the struggle to protect the silica sands in Parengarenga Harbour upon which the kūaka nest. The silica sands are mined to make glass and computer microchips. The sands are also important for growing the native pīngao grass that Ngāti Kuri use for weaving tukutuku panels in their meeting houses and for making piupiu (traditional Māori skirts). The relationship that Ngāti Kurī has with the kūaka, the pīngao plant, the silica sands, and the entire ecosystem of Parengarenga Harbour in Northland is typical of the way Māori tribes relate to their environment. However, their ability to sustainably practise their culture and maintain their traditional knowledge base is inhibited by regulations and laws that have alienated Ngāti Kurī from their lands and resources. As was made clear by a number of witnesses for Ngāti Kurī in evidence to the Waitangi Tribunal, access to their traditional lands and customary resources is vital if their culture, knowledge, and practices are to survive and flourish in the future.

Many of these traditional values of reciprocity and respect for the environment are of great significance to the modern world in which the sustainability of our natural resources is under greater threat than at any other time in human history. Although Māori and Moriori are recorded as having driven a number of flightless birds into extinction, including the oft-quoted example of the moa, they learned from these experiences and developed practices of rāhui that forbade the taking of species and resources for specified periods of time to enable replenishment and regeneration with penalties imposed for the breaches of these laws.

John Patterson, a lecturer in philosophy from Massey University describes this Māori environmental philosophy as presenting:

> *... an image of mutual dependence and harmony, in which all creatures are inter-related, in which the welfare of one is the welfare of all, in which a caring and nurturing relation between humans and other creatures is both imperative and straightforwardly natural ... . Māori philosophy is a lively philosophy, a philosophy of respect based not on insipid politeness or political correctness but on the mutual dependency of vigorous and robust creatures ...*[21]

These environmental values are at the core of the Wai 262 claim. Although current environmental legislation such as the Resource Management Act 1991 (RMA) and Hazardous Substances Act 1996[22] include provisions requiring decision-makers to 'take into account' and 'have regard to' the principles of the Treaty of Waitangi, these provisions are often read down or outweighed by scientific evidence that assumes greater significance in the decision-making process.[23]

Among the remedies that Wai 262 seeks from the Waitangi Tribunal is for Māori to have a greater say in the environmental and resource decision-making processes as was originally envisaged under the RMA legislation. The fact that this has not occurred to any significant degree is evidenced by the fact that since the RMA became law in 1991, not one local authority in the country has seen fit to exercise its powers under section 33 of the Act to transfer any powers, duties, or functions to an iwi authority, despite the many applications received from iwi over the past twelve years.

Rongoa Māori or traditional Māori medicinal knowledge

The Wai 262 claim also seeks to preserve and revive the practices of rongoa Māori or traditional Māori knowledge of native plants and their healing powers and the preparation of medicinal remedies based on those plants. Māori traditionally had an extensive knowledge of plants and their medicinal uses. The term 'rongoa Māori' refers to traditional Māori medicine, to the practice of traditional Māori medicine, and the body of knowledge behind that practice.[24] Tohunga or traditional healers had special knowledge of herbal plants and their uses. Many, if not most, of the practitioners of rongoa were elderly women. As one elderly expert on rongoa Māori explained in her evidence to the Waitangi Tribunal hearing the Wai 262 claim in 1997, 'I know the plants and they know me'[25]. She knew what time of the year and what time of the day to collect plants from the ngahere or forest. She could not just collect from any forest, it had to be the forest with which she had a close physical and spiritual relationship. She described her power to heal as a gift from the Creator and that she was just a conduit between the gods and the plants in order to aid the healing process. She never demanded payment for her services, as to do so would diminish the healing powers of the remedies she offered.

Robert McGowan, who himself is a practitioner of rongoa Māori, has spent the last thirty years working with Māori traditional healers. He records that:

One of the most consistent themes that came through in my working with kaumātua and traditional healers, is that the foundation of rongoa Māori is taha wairua 'spirituality'; not wai rakau 'herbal medicine'. The place of karakia (prayer) and tikanga (rules and protocols)—the appropriate rituals and traditions—is essential. Yet one would not gain that impression from the publications just described. There is an inclination in scientific research to reduce knowledge to terms that one can understand and then claim that that understanding is, in fact, an accurate description of the reality being investigated ... .

What is needed is an understanding of the context in which that knowledge found its origins, an appreciation of the values and customs that govern its usage, and an acknowledgement of the priorities that experience has provided. Far from being subjective and therefore unscientific knowledge, such factors provide and enshrine a depth of knowledge that is both valid and important.[26]

New Zealand law adversely impacted on the practice of rongoa Māori with the passage of the Tohunga Suppression Act 1907. Although not strictly enforced, this had the effect of marginalising the practice of traditional Māori healing and inhibited the retention and transmission of the knowledge.[27]

The reassertion of Māori identity and culture since the mid-1970s has also witnessed a co-related renaissance in the practice of rongoa Māori. A large body of knowledge of the practice of traditional Māori medicine has been retained, much of it in publications. However, as McGowan notes, the practice of rongoa Māori is quite different from the recording of its physical attributes.

One obstacle to the retention of this knowledge is the loss of traditional healers and the related difficulty in finding appropriate people to pass the knowledge on to. Another major issue identified by McGowan is the:

... separation of the vast majority of Māori from the natural world, of Tāne ... as the bush has disappeared or is greatly modified and degraded, how is something like rongoa Māori, which depends not just on knowledge of the bush, but having a living connection to it, going to survive?[28]

As regards the transmission and practice of knowledge, McGowan is of the view that:

A major effort must be made urgently to plan and establish a system to help the teaching of rongoa Māori, not just the knowledge of rongoa, but the experience of working with the people to whom the medicine belongs, those who need the healing it may provide.[29]

Concerns in relation to genetic engineering

The Wai 262 claimants have been concerned about issues of genetic engineering since prior to the lodgement of their claim in 1991. In particular the likely prejudicial effects the release of genetically modified organisms into the environment will have on whakapapa of humans, plants, and animals and on the mauri and tapu of those organisms and the claimants' responsibilities as kaitiki.

The various statements of claim of the four groupings of claimants all raise concerns over genetic engineering issues. The statements of claim filed on behalf of Ngāti Kuri, Te Rarawa, and Ngāti Wai state that:

> *GENETICS*
> The Māori world view connects humankind by whakapapa to the creation gods and to the kaitiaki of the natural and spiritual world, creating in each successive generation the obligations of kaitiakitanga.
>
> Whakapapa, and systems of knowledge about whakapapa, including systems of learning, transmission, respect for, and preservation of whakapapa are taonga within Article II of te Tiriti o Waitangi.
>
> The gene codes of indigenous flora and fauna and other natural resources are taonga within Article II of te Tiriti o Waitangi.
>
> The claimants claim that acts, omissions, policies, practices, and processes of the Crown which seek to significantly amend, destroy, or modify the genetics of indigenous flora and fauna *me o rātou taonga katoa* are in breach of the Treaty of Waitangi, and have prejudicially affected the claimants' rights of rangatiratanga and kaitiakitanga.
>
> The Crown has an obligation to actively protect the genetics of indigenous flora and fauna and other natural resources from modification which is not in accordance with the customs, laws, and values of the kaitiaki of the indigenous flora and fauna and other natural resources, including protection from the genetic modification of other species which have, will, or are likely to impact on the genetics, wellbeing and mauri of indigenous flora and fauna me o rātou taonga katoa.[30]

The phrase 'me o rātou taonga katoa' in this context also includes the whakapapa, mauri, and tapu of the physical and spiritual well-being of Māori relating, among other things, to their health, economic, social, and cultural welfare.

The expert evidence of Mana Cracknell summarises, from the Māori perspective, the in-depth knowledge that Māori have of genetics through their ancient and expert knowledge of whakapapa:

> *Whakapapa is about whanaungatanga (biogenetic relationships). It is a means of explaining and transcribing the spiritual, intellectual, social and material relationship between the claimants (and Māori generally) and the indigenous flora and fauna of this country. For example, the ancestral god Tangaroa Whakamautai is the titular holder of taonga, rights and knowledge in the sea. By virtue of whakapapa these rights (and associated responsibilities) are passed down to present day descendents of Tangaroa. Similarly, the god Tāne as Tāne Matua is the progenitor of Ngā Airihia-Tangata Māori. As Tāne Mahuta he is the lord of the forest. As Tāne-te-waananga-a-lo-matua he is the source of the wisdom knowledge given by Toi-matua. As Tāne-nui-a-rangi he is the owner of rangi (frequencies) and the proprietor of atea (space).*

> *The WAI 262 claim can be understood and explained within the above definitional context of whakapapa. Hence the claimants [sic] position today as the kaitiaki and advocates of the taonga both tapu (not tangible) and taputapu (tangible) of their ancestors including, for example, Tangaroa Whakamautai and Tāne Mahuta.*
>
> *Whakapapa, taonga and rights are inseparable, consistent and continuous. These rights are tukua iho (relayed) from distant ancestors down to the current day tribal custodians … .*
>
> *Western science often smugly assumes 'superiority' over traditional scientific knowledge. In my opinion western science is still to 'catch up' with the wisdom contained, retained and transmitted through whakapapa and traditional knowledge.*

The act of deliberately taking genes from one species and implanting into another for perceived 'economic' or other social benefits is regarded by the claimants as tampering with the sacred matrix of life, namely whakapapa.

The claimants are particularly concerned at the transgenic or horizontal transfer of genes from one species into another and the unknown and unquantifiable impacts this will have on human, plant, and animal life in the future. Science is unable to predict with any precision the long-term adverse implications of such experiments. Indeed, there is already a good deal of scientific evidence and known examples that demonstrate that horizontal gene transfer can occur between genetically modified (GM) crops and non-GM crops through cross pollination, suggesting that humans may be exposed through spores floating in the air and myriad other uncontrolled (and even unthought of) ways to genetically modified organisms.

Peter Wills, from the Department of Physics at Auckland University, supports the proposition that the Māori world-view has the potential to contribute to Western scientific understanding of genetic inheritance and the consequences of genetic manipulation:

> *Māori bring to the debate about genetic engineering a coherent and integrated perspective in which the 'intangible' world of culture cannot be separated from the description of the phenomenal world. This should challenge scientific analyses that are limited to talk about pieces of DNA and the material consequences of transposing them from one organism to another.*
>
> *Scientists are very quick to dismiss or ignore any discussion based on premises that are inconsistent with the accepted wisdom of their own disciplines. When they have to take serious account of concerns for whakapapa, mauri and tapu, whether these are expressed by Māori proponents or opponents of genetic engineering, they may find some worth in what they have eliminated from their own descriptions of the world.*
>
> *There is good reason to believe that the facts of biology (and therefore the way we define our genetic heritage) cannot be explained adequately, even from a scientific point of view, without the development of concepts akin to whakapapa, mauri and tapu.*

> *Whether we look at the level of a single cell, a whole organism, an ecological community or the whole biosphere, we find that the functionalities of the various parts are defined in terms of the integrity of the whole system. Functional interactions are the practical determinants of events and the formation of new structures, conferring on entities the capacity (cf. mauri) to act as agents of change in some characteristic way.*
>
> *The functional relationships between molecules in cells and species in ecosystems are deeply entrenched and are maintained by natural restrictions and limitations (cf. tapu). While it is true that we now have the means of setting some of those restrictions aside through genetic engineering, we should not do so with impunity because we will bear the consequences.*
>
> *By insisting on the validity of the context they use to frame their thinking, Māori can make a seminal contribution to the debate about how to deal with the world's genetic heritage, even when and where considerations of a purely technical character have been given dominance. For their part scientists need to undertake a critical analysis of their fundamental philosophical assumptions and establish new ways of thinking about biological phenomena, dropping insistence that their description of the facts is correct and complete.*[31]

Cultural and intellectual property rights: What are they and why should they be protected?

This past decade has witnessed a marked growth in international interest in 'cultural heritage tourism' and the use of Māori imagery, symbols, and designs to promote commercial products in a consumer-hungry market increasingly seeking to gain an 'edge' over their competitors. Tourists are attracted to the cultures of the indigenous peoples, and their artwork, music, and indigenous designs are becoming highly prized commodities, and powerful marketing and branding tools. The use of Māori symbolism by Telecom, Air NZ, and Adidas in promoting the All Blacks are some examples. More recently a plethora of internationally renowned companies including LEGO (use of Māori names on BIONICLE toys), Sony (the PlayStation game *Mark of Kri* uses Māori names and designs), TechnoMarine (watches and models with Māori names and imagery), Microsoft (use of Māori names and imagery in a computer game called *Asheron's Call*), a Danish restaurant (using Māori moko to promote food), and Ford Motor Company (Māori-inspired moko on a Hot Rod pick-up truck), have jumped on the bandwagon of using Māori designs and imagery to promote their products. The same phenomenon is being witnessed in other places with indigenous peoples, particularly Australia, North America, Hawaii, and Latin America.

Many more businesses in New Zealand are beginning to appreciate the 'added value' and marketing opportunities that a distinctive Māori identity, Māori place names and traditions give to New Zealand businesses operating in the international market. As Brian Richards, marketing strategist for the Māori Made Mark, observed back in 1994:

In worldwide research on New Zealand, 'sheep' and 'green' are the only two icons that stand out ... we can actually add value using our indigenous products. It will come from our Māori people, our artists, our playwrights and designers ... Māori custom and culture is absolutely wonderful. There is potential for developing Māori icons to our culture .... I would love to see New Zealand borrow from Māori elements and use them in a modern context, because they help to position us worldwide .... By drawing on Māori culture and referencing, we could produce the most stunning textiles and fabric. Nobody yet has exploited Māori graphics and upholstery and curtaining fabrics etc. ...[32]

Some may argue that it is a positive thing for Māori culture to be 'promoted' to an international audience in this way. Certainly, Māori are not against the use and development of their culture and intellectual property rights but insist that they have control over how their taonga (including in this context language, designs, symbols, and traditional knowledge) are used, for what purposes they are used and by whom they are used. It is offensive to many Māori (and certainly the Wai 262 claimants) that names such as 'tohunga' are used on plastic toys and moko are used to promote food products, watches, and Hot Rod trucks. In the case of the Ford Motor Company, they purposefully associate the 'warrior' qualities of the wearer of traditional Māori moko with their Hot Rod truck, which they describe on their web site in the following manner:

The leather-wrapped tonneau cover features a traditional Māori tribe tattoo that is die cut into the leather with black cow hair in the cutout portions. The Māori are the Polynesian people of New Zealand. In moko, a type of Māori tattooing, shallow colored grooves in complex curvilinear designs were produced on the face by striking a miniature bone adze into the skin. Tattooed designs are thought by various peoples to provide magical protection against sickness or misfortune, or they serve to identify the wearer's rank, status or membership in a group.

In Māori culture, an elegantly tattooed face was a great source of pride to a warrior, for it made him fierce in battle .... The F-150 has a great history and has consistently been the leader among full-size pick-ups - it is certainly fierce in battle. [33]

In a letter written to TechnoMarine, Kingi Gilbert, a young Māori entrepreneur and an international advocate for better protection and respect for Māori cultural and intellectual property rights had this to say about the unauthorised use of moko:

There is a large body of [Māori] fighting against popular culture to have our designs respected. The widespread use of Māori images in pop culture is watering down the core values of Māori moko, it is making it less unique, and more commercial, but mostly, it loses its 'ihi' or natural identifying force. It is seen as a commodity and not an identifying force, which a portion of it traditionally was.

Did you know that the moko was carved into the skin by bone chisel over a period of years? That it showed rank, achievements, and history of the wearer? How do you think we feel today when we see those designs as 'an identifying form' on people who know nothing about it? We don't receive any benefit from that at all, only hurt and pain. It doesn't respect our ancestors. It's like asking you to conduct a large press interview, but wear a Swatch branded hat and Mickey Mouse watch from Disneyland. Would you seriously allow yourself to be represented that way?[34]

Not only is the current intellectual property rights (IPR) system inadequate to protect Māori against the unauthorised use of their own images and designs (where those designs have not been registered), but foreign-based companies are able to register trademark rights over Māori names that prevent Māori from using those names themselves. The most recent example of this involved Moana Maniapoto, a Māori artist and performer who has won international awards. Moana, having written and produced a number of albums under her own name here in New Zealand and been a regular on the European concert circuit in recent years, was threatened in 2002 by a German company with a court injunction and damages of 100,000 deutschmarks, for daring to use her own name on an eponymous CD. The company, Media XS, registered and based in Germany had obtained a trademark for the name 'Moana' in respect of a wide range of products and services throughout Europe, which included musical products. They argued that Moana could not use her own name on her CD because it was in violation of their trademark rights. Eventually, the matter was settled out of court by her German agents by agreeing to change the name on the CD to 'Moana and The Tribe'.

This case provides a clear example of the inadequacies of the current system of IPR to protect Māori cultural and intellectual property rights. Patent attorneys might argue that any knowledge in the 'public domain' is fair game for trade marking.[35] The Wai 262 claimants and many other Māori have argued that it is not their fault that their knowledge has ended up in the public domain, but even if that is the case, there is still an on-going obligation to maintain respect for such knowledge in the way that it is represented and used. Having been deprived of most of their physical resource base, this form of intangible property (language, names, and imagery) is often the only taonga that remains for many indigenous peoples, including Māori. It is not surprising therefore that they would argue for better systems of protection and the right to control its future use.

As commercial interest in indigenous culture, artwork, and knowledge continues to grow, tribes need to retain control over, regulate, and protect their cultural heritage rights if they are not to be debased in the pursuit of commercial gain. If companies want to use Māori images and designs, they should do so only with the consent and participation of those who are the knowledge holders. This would include acknowledgment of the knowledge holders and, where appropriate, the establishment of joint venture arrangements and the payment of royalties.[36]

One of the difficulties for both Māori and private interests is the lack of any formal process for identifying where to go and who to speak to in the rare instances where commercial operators make efforts to obtain approval to use traditional material.[37] This is one of the key areas that the Wai 262 claim seeks to remedy by providing a framework and process within which these issues can be handled with efficiency and sensitivity.

International significance of the Wai 262 claim

In 1998, the Waitangi Tribunal heard from a number of international expert witnesses, both indigenous and non-indigenous, on how issues raised within the Wai 262 claim were being dealt with by other countries and at the level of the United Nations. Subjects included the Convention on Biological Diversity (to which New Zealand is a signatory), the Draft Declaration on the Rights of Indigenous Peoples and various international Non-Governmental Organisations (NGOs), such as the International Society of Ethnobiology (ISE). It became apparent over the course of the week's hearing that the issues Māori have raised within the context of the Wai 262 claim are not unique to Māori and are being grappled with by indigenous and traditional peoples and their respective countries the world over.

There are common threads that link indigenous peoples around the globe. Values such as spirituality, collective rights, and the holistic way in which indigenous peoples view and relate with the natural world. With the increasing focus on how to exploit traditional knowledge (in all its various forms) for commercial gain, it is of fundamental importance that these values are recognised and protected. The Western intellectual property system (in its current form), with its emphasis on private, economic rights is widely regarded by indigenous peoples as fundamentally flawed and therefore lacking legitimacy as a means of protecting indigenous peoples' knowledge systems.

As noted by Darrell Posey in the preface to the UNEP publication on the Cultural and Spiritual Values of Biodiversity:

> *In a world increasingly dominated by mega-modelling, global trading and consumer trends, it is easy to forget that values of plants, animals, landscapes, and ecosystems cannot be adequately measured in statistical or monetary terms—and certainly cannot be described using the languages of only a few academic disciplines and markets, no matter how politically favoured and powerful they might be. Values of biodiversity—biological, cultural, and linguistic—are intrinsic to life itself and celebrated by the myriad ... cultures and societies that have co-evolved with the natural and metaphysical worlds that surround them. Indeed, human beings are an integral part of biodiversity, not merely observers and users of the 'components of biological diversity'.*
>
> *Indigenous and traditional peoples make this fundamental principle the very core of their societies. For them, nature is an extension of society itself, and the creatures that share life with them are manifestations of the past and future generations—of their own flesh and blood. Nature is not therefore a*

commodity to be bought, sold, patented, or preserved apart from society precisely because nature is what defines humanity. The earth is their (our) mother and cannot be compromised, sold, or monopolised.[38]

In simple terms, indigenous peoples have a different 'world view' from the dominant Western cultures that place major emphasis on individualism, materialism, and capitalism in contrast to indigenous communities whose emphasis is more focused on the collective rights and responsibilities of the group.

There is considerable international interest in researching the traditional knowledge of indigenous and traditional peoples and local communities. Over the last decade and particularly in Western countries, awareness of the 'value' that traditional knowledge may offer in the fields of botanical, pharmaceutical, agricultural, biotechnological, and genetic research has significantly increased. It is estimated that about US$45 billion per annum is generated from pharmaceutical products whose origin stems from traditional knowledge of plants and medicines. This is by no means an exhaustive list of uses for which traditional knowledge is now regarded within Western science as 'valuable'.

It is, however, increasingly obvious that such cultural knowledge is not so much valued for its intrinsic worth but for its instrumental value, i.e., the commercial gains that access to traditional knowledge and associated genetic resources can add to the global economy and the development of new commercial products. It is no exaggeration to say there is a worldwide 'gold rush' mentality in the efforts being made to research, document, control, exploit, and claim intellectual property rights over the traditional knowledge and associated resources of indigenous peoples.

The two most significant processes dealing with indigenous peoples' issues at the international level is the work being carried out under the Convention on Biological Diversity (CBD) and by the World Intellectual Property Organisation (WIPO).[39] Article 8j of the CBD requires governments 'as far as possible and as appropriate' to:

Subject to its national legislation respect, preserve and maintain knowledge, innovations and practices of indigenous and local communities ... relevant for the sustainable use of biological diversity and promote their wider application with the approval and involvement of the holders of such knowledge ... and encourage the equitable sharing of the benefits arising from the utilization of such knowledge, innovations and practices.

Working groups have been established to develop policies for the implementation of Article 8j and also on access and benefit-sharing regarding traditional knowledge and genetic resources, including examining the development of elements of a *sui generis* system for the protection of traditional knowledge, innovations, and practices. Similarly, WIPO, through the Intergovernmental Committee on Intellectual Property and Genetic Resources, Traditional Knowledge and Folklore ('the IGC'), is also undertaking extensive work in these areas, including looking at the development of international regimes to accommodate traditional knowledge and intellectual property rights. The concerns expressed by most indigenous peoples (including the Wai 262 claimants) about the CBD and WIPO processes is the lack of opportunity for full and effective participation in decision-making on matters that fundamentally affect their rights and interests at national, regional, and international levels. There is also concern expressed that these international bodies, in which only governments are permitted to vote, will develop policies and processes that entrench the status quo and expose indigenous cultures to even more forms of commercial exploitation and expropriation of their knowledge and natural resources.

Conclusion

The Wai 262 claim has variously been criticised by Crown agencies and others as being too broad in its ambit and unclear about its outcomes. Originally filed in 1991, it has proven to be visionary and far reaching in scope. It has raised for discussion and public debate such complex issues as genetic engineering, the recognition and protection of mātauranga Māori in the modern world and its contribution to environmental sustainability, and the need to ensure adequate frameworks and processes for the protection and advancement of cultural and intellectual property rights in a manner that reflects a Māori cultural perspective. The developments in the international arena in these diverse but inter-related areas over the past decade illustrate the importance and relevance of the issues raised by the claimants all those years ago. Although the claim is still some way from completion,[40] there can be no doubt of the impact it has had over the past ten years in influencing the development of Crown policy across a broad range of areas; even though much of this policy would appear to be an endeavour to pre-empt the possible outcome of the Tribunal findings and recommendations.

More than anything, the Wai 262 claim is about the re-assertion of tino rangatiratanga by Māori over their culture and their resources. It is a vision that was laid down at Waitangi in 1840 and one still to be realised.

Ma wai ra, e korero	*Who will speak*
Nga piki, ngā heke	*For the ancient times*
O ngā tupuna	*Of the ancestral waka*
I runga 'i te kare o ngā wai	*On the ocean pathways*
Ma tātou ano	*We the generations*
Ma ngā uri whakatupu	*The descendants of the*
O ngā tupuna Māori[41]	*Māori ancestors*

Notes

1 The original claimants were Hema-Nui-a-Tawhaki Witana (otherwise known as Dell Wihongi) for Te Rarawa, Saana Murray for Ngāti Kurī, the late Witi McMath for Ngāti Wai, Tama Poata for Te Whānau a Rua (a hapū of Ngāti Porou), Kataraina Rimene for Ngāti Kahungunu and the late John Hippolite for Ngāti Koata. Te Rūnanga o Ngāti Porou is also now a claimant in its own right.

2 In 1988, Dell Wihongi led a delegation to Japan to bring back to New Zealand six cultivars of the New Zealand native variety of kumara that were then housed by Douglas Yen at an institute in Japan. They had been taken to Japan because the then Department of Scientific and Industrial Research in New Zealand was unable or unwilling to store them. Wihongi was roundly criticised through the media by the then Prime Minister, the David Lange, for undertaking such a mission.

3 I.H. Kawharu, 'Brief of evidence of Sir Hugh Kawharu', Waitangi Tribunal, Wai 262 K13, pp. 2–3.

4 Personal communication with the author 1997. Posey, a Fellow at the University of Oxford, presented evidence to the Waitangi Tribunal in November 1998 at a special sitting of the Tribunal in Rotorua to hear evidence from international experts. The purpose of this hearing was to hear testimony from both indigenous and non-indigenous experts from both developed and developing countries on how the issues raised within Wai 262 are also being dealt with by governments, non-governmental organisations, United Nations organisations, and indigenous peoples' groups all over the world.

5 Wai 262, Amended Statement of Claim for Ngāti Kuri, Te Rarawa and Ngāti Wai, para. 3.1.

6 Article two of the English version of the Treaty of Waitangi guarantees to Māori '... the full exclusive and undisturbed possession of all their Lands and Estates Forests Fisheries and other properties ... so long as it is their wish and desire to retain the same in their possession'. Article two of the Māori version guarantees to the Chiefs and Tribes and individuals thereof 'te tino rangatiratanga o ... o rātou taonga katoa'. This is interpreted by Sir Hugh Kawharu as meaning 'the unqualified exercise of their chieftainship over ... their treasures all.' See appendix.

7 *Attorney-General v. Ngāti Apa* [2003] 3 NZLR 643 (CA).

8 See Waitangi Tribunal, *Motunui-Waitara Report*, The Tribunal, Wellington, 1983; Waitangi Tribunal, *Manukau Report*, The Tribunal, Wellington, 1985.

9 The Treaty of Waitangi Act 1975, Schedule 1.

10 The Treaty of Waitangi Act 1975, Schedule 1.

11 See appendix.

12 See *Attorney-General v. Ngāti Apa* [2003] 3 NZLR 643 (CA).

13 C. Mohi, 'Mātauranga Māori – A National Resource', paper prepared for the Ministry of Research Science and Technology, 1993, pp. 1–3, quoted from David Williams' report on 'Mātauranga Māori and Taonga', Waitangi Tribunal Publication 2001, Wai 262 K6, p. 15.

14 L. Watson, 'Test Tube and the Kete: Science and Mātauranga Māori in the Wai 262 claim', paper presented to the Science, Culture And Fear Conference, 22 November 2002, Te Papa Tongarewa, Wellington.

15 M. Parsons, 'Māori Science', notes arising from the MAC Ministry of Research Science and Technology, meeting 15 September 1995 and personal communication with Geoff Page, Industrial Research Limited, 1995, p. 4 quoted from Williams, 'Report on Mātauranga Māori and Taonga', p. 19.

16 NZ Forest and Bird Society, Press Release, 14 May 2003.

17 Robert McGowan, personal communication, February 2004.

18 Robert McGowan, personal communication.

19 'Rekohu' is the original Moriori name for the Chatham Islands. It is also known by Māori as 'Wharekauri'.

20 Saana Murray (tribal elder of Ngāti Kuri), personal communication.

21 J. Patterson, *People of the Land: A Pacific Philosophy*, Dunmore Press, Palmerston North, 2000, p. 14.

22 Section 8 of the Resource Management Act and section 6 of the Hazardous Substances Act.

23 For example, the decision by the Environmental Risk Management Authority in approving an application for implanting human genes into cows preferred the scientific evidence of biotechnologists over the cultural and spiritual concerns expressed by Ngāti Wairere, notwithstanding that the long-term environmental effects and medical benefits of the experiments were uncertain; see 'ERMA Decision on GM Cattle Released', viewed 19 May 2004, <www.ermaNZ.govt.nz/news-events/archives/media-releases/2000/mr-20000725.a5p7>.

24 R. McGowan, The Contemporary Use of Rongoa Māori: Traditional Māori Medicine, MA thesis, The University of Waikato, 2000.

25 Evidence provided by a kuia (Māori woman elder), an expert in the practice of rongoa Māori, to the Waitangi Tribunal in support of Ngāti Wai traditional evidence regarding the Wai 262

claim. This evidence was given to a Waitangi Tribunal hearing of Ngāti Wai claims in 1997 on Wai 262 that remains the subject of a confidentiality order and is not available for public scrutiny.

26 McGowan, The Contemporary Use of Rongoa Māori, p. 20.

27 M. Durie, *Whaiora: Māori Health Development*, Oxford University Press, Auckland, 1994, p. 4.

28 McGowan, The Contemporary Use of Rongoa Māori, p. 126.

29 McGowan, The Contemporary Use of Rongoa Māori, p. 126.

30 Second Amended Statement of Claim filed on behalf of Ngāti Kuri, Te Rarawa and Ngāti Wai, Wai 262;.1.1 (g), paras 7.1–7.5.

31 Peter Wills, 'Brief of Evidence of Dr Peter Wills', Waitangi Tribunal, Wai 262 K15, paras 29–31.

32 B. Richards, 'Using the Chisel of the Mind', in W. Ihimaera (ed), *Kaupapa New Zealand: Vision Aotearoa*, Bridget Williams Books, Wellington, 1994, p. 209.

33 Ed Golden, as quoted on the Ford trucks web site, accessed 8 March 2004, <http://www.fordtrucks.com/news/newsc4.html>.

34 Email letter from Kingi Gilbert to Frank Dubarry, President of TechnoMarine, 3 September 2003. The letter expresses Gilbert's concerns over the inappropriate use of Māori designs in promoting and advertising the sale of TechnoMarine watches and suggests ways in which these issues can be addressed by proper consultation with the knowledge holders. Gilbert of Ngāti Whakaue, Ngāti Maniapoto, and Te Arawa is currently based in London and works on developing video games for Xbox and PlayStation 2.

35 The new Trademarks Act 2003 provides some limited protection.

36 For example, LEGO had indicated that it was keen to work in conjunction with Māori interests to develop a voluntary code of conduct for toy manufacturing companies wishing to utilise indigenous imagery and names on their products. They also expressed an interest in pursuing future possibilities of working collaboratively with Māori to develop products. There are also increasing signs that companies, as they become better informed, are demonstrating a willingness to engage with indigenous peoples to avoid causing offence and establish good working relationships.

37 For example, Canterbury International in seeking approval to use Māori names and designs on a new range of rugby boots had contracted with a Māori designer and spoken first with Ngāi Tahu who referred them to the Māori Language Commission, who for want of any other authority especially equipped for this purpose, gave approval to the use of the names. However many Māori still expressed concerns over the use of names such as 'Rangatira-High Chief' on a pair of rugby boots.

38 D.A. Posey, 'Preface', in D.A. Posey *Cultural and Spiritual Values of Biodiversity*, Intermediate Technology Publications for and on behalf of United National Environmental Programme, London, 1999, p. xvii. Available from, viewed 8 March 2004, <http://www.unep.org/Biodiversity/unep.pdf>.

39 New Zealand is a signatory to the Convention on Biological Diversity which has as one of its main objectives the conservation of biological diversity, the sustainable use of its components and the fair and equitable sharing of the benefits arising out of the utilization of genetic resources (article one). New Zealand is also an active member of the World Intellectual Property Organisation and regularly attends the Intergovernmental Committee Meetings of WIPO which since 2000 has been mandated to discuss and develop policies on intellectual property issues that arise in the areas of: (1) access to genetic resources and benefit-sharing; (2) protection of traditional knowledge, whether or not associated with genetic resources; and (3) protection of expressions of 'folklore' (as a subset of traditional knowledge).

40 As at the date of writing this article, the Waitangi Tribunal had indicated that a judicial conference would be held in mid April 2004 to establish a programme and timeframe for the completion of the Wai 262 claim.

41 Extract from a poem written by the claimant and kuia for Ngāti Kuri, Saana Murray, included as part of her evidence to the Waitangi Tribunal (Wai 262 D6 on the record of inquiry).

Orakei

I.H. KAWHARU

The purpose of this chapter is to trace some of the steps taken by the Orakei hapū of Ngāti Whatua since 1989 to 'recapture' the status of tangata whenua. The idea that there was such a status to be recaptured was first expressed in a response by the elders of the hapū to the news that the Crown was willing to transfer title of the Orakei marae to Ngāti Whatua on the recommendation of the Waitangi Tribunal. The Crown's announcement and Ngāti Whatua response were reported in my chapter in the 1989 edition:

> *On 1 July 1988, the Crown announced its willingness to accept the Tribunal's recommendation and to amend the Trust Board's constitution accordingly. The ministers said, 'The key to the restoration of tribal mana to Ngāti Whatua of Orakei is the marae, so it is very pleasing to confirm the vesting of the Orakei Marae, church, urupa, and access in the Ngāti Whatua of Orakei Trust Board [sic]'. The marae will now be a place where Ngāti Whatua of Orakei has standing as of right once again. For though the marae was part of Ngāti Whatua ancestral lands they have had no control over it.*
>
> *While this news was pleasing to the kaumātua, it was their belief that even with the assistance of the marae, it could take another ten years for their people to recapture fully the status of tangata whenua that their forebears had enjoyed during the first two centuries of their occupation of the Tamaki Isthmus.*[1]

As it happened, ten years was already a significant measure in Orakei's recent history. In 1978 an agreement was reached between the Orakei hapū and the Crown resulting in a statutory trust exercised over ten hectares and thirty houses, and where the beneficiaries of it were to be the living descendants of the hapū's eighteenth century ancestor, Tuperiri.[2] Its interim governing board began with a very modest portfolio, administering thirty houses occupied now by 'beneficiaries' of the trust rather than by state rental tenants on ten hectares of what had once been their 285-hectare, supposedly inalienable, trust estate established under an order of the Native Land Court in 1869.[3] The interim board controlled no marae, had no income flow, was handicapped by a rent-driven mortgage, and the hapū's historical grievances were out of reach of the Waitangi Tribunal until amendments were made to the Treaty of Waitangi Act in 1985.[4]

The prospects for Orakei, however, changed dramatically in 1986 after the hapū had submitted its successful claim to the Tribunal covering the break-up and loss of its original trust estate. In addition to the marae just mentioned, the Crown also transferred title to the Takaparawhau and Okahu parks of fifty hectares collectively known as the Whenua Rangatira, gave preferential access to state rental housing elsewhere on their former estate, and set aside a two-hectare block for commercial development on the southern margin of Takaparawhau. A three million dollar endowment was included, which went some way towards finishing the dining hall on the marae and fortuitously, was available to assist in rebuilding the meeting house, Tumutumuwhenua, after a fire almost demolished it in 1990. All these developments were incorporated into the Orakei Act 1991.

Yet there was still no cash flow and the development of administrative and entrepreneurial initiative remained hampered. In terms of the Orakei Act neither the marae nor Takaparawhau, arguably some of the finest harbour-side hectares in New Zealand, could provide an income. And among board members and beneficiaries at the time there was a low level of available professional skill and experience in law, commerce, business management, banking, and the like. On the other hand, the board could afford little professional assistance (indeed, much in the early days was acquired '*pro bono*'). Clearly, then, the rent-collecting mode of trusteeship that had characterised the pre-1991 trust boards had somehow to give place to a system of control that would protect the expanded trust's assets and develop them in the competitive environment of Auckland city.

Fortunately for Orakei the Waitangi Tribunal had foreseen such a need and had recommended that the Crown appoint a consultant on a four-year contract to assist the board as part of the Crown's reparations.[5] This was the beginning of an awareness of the need for competent planning on the part of the Board and it continued with the experience gained in the joint Auckland City Council/Trust Board administration of the Whenua Rangatira. In the latter case, developing a set of management, development, and business plans led to the Board turning to their consultant to draw up a strategic plan for all their operations covering:

- socio-cultural development (in housing, education, health, and marae-related activity)
- economic development (especially joint ventures where external finance and development expertise would be joined to hapū land), and
- political relations (for example, agreements with central and local government and regional institutions and organisations).

Housing

The trust board's experience in administering its own housing estate, in the first ten years of its existence, had been limited to rent collecting. The land itself was held in one title and could not be mortgaged. Despite, or perhaps because of these constraints, the hapū generally had not lost sight of the principles of whanaungatanga (kinship) in their dealings with each other. First, there was acceptance of the proposition that the occupants of the houses at the time (1978) were there as of right and needed only to have that right confirmed and protected by an agreement with their board. This right of particular families to continue to occupy the houses they had earlier been renting from the state extended from their eviction from their village and marae in Okahu Bay in 1951–52. Although the land was now held by the board on behalf of all its hapū beneficiaries, first priority was given to existing occupants in recognition of the fact—and the trauma—of their eviction twenty-five years earlier.

Second, while the Crown agreed to return land equivalent in area to that which it had not used, it nevertheless intended to debit the hapū $200,000 for the cost of the improvements on that land (roading and services). At this point the Māori Trustee came to the 'rescue' with the offer of a thirty-year mortgage for which annual repayments of $15,000, it was assumed, could be met out of rent. In grappling with this the community decided that the rent would be calculated not on the basis of income, age or status in the hapū, quality of harbour view, number of occupants per house, and so on, but simply on the number of bedrooms (all houses being of the same age, type of construction, and design). To be at Orakei now was a privilege, no longer a mark of humiliation, a privilege willingly paid for by those fortunate enough to live on their ancestral land once more.

As noted, the settlement following the hapū's successful Treaty claim later in 1986–87 included a preferential allocation of state rental tenancies located elsewhere on the former Orakei Block. However, when the Housing Corporation changed to Housing New Zealand as the state housing agency, it cancelled the hapū's preferential rating, and instead gifted fifty houses to the board and offered to sell it another fifty-two for $5.8 million. The board accepted this alternative, obtained a bank loan, and secured it with a five-year rent lease from Housing New Zealand. At the time of writing, the board had begun discussing future options with the state agency, especially since many of the fifty-year-old houses were in poor condition thus presenting the board with the decision of having to repair or replace them. Apart from this there was the need to make more efficient use of the housing land, since the land itself was still escalating in value.

Meanwhile, the increase in the number of locally resident beneficiaries was augmented by the construction of twenty owner-built houses on the southern margin of the land returned in 1978. Expansion continued into the new millennium with further development planned for the papakāinga.[6] For example, a beneficiary newsletter reported in December 2001 that eleven sections cut out of the papakāinga were to be balloted to qualified beneficiaries subject to various criteria such as:

1 A $10,000 application fee, refundable in the event of an unsuccessful application.
2 Approximately $7000 of the application fee being required to pay for the common infrastructural costs including resource consent, sub-division, right of way, and services access such as power, sewerage, and stormwater.

3 The Trust Board would confirm whakapapa entitlement and approve housing design, materials, and certain other quality covenants.
4 The price of house construction would be not less than $150,000 for each house and applicants had to be able to meet Housing New Zealand lending criteria since banks were unlikely to approve lending on papakāinga leasehold land.
5 The fact that the Trust Board would be unable to provide any financial assistance, although it would provide the land and a licence to occupy to the successful qualified applicants.

In short, some progress had been made since the 1980s in the task of housing more beneficiaries on the hapū's ancestral land, improving the existing housing stock, and using the land to best advantage. Yet as with other board portfolios, continuing limits on cash flow tended to frustrate plans and elicit occasional complaints about delays from beneficiaries. Nonetheless, the board was at least gaining a better appreciation of the role that Housing New Zealand could play in helping it improve the rate of progress in development. Meanwhile, the community continued to grow in size and to express its revitalised sense of identity.

Health

In 1996 the Ngāti Whatua tribal trust board, Te Runanga o Ngāti Whatua, entered into an agreement with the Crown to co-purchase and monitor health care services for all Māori people (at the time approximately 76,000) resident within the tribal district (see M. Kawharu's chapter). It was an innovative Treaty-driven scheme, shared with the Tainui and Tai Tokerau tribes and known by its acronym Māori Co-purchasing Organisation (MAPO). The Ngāti Whatua MAPO was called Tihi Ora.[7] Contracts were entered into between Tihi Ora and providers of health care services ranging from small clinics to hospitals. It was at this time that the Orakei Clinic was established by the Trust Board, adjacent to the Orakei marae. As a hapū-owned and marae-based health service, its priority target was the Orakei hapū itself, particularly those living locally or at least in the Auckland District Health Board region. Next in the range of priorities were other Māori, Pacific Island people, recent immigrants, and low-income populations generally. It was the aim of what became known as the Ngāti Whatua o Orakei Health Services (NWOHS) to provide this clientele with general practitioner and practice nurse services, together with a range of community services such as dental health, asthma support, and a smoking cessation program.

By 2001, it had become clear that many who lived five kilometres or more away in Glen Innes were not making regular use of the clinic's services and accordingly, a second clinic was set up in that suburb. It was financed as a result of skilful management of the bulk funding received for the Orakei clinic.

In 2003, NWOHS joined a Primary Health Organisation (PHO) called Tamaki Health Trust, together with seven other providers having a combined patient register of some 20,000. The government established PHOs that year primarily to benefit Māori and Pacific Island people, categories deemed to have the greatest need for improved levels of health. Indeed, to qualify for government funding a practice/provider register had to reflect a Māori and/or Pacific Island population of at least fifty per cent. With that prerequisite the actual budget would then be based on the number of registered patients (where previously under Primary Health Care contracts Māori providers were funded regardless of the number of patients registered).

In July 2003, NWOHS also purchased the Otahuhu Union Health Centre. The strategy behind this particular initiative was to attempt to cement Orakei as the Māori lead provider within the PHO, to build up the existing patient register, and to offer the same services, including community services, to more widely dispersed hapū members and other Māori in South Auckland.

At the time of writing, the relatively new NWOHS had developed core competencies and strengths that were contributing to the delivery of successful health services to an increasing number of patients. Community staff, the majority of whom were Māori and experienced in working among 'hard to reach' communities, likewise contributed in full measure to the programme: referrals made from each of the clinics to the community services sector were providing a seamless integration of patient care. Ongoing workforce development included information technology competence, leadership roles, and professional development that were offered to staff with monitoring advice from both the Ministry of Health and the Auckland District Health Board.

The onset of PHOs meant changes for NWOHS. The organisation had to adopt a new emphasis since the PHO environment, with its per capita funding, appeared to be bringing Māori Primary Health Providers closer to mainstream providers. The PHO environment was said to be competitive and 'relentless' in its demands, but with the right support, NWOHS were confident that they would sustain the delivery of improved health services to the hapū and to the wider community without losing their Māori ethos. The trust board had no reason to doubt that confidence.

Education

The Orakei hapū's interest in fostering (European) educational development can doubtless be traced to their invitation to Governor Hobson to relocate and establish his seat of government on their land in Tamaki in exchange for the opportunity, among other things, to learn to read and write. While the hapū lands eventually helped fund schools and hospitals in Auckland, no education programme found its way into the community until after World War II. This was the Play Centre Movement of the 1960s. It mobilised thought and action in Orakei itself and also saw educationalists from outside the community coming to help establish a play centre, train mother helpers for preschool activities, develop a homework centre and library and so on as well. These were major initiatives for a community that at the time had no university graduates and few members with any tertiary training at all.

There was also a lack of a marae and thus a lack of a Ngāti Whatua cultural focus to act as a counterpoint to the individualistic skills required of students in school and beyond. While a good start had been made, it did not lead to an on-going, autonomous community structure promoting education. And when outside voluntary help diminished with time, nothing of lasting substance came to take its place and Orakei youth once again made their way as best they could. However, the community found itself in 1978 with a statutory trust board, and then a decade later, with a three million dollar 'endowment fund' in part compensation for the dissolution of its former trust estate. This enabled the board to set aside a few thousand dollars per annum from which to offer small grants in aid to students, graded from primary school to university. This was never sufficient; for example, it did not to cover all tertiary fees. However what was important was the idea of support itself: the hope for a student's success held in the community and that however modest, a grant to the individual was a right by birth and of belonging to the Orakei hapū of Ngāti Whatua. An education update circulated to beneficiaries at the time of writing carried a 'vision' statement. It said:

> *We see education as a priority for enhancing individual, whānau and hapū well-being. The Ngāti Whatua o Orakei Trust Board engages in educational programmes to support the achievement of its descendants. Our primary focus is to protect and affirm hapū identity; support, encourage and contribute to the life-long development and well-being of Ngāti Whatua; promote and assure educational excellence among Ngāti Whatua and promote opportunities for professional input into hapū development.*[8]

As was the case with the Play and Education Centre enterprise in the 1960s, Orakei was fortunate in the friendly interest shown by sections of the wider community in their children's education. Perhaps the catalyst for a new three-school relationship with Orakei (Kings School, St Cuthberts College, and Kings College) was a genuine interest on the part of these schools in Ngāti Whatua o Orakei as tangata whenua. It has led to visits to the schools by Orakei representatives, and by school representatives to the Orakei marae. In one instance, Orakei was engaged in tutoring the students at Kings School in kapa haka and offered the school an inscribed boulder as a symbol of friendship animated by common interest in the goal of learning. If silent, it is nonetheless eloquent in its stance inside the school gates.

Currently, Kings School, Kings College, and St Cuthberts offer Endeavour Scholarships for Māori and Pacific Islands girls and boys. The scholarship programme aims to provide eight scholarships each year—four to boys and four to girls starting year seven (form one). The girls' scholarships cover education at St Cuthberts College through years seven to thirteen (forms one to seven). The boys will start their intermediate education in years seven to eight (forms one and two) and then move to Kings College for their secondary education in years nine to thirteen (forms three to seven). These scholarships cover all costs of fees, uniforms, laptops for every student, school trips (national and international), and sports costs. While only a fortunate few will gain directly, the assistance of the scholarship will set standards of educational excellence and provide an incentive for the hapū as a whole to achieve them. It is seen as a welcome addition to the long-standing and active interest in the hapū and its children held by the local primary schools and Selwyn College.

There is also a homework centre that began in February 2003. It operates every Monday and Wednesday between 3.30 pm and 5.30 pm for students in years one to eight, and whānau are encouraged to support the kaupapa. The centre started with twenty-five to thirty children attending each session, with numbers growing. At the same time that the homework centre began, the Trust Board was establishing 'Te Puna Reo' at the marae, an early childhood centre where the principal language was to be Māori.

However, this was not the only hapū initiative within the marae precincts. Holiday programmes have also operated at the marae (one for children under seven, three for primary school children and one for secondary school pupils) focusing on Ngāti Whatua history and language. The early success of these holiday programmes has led to the introduction of wananga aimed at giving tertiary students a perspective on Ngāti Whatua development needs. It was reported that in 2003, the concluding education hui was attended by more than 400 members of the hapū and their families, who came from throughout Aotearoa.

But there were also external linkages underpinning the trust board's efforts to augment local organisation. First to capture attention was the launch of the Crown's Tertiary Education Strategy 2002–07. The trust board was impressed by a number of the strategic objectives closely comparable to its own, such as a clear accountability of Crown/iwi/hapū educational programmes to the 'target' community; programmes that recognise te ao Māori perspectives and support the revitalisation of te reo Māori; and a tertiary education system that contributes to hapu and iwi development.

Another major initiative was the signing in 2003 of a memorandum of understanding between Ngāti Whatua o Orakei and the University of Auckland. Under the memorandum the two parties will discuss joint projects 'focusing on the benefits to each party and the availability of the necessary resources'. For its part, the Orakei Trust Board undertakes to 'use its best efforts' to support the university's aims and objectives. In return, the university will use its best efforts to conduct research to assist the Orakei Trust Board 'to realise its goals for its beneficiaries, including consolidating their cultural heritage, developing an economic base and administering a comprehensive social welfare programme with particular reference to their health and education needs'. The university believes that the memorandum gives 'formal status to—and takes to a new level—the long-standing relationship between the university and Ngāti Whatua as mana whenua'.[9]

Culture

If housing and health have an education dimension, then so too do activities regarded in the community as 'cultural', especially if they have a focus on, or derive from, the marae. This has been especially evident in efforts to restore the meeting house, Tumutumuwhenua, of which all but the shell had been destroyed by fire in 1990.

Meeting house

A 2003 beneficiary newsletter reported that first attention was being given to replacing the woven tukutuku panels.[10] And it was here that two of the primary ingredients in the panels, pingao *(Desmoschoenus spiralis)* and toetoe (*Cortaderia spp.*), have been found to be in diminished supply in their natural habitat. Toetoe in particular is struggling to compete with introduced exotic weeds such as purple and white pampas or 'cutty grass'. To help cope with this, over 3000 toetoe have now been grown from seed by hapū workers for planting. Requests have also been made of beneficiaries, 'to find out how you can restore our whenua and with it too our tikanga and mātauranga'.[11]

At the same time, those working on the badly scorched carvings had to turn their minds to the complex network of whakapapa that had inspired the original symbolism of the house, the better to appreciate the purpose of their labours. This too, became an ongoing mental and spiritual exercise in its own right.

Whenua Rangatira

While the securing of title to the marae by the Orakei Act was the primary 'mana dimension' of the Orakei settlement for the Orakei hapū, the award of title to the Whenua Rangatira provided it with the means to act on its manaakitanga obligations as well. In law, the land was set aside as a Māori reservation 'for the common use and benefit of the members of the hapū and the citizens of the City of Auckland'.[12] It was to be administered jointly by the hapū and the Auckland City Council (ACC) through a body known as the Orakei Reserves Board. Almost fifty hectares in extent, it comprises the large upland Takaparawhau Park and the smaller Okahu Park and part of the foreshore encompassing the original papakāinga. Both the hapū and the wider community have expressed a desire to see the Whenua Rangatira used for informal recreation pursuits, with additional appropriate facilities for public enjoyment.

Much of the land is oriented westward towards central Auckland and the harbour area, and northward towards Rangitoto and the Hauraki Gulf beyond. Vistas to the east of the marae extend over Mission Bay towards Waiheke Island. They continue unimpeded across the sea approaches to Auckland and back around to the city hinterland. One of the main objectives of Ngāti Whatua and the ACC is to ensure the character and quality of the existing natural landscape is maintained and enhanced by achieving (i) an appropriate balance between forested and grassed areas and (ii) the selection and planting of native flora where revegetation is identified as being needed, for example, to control cliff erosion.

When the latter objective became known in the hapū it responded with enthusiasm—and they were not alone. Children from the Orakei Primary School and later students from St Cuthberts College took part in planting days with as many as 1000 plants being put in, in a given day. Elders contributed to these occasions as well, helping and sharing their knowledge of Ngāti Whatua history and lore. Enthusiasm was not the only ingredient, however. A Whenua Rangatira landscape plan developed by the staff of the trust board and approved by the Reserves Board had resulted in the planting of more than 30,000 plants in the three years prior to 2003, followed by the appointment of four full-time workers engaged in daily planting, weeding, and maintenance activity. The objective for the period 2003–06 is to plant more than 100,000 plants on the Whenua Rangatira. The scale of such an operation inevitably led to a proposal for a nursery and resource centre. At the time of writing the hapū community endorsed a name chosen by kaumātua for the centre: 'Pukaki', taken from a Ngāti Whatua planting karakia. The primary role of the Pukaki centre is the growing of plants for the Whenua Rangitira, with the intention of supplying plants on a commercial basis to the market in the future. Education programmes for beneficiaries and the wider community, covering plant propagation, ecological restoration, and native plant use, will be available at the centre. The centre will provide the hapū with a significant resource to enhance its ability to exercise kaitiakitanga (resource management, guardianship) over the Whenua Rangatira and in time, the isthmus more generally.

In February 2002, the hapū hosted the Aotearoa Traditional Performing Arts Festival. Thirty-five teams came from as far as Australia and the South Island. The performances reflected the pursuit of excellence in Māori traditional dance in Aotearoa. The hapū provided a skilled workforce for all the management, administration, corporate hosting, television and stage direction, security, and maintenance operations. Complementary attractions at the festival included an arts village with whakairo (carving) and ta moko (tattooing). A variety of stalls added their flavour of kai, display, and a fashion show to the mix. The Orakei Medical Clinic's team supported the St Johns Ambulance in the mobile clinic and volunteers put the seal of success on arguably the most ambitious and high-profile festival Orakei had ever seen.

Economic development

Negotiations with the Crown began in 1992 to purchase the railway station site and 20.8 hectares of former rail yards surrounding it and were completed in August 1996. Rather than pursue a Treaty claim over the reclamation of the former harbour bed, the board decided to raise the purchase price of the land (by on-selling the leasehold to development partners) and buy it. The leasehold was sold for 150 years with the first fifteen years of lease revenue being capitalised to provide the purchase value. After 2011 Ngāti Whatua will thus receive ongoing cash revenue from ground leases at commercially valued levels for the remaining 135 years of the lease.

The developers financed the land on the basis of the difference between the relative leasehold value at the time of purchase and the price paid to the Crown.

Over the years there has been much interest, both national and international, in investing in the railway lands. However, market contraction and investors' own constraints have seen deals that were very close to being secured fall over. This applied in Orakei's case and defensive action had to be taken, resulting in Ngāti Whatua becoming an investor. With land close to subdivision completion and millions of dollars of unconditional sales having been achieved and settled in the first year, the board decided to support an investment in one part of the land (where the old Chinese markets were once located) in order to ensure that a forced sale did not occur and precipitate a reduction in land values in the other part (the neighbouring rail yards). The decision to invest thus moved Ngāti Whatua from a role as landlord of the freehold to that of active investing participant in the development of the land.

One positive and direct effect of this decision was illustrated within months when, with the intervention of Ngāti Whatua, Auckland City was convinced of the viability of the land for a stadium and purchased the leasehold interest. Construction of this stadium is due to begin in mid 2004.

Even though by the end of March 2000 total sales of the former Chinese markets land approached the level of the initial purchase price excluding the cost of finance, difficulties with the remainder persisted. In May 1999 the lease of this land was eventually on-sold to another developer at a level sufficient only to cover the remaining debt of registered security holders. This did not include the value of the Ngāti Whatua investment made in 1997, which has since been written off by the Trust Board.

Ngāti Whatua continues to own the land, which has trebled in value from the time of purchase in 1996 to 2004, thus increasing the potential cash flow from ground leases commencing in August 2011. It has serviced its initial investment from other successful commercial development activities undertaken by the Trust Board.

At Orakei, of the sixty hectares returned to hapū ownership under the 1991 Orakei Act, three hectares (less than five per cent) was zoned for commercial development. The current and previous three boards since 1991 considered a range of options to develop this land and found a rest home/retirement village to be the most attractive. The three levels of approximately 100 units of premier lifestyle living are now fully occupied. Stage two of the village consists of building over sixty townhouse units and is to be completed in 2004. It has the brand name of Eastcliffe.

Whatever the outward character, the project fits Ngāti Whatuatanga principles well, i.e., the freehold title of such land will never be sold and the development will provide continuing financial benefits for future generations of trust board beneficiaries. In addition to the employment and training opportunities provided by the project, profits from the investment are to be invested in the education, training, and housing needs of hapū members. Very little equity investment was required from the board, but their provision of land together with the financial investment and proven management skills of their partner has already ensured financial success. It is a success, which is expected to continue.

The board has looked at replicating the formula outside of Orakei. For instance, the old Tamaki Girls College site in Glen Innes purchased by the Board from the Crown in the mid 1990s has been identified as a potential opportunity for building a less exclusive retirement care complex. Management and development expertise would be transferred from Eastcliffe, but the target market would be those interested in $200,000-townhouse units rather than the $700,000-units of Eastcliffe.

Another significant development has been the hapū's involvement in the suburb of Mt Albert. In 1992 the Crown returned to the Orakei hapū 3.5 hectares of land lying immediately adjacent to the tertiary institution 'Unitec'. This was in recognition of the hapū's gift of 3240 hectares to the Crown in 1841 made in expectation of receiving medical and educational services.

The Auckland District Health Board (ADHB) had for some time leased the land and buildings for a mental health facility. Both the ADHB as tenant and Ngāti Whatua as landlord agreed to a temporary two-yearly lease arrangement with minimal capital maintenance upkeep. A longer-term plan was agreed to whereby the landlord would commit to capital improvement of the buildings and the tenant would commit to a long-term lease at negotiated rental.

In 2000, Ngāti Whatua engaged a property developer/consultant group to investigate a long-term plan for the site. In the event, Ngāti Whatua entered into a joint venture with the group and presented a proposal to the ADHB for developing a larger residential facility and refurbished administration and catering facilities. After lengthy consideration, the ADHB declined the proposal in early 2001 and also agreed to end its tenancy on the site at the end of the lease period (31 December 2003).

The initial setback in fact offered a new opportunity. If a health purpose was not to succeed, then an education purpose seemed an obvious choice with a neighbour such as Unitec. Opportunities could also be seen by Unitec and in February 2003 a 133-bed student apartment development was opened by Ngāti Whatua and their joint venture partner Townscape, as stage one of a larger plan confirmed by the three parties (including Unitec) to develop the site to accommodate up to 1000 beds over the following eight to ten years, subject to continued student demand.

Ngāti Whatua of Orakei have been involved in yet other kinds of resource development closer to home in Okahu Bay. Their satellite-fishing village on the bay once supported their other main settlements at Onehunga, Mangere, and elsewhere in the northern Manukau Harbour and the Waitemata Harbour itself. Eventually Okahu Bay and the Orakei Block behind it became the hapū's main centre after the alienation of nearly all the rest of their Auckland lands by 1845.

However the hapū's customary reliance on kaimoana (shellfish) collected from Okahu Bay became severely restricted once the city sewer began discharging sewage into the Bay in 1914. Regular sewage discharges continued over the years while stormwater runoff from Tamaki Drive and the wider catchment added to the pollution. Unfortunately it was not long before outbreaks of typhoid claimed the lives of several members of the hapū who had harvested and eaten shellfish from the bay. The sewer and then Tamaki Drive prevented, and continue to prevent, direct access from the former papakāinga to the foreshore and harbour; and kaimoana has not been harvested from Okahu Bay by the hapū for at least two generations.

Despite this background and their eviction in 1951, the hapū still regard the Okahu Bay papakāinga as their spiritual home. Thus when they became engaged in 2001 in a marina development project in Okahu Bay they were determined to ensure that they did so in ways that would enhance rather than compromise their customary values and their tangata whenua status. Orakei Marina Ltd and the Trust Board are a joint venture enterprise responsible for the construction of a 172-berth marina in the bay. Benefits for the hapū from the project include employment for beneficiaries, funding for restoration projects, marine-related education scholarships, plus a mechanical dry-docking facility for tribal waka. On the operational side, the marina will provide sewage and pump-out facilities to each berth, swing moorings will be reduced to provide a clear channel for waka launching and landing, and material dredged for the marina will be disposed of elsewhere within the Ngāti Whatua tribal district. At the level of governance, the hapū will provide input through representation on a trust that will own and manage the marina.

Also concerned with the harbour, Ngāti Whatua were involved in a government and private sector-funded consortium together with Auckland New Ventures Trust, Poutama Trust and Tourism Auckland to facilitate Māori participation in the business opportunities directly and indirectly associated with the Louis Vuitton and Americas Cup regattas in 2002–03. Events involving the international media, brief cruises on the ocean-going twin-hulled canoe *Te Aurere*, and Māori cultural performances were all part of a continuous promotion of Māori business flair, expertise, and networks throughout the regatta. Although Ngāti Whatua business initiatives themselves were not directly involved in the consortium's activities, Ngāti Whatua played a key role in fulfilling its manaakitanga responsibilities.[13]

Political relations

The 1978 Act restored some limited sense of turangawaeawae to the hapū insofar as it gave back title to the land on which their houses stood and confirmed title to their urupā. The 1991 Act went much further and allowed recognition of their Trust Board's mana whenua not only over their former remnant holding and marae in the Tamaki Isthmus (i.e., the Orakei Block), but also over the Isthmus itself.[14] Yet it attracted little attention in the public domain at the time it was passed into law. In any event, the concept of mana whenua over the Tamaki Isthmus as it appears in the Orakei Act could have application in at least three different city jurisdictions and levels of interpretation (Auckland, Waitakere, and North Shore).

Nevertheless it was not long after the formation of the Orakei Reserves Board in 1992 that its operations did begin to raise the hapu's profile at least in the governance of Auckland City. It was also in that year that Orakei began the lengthy process of negotiating with the Crown over the purchase of the former railway station and twenty hectares of surrounding land (see above). In the end, the Trust Board's purchase was an event of some significance for the City of Auckland as well since it led, as noted, to the council becoming a tenant of the Trust Board with plans to build an indoor stadium and convention centre on a part of this land.

This increase in the scale of Orakei–Auckland City Council unity in the hospitality/recreation field took place at the same time as the hapū was assisting the council and central government in hosting national and international conferences in the city beginning, for instance, with the Commonwealth Law Conference in 1990, the Commonwealth Heads of Government Meeting (CHOGM) in 1995, and Asia Pacific Economic Co-operation (APEC) forum in 1999.

Finally, at the end of the decade the hapū was invited by council to contribute to a joint Arts Agenda—a strategy for arts and cultural development for the city—followed up later with representation on the inaugural Auckland Festival Trust, and a seat on 'The Edge' Board (responsible for the Aotea Centre, Town Hall, and Civic Theatre).

On a more sombre note in 2001, the Orakei Trust Board joined forces with Auckland City and Auckland District Police in a 'Safer Auckland City' (SAC) partnership in crime prevention. In its explanatory document the council described its role as sponsoring a nationally designed and locally implemented Safer Community Council model for achieving crime prevention in the City of Auckland.

SAC adopted a bicultural approach to crime prevention as part of a methodology that took into account the wider social context in which crime occurs. As the sole tangata whenua organisation in the heart of the city, the trust board provided its city council and city police partners with a ready means of linking with Māori interest groups and government departments in central Auckland generally. Aside from the SAC kaupapa and on a less formal, structured basis, Orakei kaumātua have also been engaged in supportive roles with the Justice Department, particularly with judges and police officer training.

The same network-linking philosophy permeated relationships with the service industry that the trust board began to develop through the latter part of the 1990s. Memoranda of understanding were concluded, for example, with Transit New Zealand and with Metrowater (with respect to the protection of cultural sites and customary values), while discussions were held with Ports of Auckland (with respect to the exchange of information in areas of common interest, such as reclamation of the seabed and so on). And as for the concept of 'network' itself, Orakei joined an ad hoc group of individuals called a 'Committee for Auckland' representing a broad spectrum of commercial, industrial, media, and educational interests in the city oriented to making best use of Auckland as the 'ideal place in which to live and work'. At the very least, the group attempts to keep disparate interests in touch and forward looking.

Relations with iwi

For the Orakei hapū, relations with iwi have been on a different plane from the relationships described above. To begin with the Ngāti Whatua iwi itself, it might seem anomalous that there should be two statutory trust boards within its borders and indeed where one is, to an important extent, part of the other. However, each has a different history of origin and purpose and are, in these terms at least, mutually exclusive.

Orakei owes its board's origin to the agreement reached over the return of land in 1978 equivalent to that taken under Public Works Act but not used for the intended purposes (see above).

The Ngāti Whatua board on the other hand, Te Rūnanga o Ngāti Whatua, was established by an Act passed in 1988, when devolution to iwi of Department of Māori Affairs' responsibilities was then government policy. The Act enables contracts to be entered into with the Crown on behalf of the tribe as a whole. The defining tupuna is an ancestor of Tuperiri, Haumoewarangi. The governing body of Te Rūnanga consists of up to eleven representatives from thirty-three marae, divided into five wards. Orakei alone constitutes one ward and has one representative. The relationship between the two boards has proved effective in such fields as the administration of Treaty-driven health and education programmes, the protection of fisheries interests, the preparation of Treaty claims, and the preservation and promotion of Ngāti Whatua lore. Yet it is the Act's requirement of Te Rūnanga to preserve local autonomy wherever practical that appears to be the key to the ongoing vitality of Ngāti Whatua iwi. In so far as Orakei itself is concerned this is 'integration' in both theory and practice.

Other iwi

In 1996 amendments made to the Auckland War Memorial Museum Act included the formation of a Māori committee to give advice to the governing trust board on matters of Māori protocol, both with respect to the custodial care of taonga and to relations with iwi. When consulted, Ngāti Whatua o Orakei proposed a five-member committee, a proposal that recognised both their mana whenua over the museum site and their pre-Treaty historic relations with Tainui and Ngāti Paoa lying beyond their immediate southern border. The accepted proportion of representation was three representatives of Ngāti Whatua, one Tainui, and one Ngāti Paoa. The committee became known as the Taumata-a-Iwi. Since 1996 the arrangement has worked well in the face of frequent testing 'issues'. This experience has led to the formulation of a kaupapa—set of principles—against which further issues can be considered, as well as the refinement of the principles themselves, and the clarification and consolidation of the ongoing trust board/committee relationship.

The Ngāti Whatua, Tainui, and Ngāti Paoa relationship has been duplicated in another context altogether. An eighty-hectare block of land in Crown title administered as a trust lies in a contestable zone of interest for all three tribal groups. The land is part of a once much larger block in the South Auckland/ Penrose area acquired by an early CMS catechist, James Hamlin, and used in recent years as temporary grazing for cattle bound for a nearby abattoir. Were it not for the trust control, however, the land might well have become the subject of a Treaty claim brought by each tribal group. As it is, each has one representative on the trust and the three are joined by representatives of the Crown and Auckland Regional Council in maintaining the land as a park for public enjoyment. Treaty claim contests have, by common consent, been set to one side for an indefinite period.

Treaty relations with the Crown

While the Orakei Act 1991 settled Ngāti Whatua o Orakei's grievances arising out of the break-up and sale of the former trust established by the Māori Land Court over the Orakei Block, section 19 of the Act also enabled the trust board to negotiate with the Crown beyond the borders of the Orakei Block over matters of common concern. On this basis, the board lodged a Treaty claim against the Crown on behalf of its beneficiaries in 1993, prepared its case over the following ten years, and entered into direct negotiation with the Office of Treaty Settlements in May 2003.

In brief, the claim covers the loss of a total area in excess of 32,000 hectares in the Tamaki Isthmus, parts of North Shore, and West Auckland, plus the seabed, foreshore, and reclamations in the Waitemata Harbour, and northern parts of the Manukau Harbour. This was the area throughout which, at the time of the signing of the Treaty of Waitangi, the various sections of the hapū had been working their gardens and fishing grounds, backed by supporting settlements and bases.

The specific claims of Treaty breaches related to the failures: (i) by governors Hobson and Fitzroy to fulfil Colonial Office instructions that fifteen to twenty per cent of Crown on-sale funds were to be employed for the direct benefit of Ngāti Whatua, (ii) Governor Fitzroy's unilateral abrogation of the Crown's right of pre-emption clause in article two of the Treaty and his failure to execute protective measures, including:[15]

- the prevention of sale of wāhi tapu
- the requirement of surveys of land before sale
- the establishment of a trust based on ten per cent of all land purchased from Ngāti Whatua in Tamaki
- Governor Grey's cancellation of the 'tenths' promise after Ngāti Whatua had already transferred their lands; and his withholding of land from Ngāti Whatua (after his land commissioners had failed to ratify many settler purchases for irregularities) and keeping it for the Crown, without notifying or compensating Ngāti Whatua.

This is an urban claim with a number of features, which lend it special character. For instance, (i) land values were greater than non-urban values as much in the 1840s–50s as in modern times; (ii) as a result Crown profits from Treaty breaches and the impact of losses on Ngāti Whatua were proportionately greater than elsewhere and on other iwi; (iii) likewise, iwi other than Ngāti Whatua in Tamaki were unaffected, or less affected, by breaches of Normanby's instructions, as these occurred in the first twelve years of colonisation 1840–52; (iv) while potentially a New Zealand-wide matter, the 'waiver' breaches in practice were virtually an Auckland matter alone.

The harbour bed and foreshore aspect of the claim will doubtless set precedents for ongoing debate over this matter. Certainly there was no existing formula or Treaty settlement to guide negotiations at the time they began. Perhaps yet another ten years must elapse for Crown and Ngāti Whatua to find the partnership and protection so earnestly promised when Ngāti Whatua signed the Treaty on the shores of the Manukau harbour on 20 March 1840.

Conclusion

In pre-contact times Ngāti Whatua, like all tribal groups, faced constant threats to survival from hunger or military defeat. Accordingly, after the raupatu (conquest followed by occupation) of 1740, the evolving Ngāti Whatua/Waiohua amalgam, known by the several segments of Te Taou, Ngaoho, and Te Uringutu, was to be found in varying proportions throughout the Tamaki Isthmus working and protecting its circuits of gardens and fishing grounds. Its viability and integrity as a collective subgroup of Ngāti Whatua was therefore dependent on effective measures of internal social control and welfare, and external measures of defence, including strategic alliances.

When translated into contemporary times, the practice has changed, but not the purpose of protecting the viability of Orakei as a hapū of Ngāti Whatua. Thus, the Board's basic policies since 1991 have focused on land use, education, skills training, and health care; and on establishing relations of mutual benefit with organisations having complementary goals. It was hoped that the more success attended these efforts, the more secure the Orakei hapū would become in their cultural and political environment and the greater the likelihood of their being able to support the interests of the wider community in the name of Ngāti Whatua. More than that, it seemed the most constructive way by which they might recover the status of tangata whenua—the very status that had once entitled their chiefs to sign the Treaty and to invite Captain Hobson to share the Tamaki Isthmus with themselves in 1840. They might not have achieved it in the speculative 'ten years' quoted at the beginning of this chapter, but it was well within sight at the time of writing.

Notes

1 I.H. Kawharu, 'Mana and the Crown: A Marae at Orakei', in *Waitangi: Maori and Pakeha Perspectives of the Treaty of Waitangi*, I.H. Kawharu (ed.), Auckland, Oxford University Press, 1989, pp. 211–33.

2 Orakei Block (Vesting and Use) Act 1978.

3 Re 1869 decision, see Waitangi Tribunal, *Report of the Waitangi Tribunal on the Orakei Claim, Wai-9*, The Tribunal, Wellington, 1987, ch. 5. The original 1869 decision by Chief Judge Fenton was published in F.D. Fenton, *Important Judgments Delivered in the Compensation and Native Land Court*, published under the direction of the Chief Judge of the Native Land Court, [Auckland], 1879.

4 Extending the jurisdiction of the Tribunal to cover events from 1840 rather than from the date of the Act, 1975.

5 Waitangi Tribunal, *Orakei*, s. 15:5, Endowment Contribution, p. 278.

6 The papakāinga includes the Orakei community's housing estate in Kitemoana, Reihana, Kupe, and Ngaoho streets. The hapū land includes the reserve land (marae and Takaparawhau or 'Whenua Rangatira') and papakāinga, while the development land includes that part of Takaparawhau set aside for commercial ventures (and presently includes the retirement village): Orakei Act 1991, ss 4–6 and Schedules.

7 The full name is Te Tihinga Ora o Ngāti Whatua.

8 *E Wawa Ra*: Newsletter of the Ngāti Whatua o Orakei Māori Trust Board, November 2002.

9 University of Auckland, *University News*, April 2003, vol. 33, no. 3.

10 *E Wawa Ra*, March 2003.

11 *E Wawa Ra*, March 2003.

12 Orakei Act 1991, section 8.

13 I am glad to acknowledge help received from Patrick Snedden and Tiwana Tibble in interpreting certain aspects of the trust board's portfolio. Responsibility for presentation of these aspects, however, is entirely my own.

14 The board has exclusive authority to negotiate with the Crown or any other authority on behalf of its beneficiaries throughout the Tamaki Isthmus—though not 'exclusive' vis-à-vis other iwi or non-Orakei hapū of Ngāti Whatua (see Orakei Act 1991, section 19).

15 The right of pre-emption was the Crown's exclusive right to purchase land from Māori.

READING 7

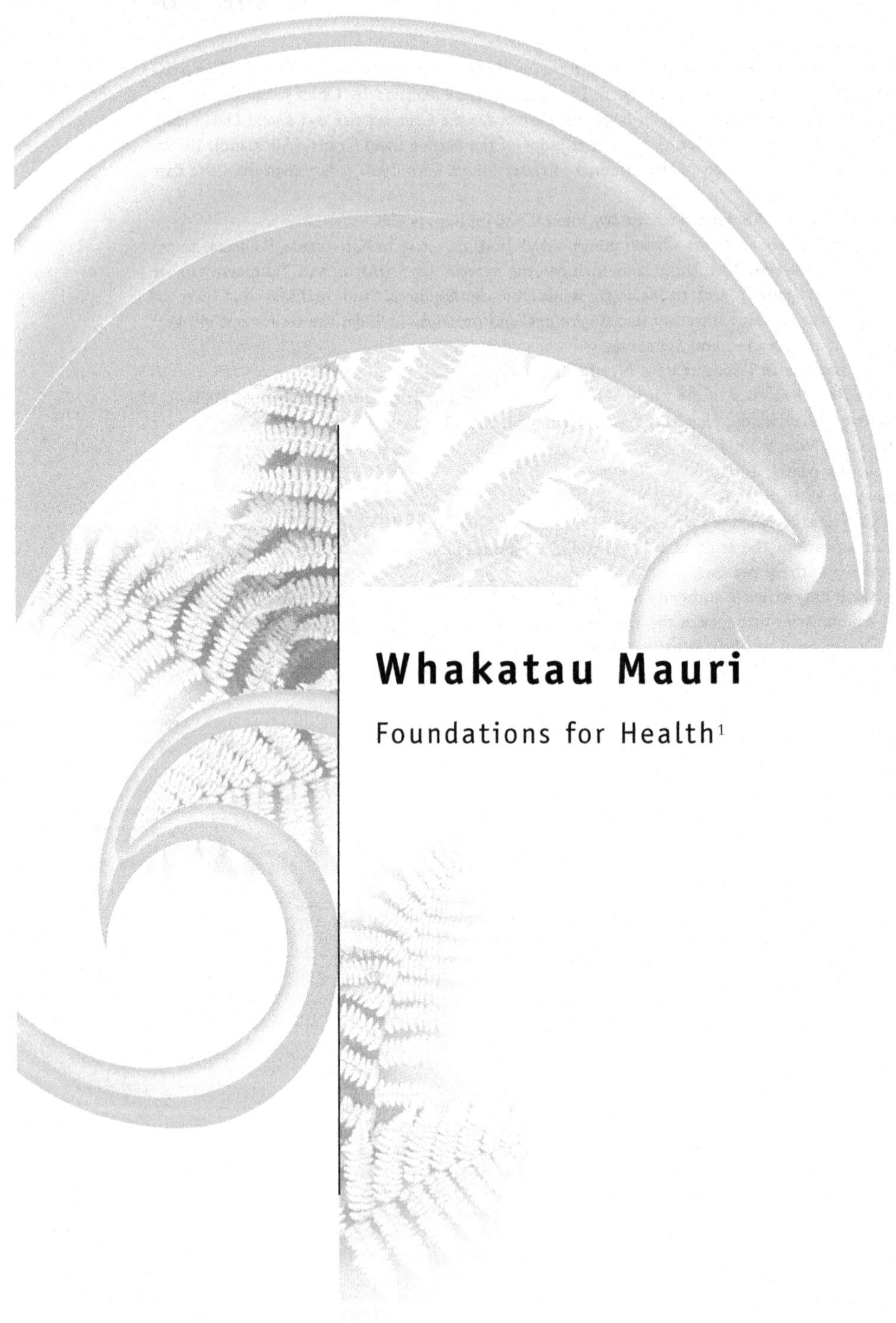

Whakatau Mauri

Foundations for Health[1]

The foundations for health are complex, often ill defined, and not necessarily linked in a direct way to either physical or mental disorders. But it is impossible to address Māori health without understanding the wider environments within which health status takes shape. There is some debate as to whether improvements in health are the result of advances in medical science and the delivery of quality health services, or whether change owes more to improved living conditions and higher levels of personal support. And are the foundations of health the same for Māori as for other New Zealanders or are there specific factors that must be taken into account? While Māori and non-Māori live side by side they do not always share the same environments nor the same narratives, and neither do they subscribe to identical values or aspirations.

Yet for all people, although the mix might be different, health is the product of a range of interacting determinants. There is seldom a single causative explanation for any illness or accident; instead health outcomes reflect complicated combinations of past and present, individual and group, home and nation. History has brought many lessons for health, including the catastrophic population collapses that occurred in the South Pacific during the colonisation of Polynesia.[2] Culture too plays a significant role in both determining and shaping clinical presentation[3] and there is a relationship between changing epidemiological patterns and the broad range of social policies.[4] Increasingly it has been recognised that in order to understand indigenous health it is necessary to consider historical, cultural, and political forces and to appreciate the dimensions of adversity.[5] Threats come from many quarters often traceable to the process of colonisation and its almost universal accompaniments: depopulation, violence, dislocation, poverty, and cultural repression.[6]

Mental health is even less likely to be determined by only one or two aetiological forces. Psychological well-being is related to personal encounters, developmental experiences, societal values and equity, stress, genetics, culture, standards of living, physical health, and political influence.[7] In short, the foundations for mental health are to be found as much outside the mind and the body as within. They lie with families, communities, jobs, decent homes, schools that value children, reliable transport, policies for health, equity and fairness, access to goods and services, safety and security, and experiences carried over from earlier times.

Māori health is built on platforms that are not dissimilar to the foundations underpinning the health of other New Zealanders. But they are not the same. Platforms for Māori health are constructed from land, language, and whānau;[8]

Table 2.1 Foundations for Health

Foundation	*Indicators and Risks*
Te ao hurihuri Society and the economy	housing education employment and income justice
Te Ao Hou Lifestyles	smoking gambling injuries recreation and leisure nutrition alcohol and drug use
Hikoi tāngata Journeys	collective histories the forces of colonisation terms of participation in society
Te ao Māori Identity	access to the Māori world culture heritage whānau
Mana ake Uniqueness	genetic endowment personality and temperament personal journeys

from marae and hapū;[9] from Rangi and Papa;[10] from the 'ashes of colonisation';[11] from adequate opportunity for cultural expression;[12] and from being able to participate fully within society.[13] Like other New Zealanders Māori are not immune from the effects of unhealthy policies, nor from unacceptable standards of living, but all too often Māori have encountered expectations that they should abandon a Māori base. Yet being Māori is itself a foundation for health.

In Table 2.1 the broad foundations for health are listed: society and the economy, lifestyle, journeys, identity, and uniqueness. Together, and under ideal circumstances, they have the capacity to endow individuals with key prerequisites for health. The first four foundations reflect the contributions that come from influences beyond the individual. They can be critical for shaping health outcomes. However, even when they are able to contribute in an optimal way, they may not be able to counter influences that arise from within. Every individual has a uniqueness that can turn an external hazard into a non-event or a minor happening into a life-threatening incident. The determinants of health are sometimes classified as person variables (such as genetic endowment, personal life experiences) and contextual variables (such as housing, access to health services). But those distinctions are not easily separated, nor should it be supposed that they operate in isolation of each other. In that respect the earlier debates about whether poor health was a product of nature or nurture failed to take account of the interaction between both sets of determinants.

TE AO HURIHURI: SOCIETY AND THE ECONOMY

A causative relationship between health and socio-economic conditions is well established.[14] Generally, where there is greater choice in housing, education, leisure activity, and employment, standards of health are higher. Ill health is more likely to occur when there is less choice, and the poorest and least educated people have the lowest health status in any society. 'They fill the prisons and dole queues, occupy the low standard-housing and are hospitalised more frequently.'[15] Moreover the pattern of disadvantage is circular. Those with the worst mental health, for example, have the greatest unmet housing needs.[16] Similarly, disparities in standards of health between Māori and non-Māori are strongly influenced not by genetic factors or increased predisposition to illness but by environmental factors, most of which are amenable to change.[17] By implication, therefore, gains in health are more likely to come from improved standards of living than simply from improved health services.

Indicators

While several indicators have been used to measure socio-economic status in relation to health and well-being, the factors shown to have the greatest influence are income and poverty, employment and occupation, education, and housing.[18] Social cohesion or interconnectedness also appears to be important in its own right. Three broad categories of indicators have been used to describe the social well-being of New Zealanders and their significance for social policy planning: family and household circumstances, occupation and work, health, security, and well-being.[19] Personal and household income, household composition and family type, and legal and social marital scale are measures of family and household circumstances, while participation in education and training, the labour force and domestic and caring work are useful to describe occupation and work. The third category, health, security and well-being, incorporates measures such as lifestyle, smoking, alcohol and drug use, accidents, disability and hospital attendance.

Occupational groupings have been the most frequent way of linking health with socio-economic status, but for women, the elderly, and the unemployed the measure was unhelpful. The development of the New Zealand Index of Occupational Status (the NZSEI) goes further, linking education and income with occupation and providing a more robust scale than the Elley-Irving Scale of male occupations. It includes women in the workforce and those in part-time work. High scores are linked to occupations that are better paid with less manual work.

Measures of socio-economic well-being derived from census data have also been developed to identify disadvantage at community, rather than household, levels. A New Zealand Index of Deprivation (NZDep96) links higher mortality rates, increased hospitalisation, and increased registration for lung cancer with reduced access to a range of goods and services. It is based on nine variables selected from census data and applied to mesh blocks (i.e. geographical units containing about 90 people used for collating statistics). The nine variables are communication (telephone), income (benefits), employment, income (equivalised income), transport (car), support (single parent), qualifications, home ownership, and living space.[20] The NZDep96 enables each mesh block to be given a deprivation score—from which the likely health problems of an individual living in a particular residence (within a defined mesh block) can be anticipated. Smoking, for example, is more likely to occur where there is a high deprivation score.[21] However, there is no clear relationship between NZDep96 and health status measured by Short Form-36 profiles (SF-36). The most deprived group of Māori males, for example, had a significantly lower self-reported health score than the least deprived group on one scale only (physical functioning).[22] In other words differences in health status between Māori and non-Māori cannot be totally explained by socio-economic indicators; cultural factors also play a role. Likewise Māori and non-Māori who share similar NZDep96 scores experience different standards of health, suggesting that socio-economic factors do not operate independent of cultural and structural constraints.[23] But there is still controversy about the implications of the deprivation index (are areas of deprivation a cause of poor health, or do people with poor health congregate in particular areas?), and health policy needs to target populations as well as places of residence.

Disparities

In 1998 the National Health Committee published an evidence based report which confirmed the importance of socio-economic circumstances for health.

The report drew attention to national inadequacies in income, employment, education, housing, and the ways in which culture can positively and negatively influence health. On most measures, such as those already outlined in Chapter 1, Māori performance was low, especially in employment, education and income levels. Poverty itself is a health hazard. In South Auckland, for example, a third of the population over 15 years is receiving income support, 20 per cent of households have no car and 11 per cent have no telephone. Rates of disease are higher there than elsewhere in the country, and children in the most deprived areas are twice as likely to be admitted to hospital as children in the most affluent areas.[24]

National economic growth predicted by the year 2000 is unlikely to have an immediate or major effect on reducing disparities between Māori and non-Māori employment status and income levels. An analysis by Te Puni Kokiri suggests this is because the demographic and socio-economic characteristics of the Māori labour force promote unemployment in times of economic recession and inhibit employment in times of recovery. The characteristics include a youthful age structure, low levels of educational attainment, under-representation in formal systematic training, over-representation in low skilled occupations, under-representation in high growth industries, and the presence of a comparatively high proportion of long-term unemployed.[25]

In addition to socio-economic effects, the level of social cohesion can affect health. Strong ties with family or whānau, high levels of civil and political participation, good public transport, good social networks and a strong community identity can overcome some of the ill-effects of deprivation. Unfortunately, social cohesion and deprivation are linked; poor housing conditions, for example, contribute to social exclusion, while the absence of a telephone (and consequent reduction in networking opportunities) is more likely to be associated with low income. In 1996, 15 per cent of Māori households were without a telephone compared to 5 per cent of New Zealand households.[26] Housing is a critical determinant of good health. Yet Māori are twice as likely as non-Māori to live in rental accommodation and are more likely to pay a greater proportion of income as rent. Home ownership appears to be declining among Māori; by the time the 1996 Census was carried out only 50 per cent of Māori owned their own homes compared to more than 70 per cent for non-Māori. Implications of these disparities have been highlighted in a report by Te Puni Kokiri and a series of recommendations were made to the Ministry of Housing to formulate more effective housing policies.[27]

Pathways to and from Health

Pathways between socio-economic hardship and health are two-way: poor health can contribute to lower standards of living; but more than that, social and economic hardship leads to poor health. Interventions that aim to improve the underlying socio-economic position, such as income and education, are therefore likely to increase an individual's opportunity for good health. However, the wider political climate may not favour an increase in social payments either through benefit payments or the level of tertiary educational subsidies. A level of unemployment may even be considered necessary to maintain incentives for productivity. Māori political views are not uniform but there is widespread concern about the number of people whose health is compromised by low standards of living with little prospect of significant change. To that extent, the presence of fifteen Māori members of Parliament after the 1996 general election was greeted as a unique opportunity to address unemployment and related consequences of socio-economic disadvantage. Towards the end of the three-year term, however, there were few signs of improvement. In fact a report from Te Puni Kokiri released in 1998 suggested that the gaps had increased in a number of areas.[28] Moreover, in 1999 there were fresh concerns about the deteriorating position of Māori women,[29] and an updated report from Te Puni Kokiri in 2000 painted 'a disheartening picture' of continuing disparities.[30]

Apart from addressing the fundamental socio-economic inadequacies, gains in health might be secured by targeting the factors that are intermediary between standards of living and poor health.[31] Smoking, for example, aggravates poor health and even in adverse economic circumstances, its cessation will lead to better health. Some caution is needed, however, before presuming that all sections of the community will respond to health promotion in the same way. Higher socio-economic groups are more likely to act on health education messages and may capture the benefits, leading if anything to a widening of disparities. While all groups should be encouraged to adopt healthy lifestyles, not all groups will be able to make the same use of advice. Blaming the victim is a possible backlash reaction; it could lead to penalties against parents who do not have their children vaccinated; or adults who suffer from respiratory diseases but continue to smoke. Behavioural change is dependent on many variables, including the socio-cultural factors that characterise a particular group. Targeting Māori behaviour patterns requires an understanding of both cultural and social factors so that the message is not received as an injunction imposed from above without any reference to local feelings or realities.

Health interventions can also be targeted towards those who suffer from poor health so that their socio-economic disadvantage does not deteriorate. Reduced prescription charges, subsidised medical costs, compensation for accident-related loss of earnings, and favourable employment conditions can minimise the socio-economic consequences of illness and injury. People who have experienced poor mental health are over-represented in those groups that are traditionally disadvantaged in the housing market, and there have been recommendations for a combined approach involving income support, the mental health sector, and housing agencies.[32] However, 'reverse causality'—socio-economic disadvantage arising from illness or disability—is not a major contributor to socio-economic inequalities in health,[33] and there is a risk that excessive support will simply foster a sick role.

Disadvantage

The impact of socio-economic disadvantage on Māori people has been recognised as a major impediment to further health gains. In a review of Māori standards of health between 1970 and 1991 Pomare et al. concluded that socio-economic factors were strongly related to health and that over the previous decade Māori had become relatively worse off compared to the non-Māori population.[34] Similarly in the report *Ngā Ia o te Oranga Hinengaro Māori* a strong association was drawn between the patterns and diagnosis of mental disorder for Māori, and social, cultural and environmental factors.[35] Furthermore, when the Public Health Commission proposed a strategic plan for Māori public health, emphasis was placed on the major social indicators, including unemployment, housing, income levels and educational status. The first goal for improving whānau well-being was 'to promote a social and physical environment which improves and protects whānau public health'.[36] However, a longitudinal study in Christchurch, although revealing a high prevalence of mental disorders among Māori youth, failed to demonstrate a strong causative link with socio-economic conditions. Instead the strongest predictors of disorder related to the individual's immediate social environment (family, school, and peers). As a consequence it was considered that attempts to reduce rates of disorder in adolescence by focusing on general socio-economic change were less likely to bring improvements than a focus on more proximal families, schools, and peers.[37]

But a study into the effects of the closure of two meat-processing plants, Whakatu and Tomoana in 1986 and 1994 respectively, has shown that there have been serious effects on both mental and physical health for the many Māori employees whose jobs were abruptly terminated. An ongoing process akin to grieving was common and stress was a major consequence as workers struggled to maintain family functioning.[38] On the basis that environmental factors are highly relevant to Māori mental health, Lorna Dyall has recommended the development of structures for rebuilding cultural, socio-economic and political positions.[39]

For every example of disadvantage that can be attributed to contemporary socio-economic policy, there is likely to be an example of advantage accruing from those same policies. The health consequences of modernisation can therefore be seen in two lights. First, improvements in standards of health with increased life expectancy and demographic growth suggest that the impact of modernisation has been beneficial. But from another perspective modernisation is seen as the root cause of individualism, stress, cultural destruction, and alienation.[40] Unhealthy lifestyles are the result. While there is some merit in comparing past and present standards of health—traditional and modern—some caution is also needed not to idealise the distant past, nor to define the Māori position according to deficits in Western lifestyles. To the extent that Māori are disadvantaged by inequalities in standards of living, consequences for health must receive adequate attention. But it is probably too simplistic to argue that socio-economic disparities by themselves are the cause of ill-health.

TE AO HOU: LIFESTYLES

Lifestyle and Disease

During the nineteenth century, the major threats to Māori health came from influenza, whooping cough, pneumonia and typhoid fever. They contributed disproportionately to mortality rates. Tuberculosis was also a threat and even into the middle of the twentieth century was endemic within many Māori communities. Although lack of natural immunity was probably a determining factor, the high toll from infectious diseases was also related to changes in lifestyle—a move to low-lying villages, different foods, association with European immigrants, less exercise, and overcrowding. Following urbanisation in the 1950s, additional health risks emerged in parallel with the adoption of newer lifestyles again. Reduced whānau support, alcohol and drug misuse, smoking, high-risk leisure pursuits, over-eating, long term unemployment, and substandard housing were all to become the new major risks to health.[41]

The contribution of lifestyle to health is well documented, though the reasons why certain lifestyles are pursued is less clear. Social and economic factors are important but cultural factors also play a part, and despite an element of choice, many Māori are introduced to lifestyle practices well before the exercise of mature choice is possible. Trapped lifestyles are a response to socio-economic restraints and the uncensored expectations of peers and communities. As a result, information to guide healthier modes of living must compete with worldwide behavioural norms that make sense to individuals and groups and offer more immediate rewards. Quite apart from income levels or educational attainment, or housing standards, lifestyles are moulded by television, international magazines, websites, and the impact of global trends.

Lifestyle Risks

Māori lifestyles reflect patterns common to all New Zealanders and, in turn, need to be seen within the context of national policies and practices. Alcohol misuse among Māori has escalated in proportion to changes in licensing laws and an increase in alcohol outlets.[42] Similarly gambling addiction has emerged as a serious lifestyle risk—worse, according to West Auckland community leaders, since the establishment of the Auckland gambling casino, Sky City, under the Casino Control Act 1990.[43] Māori are three times more likely to become problem gamblers compared to non-Māori. In 1998, for example, of those 20 years of age and over who received personal counselling or telephone helpline services for problem gambling, 20 per cent were Māori even though Māori made up only 11 per cent of that age group.[44] The new forms of gambling (casino based) are expected to lead to greater crime and violence, co-addictions (drinking and smoking), poverty, and worsening mental health.[45]

Recreational drug use is another modern lifestyle health risk. Increases in the use of cannabis among Māori have led to public outcries in two directions. First, there has been pressure from a lobby groups, including the Green Party and some Māori elders, to legalise or at least decriminalise marihuana because its use is so widespread.[46] They argue that it makes little sense to regard the habit as criminal. But others, including large numbers of Māori health workers, predict that Māori would quickly become the victims of decriminalisation and they caution against any liberalisation of the law. In the light of the evidence received at a Select Committee hearing, the government declined to reconsider the legal status of cannabis. 'The legal status of cannabis is not an issue that the government intends to review.'[47] Legalities aside, lifestyles that revolve around cannabis are threatening the health and social structure of many Māori communities and need to be addressed at community, tribal and governmental levels.

Tobacco smoking among Māori is a longer standing lifestyle pattern. Although there was no tobacco in New Zealand prior to colonisation, even by 1850 nicotine addiction was firmly established.[48] In the 1996/97 New Zealand Health Survey, nearly half of all Māori adults 15 years and over reported that they were current smokers, compared with nearly one-quarter of Pākehā adults and a little over one-quarter of Pacific adults.[49] A higher proportion of women are smokers, to the extent that it is often regarded as a 'cultural norm',[50] and they tend to be younger than Māori male smokers. Nearly 60 per cent of Māori women aged between 15 and 44 years were smokers.[51] Maintenance of the habit may be linked to marketing campaigns that specifically target young Māori and seek to benefit from a lucrative Māori market.[52] But it is also linked to peer pressures, socio-economic status, and the addictive nature of smoking itself. Moreover, if an adult in the home smokes then it is quite likely that younger members will smoke as well.[53] There is some evidence that smoking uptake has reduced for males, and there are probably proportionately more non-smokers now than a century ago. But any downwards trend in the number of smokers may be arrested as more and more young Māori, especially women, take up the habit. The phenomenon has been remarkably unresponsive to educational and promotional efforts. Despite knowledge of the risks, smoking remains endemic. Moreover, smokers are also more likely to drink alcohol in a potentially hazardous manner.[54]

Risks of an another kind are also apparent from claims to the Accident Compensation Commission. Māori may be inclined towards risk-taking behaviour as part of an excessively physical lifestyle. Certainly their rates of sports injury and work related injuries are higher and hospitalisation for motor vehicle injuries is around twice that for non-Māori.[55] Motor vehicle crashes are a major cause of admission to hospital for Māori people and the leading cause of death for all males and females aged 15 to 24 years.[56] In implementing a strategic plan for injury prevention, the Accident Compensation Commission has recognised the importance of addressing cultural factors and employing Māori staff to influence Māori networks. But high occupational injury rates also reflect the concentration of the Māori labour force in manual and high-risk jobs. Nearly 30 per cent of the Māori workforce is employed in the five most dangerous industries (mining; manufacturing; electricity, gas and water supply; transport and storage; and construction).[57]

Injuries within the home are a matter of even greater concern. Whānau violence and its impact on Māori children has been identified as a significant health risk and this is reflected in the high numbers of admissions for Māori women and children in women's refuges. In 1997, 45 per cent of women and 53 per cent of child admissions were Māori.[58] A return to a traditional understanding of the role of Māori children in the family and revaluing the importance of this role has been recommended as the basis for a preventive strategy. Ensuring that family policies are culturally relevant and including Māori perspectives in whānau policies is also seen as necessary.[59] Te Korowai Aroha and Kokona Whānau are examples of Māori community programmes that focus on strengthening relationships through whānau restoration using Māori communication styles and preferences. Programmes such as Strengthening Families and Whaiora Whakaruru are designed to improve the quality of parenting, taking into account the cultural and other needs of Māori parents.

Excessive rates of sports injury suggest high levels of Māori participation in sport, but there is also concern about lifestyles that are too sedentary. Apart from reducing the likelihood of some bodily illnesses, physical activity has also been recognised as important for good mental health; people who are physically active have fewer depressive episodes, higher self-esteem, greater confidence in their ability to cope, and better cognitive functioning than sedentary people.[60] In the 1996/97 New Zealand Health Survey, 20 per cent of Māori were sedentary, compared to 14 per cent of Pākehā.[61] A number of factors that reduce involvement in physical leisure activities have been identified. Costs (fees, suitable clothing), transport difficulties, competing whānau commitments (especially for women), inadequate childcare arrangements, and lack of self-motivation are significant barriers. In addition there may be specific cultural barriers such as whakamaa (a sense of embarrassment) and lack of whānau support.[62]

Lifestyles are closely linked to nutritional patterns and these create significant health risks for Māori. Diabetes is a relatively frequent consequence. Whereas for all New Zealanders diabetes affects 2 to 5 per cent of the population, between 5 and 10 per cent of Māori are affected. In a South Auckland prevalence study the Māori rate was found to be two-and-a-half times the rate for European New Zealanders, and the increased risk was independent of household incomes but partly dependent on obesity. As a proportion of all types of diabetes, non insulin-dependent diabetes mellitus (NIDDM) is more common in Māori than any other ethnic group in New Zealand and obesity is a known risk factor. Reductions in refined sugar intake are probably less important than reduced intake of total fat, reduction and prevention of obesity, increased fibre intake and more physical activity.[63]

Lifestyle Changes

Although Māori health status warrants concern about lifestyle, it should also be recognised that Māori are increasingly successful in competitive sport, have made significant dietary adjustments, and are more aware of health issues than at any time in the past. There have also been a number of successful interventions aimed at changing maladaptive lifestyles. Smokefree Marae for example seeks to turn marae—land and buildings—into smokefree zones. The programme appeals to cultural pride and uses visual and aural messages that are designed for Māori eyes and ears.[64] As part of a wider national smoking cessation campaign, a Quitline telephone service is able to arrange Māori advisors.[65] Māori value systems are essential for such programmes and they need to promote Māori well-being, not alien desires, using concepts that are easily understood and transferable.[66] In that respect, to be consistent with Māori views on health, injury prevention needs to go beyond physical injury to embrace wider perspectives. Kia tupato (taking care) rather than injury prevention might be a more acceptable term to add relevance to the message.[67]

Marae-based health-promotional programmes have been used for smoking cessation, alcohol use and misuse, nutrition, fitness, and first aid. The 'Health through the Marae' project was initiated by Ngāti Te Au in 1990. Customary practices such as karakia (incantations), rongoa (traditional healing), wai tapu (water immersion), and observance of tikanga (tribal lore), have reinforced health messages within marae settings. Health 'live-ins' have attracted support on many marae, and have played some part in increasing health awareness and, in some instances, changing lifestyles in a dramatic way. Existing Māori heath practices are acknowledged and new Māori health codes are drafted to meet modern situations.[68] In the far north Te Hauora o te Hiku o te Ika launched a health promotional programme during 1999 on several marae in the Kaitaia area. It focuses on smoking cessation, diabetes management, home security and self-defence but is tailored to suit the particular needs of each marae.[69]

Nutritional workers have also been active in the promotion of Māori health at community levels. Although making up a relatively small part of the total nutrition workforce, Māori workers have pioneered significant lifestyle changes through a focus on healthy patterns of eating. While using conventional methods such as information about food values and advice about the relative merits of food types, Māori nutrition workers, nutrition kai awhina, have also explored other dimensions, including a whānau focus, partnerships with Māori community groups, marae based actions, and the training of a workforce that is linked into Māori networks and societal structures.

Prior to 1995 information-based persuasion was the main approach used by dietitians and nutritionists, but results were disappointing and behavioural change was minimal. Since then the approach has shifted to focus on Māori communities and alignment with whānau, hapū and iwi.[70] Kai o te Hauora Scholarships have enabled a new group of Māori to gain knowledge in nutrition, but they have also helped to develop strategies for interventions within Māori communities. They have become part of a wider health promotional workforce and have been able to influence not only improved dietary patterns but also healthier lifestyles in a much broader sense.

In 1988 the Māori Womens Welfare League launched a Healthy Lifestyles Programme centred largely on netball as a medium for attracting young Māori women and then promoting health. Abstention from smoking and alcohol consumption formed significant parts of the wider message.[71] The League was able to demonstrate that a key to the success of health promotional programmes is Māori participation and ownership. Control of violence illustrates the point further. Groups such as Taihoa Tane and Ngā Tāne e Mahi ana i roto i Tēnei Ao Hurihuri have been formed by Māori men for Māori men. Their message is direct: that men should own their own violence. But their group approach creates a supportive whānau environment within which alternate strategies can be developed, while at the same time strengthening cultural identity.[72] Māori Christians have also developed remedial programmes for male aggression, sexual abuse, and misappropriated mana (power). Kahui Tane is a programme of educational and attitudinal change based on tikanga Māori (Māori lore) and Christianity. Fifteen kete (baskets) make up a package to address aspects of family life such as managing aggression, achieving communication, practicing aroha (love), and managing whānau affairs.[73]

Dealing with problem gambling provides another example of Māori initiative. A group of volunteers have joined forces to address addictive gambling and assist Māori gamblers. 'Māori Action Against Problem Gambling' provides individual support and information written in a style that makes sense to Māori. Like other similar promotional programmes, it builds on cultural affinities and recognises the socio-economic realities within which Māori live.[74]

Successful Māori health promotion requires that interventions should not only be culturally relevant; they should also be owned by Māori, should empower communities, and should emphasise opportunities for positive participation in Māori society and society at large. For its part the State needs to ensure that policy frameworks are also consistent with good health. There is no great virtue in encouraging healthy lifestyles in poor areas without also attempting to redress the structural inequalities that limit human lives and aspirations. 'We should do more than try to turn poverty into a healthy experience.'[75] In short, health promotion will be of limited value if it is not accompanied by fundamental changes that guarantee human dignity and full inclusion in society and the economy.

HIKOI TANGATA: HUMAN JOURNEYS

Health is determined by the past as well as the present. While socio-economic circumstances and modern lifestyles have more obvious and immediate effects, the health status of indigenous peoples has been strongly influenced by the experience of colonisation and the subsequent efforts to participate as minorities in contemporary society while retaining their own ethnic and cultural identities. Colonial journeys may have led to innovation and adaptation but they also created pain and suffering from which full recovery has yet to be felt. When there is a loss of the resources necessary to sustain well-being and a loss of standing in terms of full participation in society and the economy, health too is threatened.

Confrontation with the West

By 1800 sufficient encounters between Māori and Europeans had occurred to indicate that a new order was close at hand. At first it was a novelty. Whānau (family groups) vied with each other to have a Pākehā retainer and to marvel at a range of new technologies and home comforts. But as the numbers grew and the hunger for land increased, the novelty wore off. The traditional tribal laws of tapu had little effect against soldiers, muskets, legislators and missionaries. By 1857, the population had already declined to around 56,000.[76] A diet of potatoes and little else was simply not compatible with life and gave scant protection against new infectious diseases such as measles, tuberculosis, and influenza. The decline was swift and relentless, and as mortality rates soared so, in parallel fashion, land holdings decreased.

Convinced of the inevitability of Māori demise, in 1874 the *New Zealand Herald* maintained: 'That the native race is dying out in New Zealand there is, of course, no doubt... The fact cannot be disguised that the natives are gradually passing away; and even if no cause should arise to accelerate their decrease, the rate at which they are now disappearing points to their extinction in an exceedingly brief period.'[77]

The prediction seemed to match the demographic facts. By 1896, the population reached its lowest ebb. At 42 000 there was every reason to believe that survival had come to an end and that the next millennium, if not the next century, would see the passing of the Māori.[78] A combination of disease, musket warfare, and starvation contributed disproportionately to the near disappearance of the race. Moreover depopulation was greatest where land alienation had been most extensive. Loss of land had more than economic implications. Personal and tribal identity were inextricably linked to Papatuanuku—the mother earth—and quite apart from loss of income and livelihood, alienation from land carried with it a severe psychological toll.

Land and Health

Two methods were used to separate Māori from their land. The most unjust was confiscation, legalised through two Acts of Parliament, the New Zealand Settlement Act and the Suppression of Rebellion Act, both passed in 1863. They gave the government wide ranging powers to confiscate three million acres of traditional lands. Tribes who actively or passively resisted surveyors or sales were regarded as rebels and their lands were confiscated; even if there were little more than a suspicion of 'rebellion', land could be taken. Other laws were passed with the express purpose of speeding up sales and transferring ownership from tribal collectives to individuals. The Native land Act 1862 and the Native Land Act

1865 largely did away with customary land titles, freeing up land for sale and in the process undermining the social links between families and within tribes. Māori society had depended on common interests in traditional lands for cohesion and purpose. As land was transferred, through one means or another, so Māori identity and well-being were rendered vulnerable until eventually even survival appeared unlikely. Out of nearly 66.5 million acres, by 1896, only 11 000 acres remained in Māori ownership. By then, in like fashion, the Māori population had declined to less than 42 000.

Recovery

Extinction may well have followed were it not for two Māori strategies each of which played an important role in transforming an expected genocide into an unexpected recovery. One approach to the problem of Māori dispossession advocated adaptation to Western society but with the retention of a strong Māori cultural identity; professional Māori leadership and government accommodation of Māori interests was to be the key. The other approach also supported the acquisition of Western knowledge and skills but placed greater emphasis on Māori control and autonomy and less dependence on government goodwill.

The call for acceptance of a predominantly Western world was first made by a small group of Māori students from Te Aute College in 1887. During the summer vacation they travelled to rural and often remote communities bringing new messages—messages about education, ventilated housing, agriculture, economic development, and health and hygiene. Two of the Te Aute group, Maui Pomare and Peter Buck (Te Rangi Hiroa), were to become medical graduates before entering politics. A third, Apirana Ngata, achieved distinction in law, politics, literature and land reform. Māori social, economic and cultural revival is often credited to this trio and their select band, the Young Māori Party. Their philosophy was simple enough; create pride in a Māori identity and Māori culture and use that as a platform for accessing the best of Western technology and education. Because they were able to address their audiences in Māori and employ Māori metaphors to make key points, their task was so much easier and, more importantly, they had a level of credibility that non-Māori could never possess.

Ngata, Pomare and Buck were in no doubt that the answer to Māori survival lay in the need to adapt to Western society and to do so within the overall framework imposed by the law. Though strongly and emphatically in support of

Māori language and culture, they were equally passionate advocates of Western democracy, education and modern health practices. They believed it was possible to retain a secure Māori identity while embracing Pākehā values and beliefs.

In contrast, other Māori leaders considered that a dual identity was not only impossible but that it had contributed to the dramatic population decline in the nineteenth century. For them the answer to dispossession and disease was Māori sovereignty. While sharing the belief of the Young Māori Party that reformative measures were needed if Māori were to survive, the approach of the Māori sovereigntists was to use the new tools of education and technology but to focus Māori energies on building an identity that not only lauded Māori language and culture, but also included a sense of ownership and control. The emphasis was on Māori autonomy and authority, even if it meant defying the law. This group was less convinced about the need to adapt to colonial frameworks; they considered that it ought to be the settlers who made the adaptations. Some, like Rua Kenana, went further, advocating the expulsion of all Europeans from the country.

Not surprisingly government sympathies were with Ngata's approach, and legislation was introduced to bring Māori within the orbit of colonial New Zealand. The 1900 Māori Councils Act, for example, established local Māori committees, but it gave them little real power. The second part of the Young Māori Party's prescription—a strong Māori identity—was not only sidelined in legislation but in one way or another it was actively discouraged. It became policy, for example, not to allow Māori children to speak Māori in the school grounds. Those who did were punished.[79] And Māori adoption practices, based on a collective approach to child care, were all but prohibited. So too was the practice of traditional Māori religion. Even the new Māori Christian churches such as Ratana attracted scorn and were promptly labelled by other churches as heretic. But the greatest blow to the organisation of Māori knowledge and understanding occurred in 1907 when the Tohunga Suppression Act was passed. By outlawing traditional healers, the Act also opposed Māori methodologies and the legitimacy of Māori knowledge in respect of healing, the environment, the arts, and the links between the spiritual and the secular—te kauae runga and te kauae raro.

In defiance of popular expectations, however, the passing of the Māori did not occur; the population decline was halted and whānau again began to grow in numbers. Even by 1936 there was evidence of a substantial reversal (82 000) and by 1996 the population had reached an all time high, 579 714 New Zealanders claiming Māori descent.[80] True, the face of Māori had changed, some were fairer and even blue-eyed, there were very early signs of an increasing number of people over the age of 75 years, and many Māori, perhaps 20 per cent, had lost any link to a hapū. What remained, though, was a strong sense of whānau and a positive feeling about being Māori.[81]

Legislation and the Enhancement of Identity

Since 1975, when the Treaty of Waitangi Act was passed, there has been increased recognition of Māori aspirations for greater participation in society and the economy. Paternalism and assimilative laws have been confronted and there has been a degree of acceptance that Māori not only have legitimate claims based on the Treaty of Waitangi, but also have rights by virtue of being indigenous to New Zealand, including the right to be Māori.[82] Change has not come easily: litigation, confrontation, and the mutual exchange of accusations and bitterness have characterised progress. But there has also been a demonstration of goodwill, patience, and a desire to move beyond the injustices of the past and on to more positive developments.

Slowly some of the laws of the land have come to reflect Māori perspectives and values. The Resource Management Act 1991, for example, requires that Māori environmental values be taken into account along with the recognition of cultural values pertaining to any building permit, land or water usage or resource utilisation. Te Ture Whenua Māori Act 1993, an Act about Māori land, is based on traditional Māori attitudes to land and its importance for future generations. Whereas earlier land laws, even as recently as 1967, were largely written to speed up the alienation of Māori land, the 1993 Act now makes it extremely difficult for Māori land to pass out of Māori ownership.[83] Multiple ownership, once decried as inconsistent with economic development, is now actively encouraged through provisions for a variety of trusts and incorporations. The new Act also provides for improved management structures to enable better commercial returns on tribal land. In the process trade-offs have been made between individual rights and collective rights, so that greater power is now vested in collective decision making, as it was before the imposition of British law. At the same time Māori individuals are no longer as free to dispose of Māori land as they might wish. Their task, according to the legislation, is to practise wise stewardship for the benefit of future generations.

Social policy legislation has also incorporated Māori values, beliefs and practices. The Children Young Persons and Their Families Act 1989 requires social workers to recognise tribal arrangements and Māori family relationships, especially those of whānau. Far from encouraging Social Welfare custody over Māori children, a common approach up until the mid 1980s, the philosophy now rests on the assumption that children are best raised within their own cultural context and with their own people. Leaving aside difficulties with resourcing and not infrequent uncertainties about the rights (and welfare) of the child as against the rights of the family, the Act appears to support a positive Māori identity. It allows for tribal elders to take active leadership roles in family group discussions and requires professional workers to observe—or at least not to ignore—cultural preferences and custom.

In the health sector, the Health and Disability Services Act 1993 is less explicit about Māori culture or identity, but government health policy, even without legislative backing, recognises the importance of taking Māori culture and society into account when programmes for improving Māori health are being developed. In identifying Māori health as one of four health gain priority areas, there is active encouragement for more Māori health providers, and tribal and Māori community health programmes are rapidly increasing. In addition, providers in hospitals are asked to indicate how their services will contribute towards improved health outcomes for Māori. The Mental Health Act 1992 similarly recognises the significance of a Māori cultural identity. Section 5, reinforced by section 65, requires that any court or tribunal which exercises power under the Act must have respect for a person's cultural and ethnic identity, language, and religious or ethical beliefs. They must also show proper recognition of the importance to the patient's well-being of family ties, as well as whānau (extended family), hapū (subtribe) and iwi (tribe).

With the 1996 move to a new system of parliamentary representation, mixed member proportional representation (MMP), there is legislative provision for the number of Māori seats in Parliament to be determined according to the size of the Māori electoral roll, rather than fixed at four, as they were from 1877. Under the new formula the number of Māori seats rose to five in the 1996 general election and to six in 1999. As well, the inclusion of Māori candidates as list members led to a greatly increased Māori representation in Parliament from 1996, when fifteen members took their seats in a 120-seat Parliament. Following the 1999 election, the number had risen to seventeen.

Māori journeys towards active participation in society are important for health. Good health is not compatible with political marginalisation any more than it is with socio-economic deprivation; the Ottawa Charter's emphasis on community empowerment sits comfortably with Māori expectations arising from the Treaty of Waitangi.[84] Both are concerned with self-determination by communities of interest, and both anticipate fairness and equity in society. Although signed in 1840, and observed in an inconsistent manner by the Crown, the Treaty remains the founding document of modern New Zealand and, in article three, guarantees that Māori will share equally in the benefits of modern society. Some progress has been made towards meeting that goal, though the continuing disparities in standards of health between Māori and non-Māori are clear indicators that much remains to be done. At community levels, powerlessness, both in economic and political terms, effectively blocks many Māori men[85] and women[86] from having any meaningful sense of control over their own health. It is a reminder that the achievement of good health, and especially good mental health, requires approaches that go well beyond the provision of health services.

TE AO MĀORI: IDENTITY

Identity is a necessary pre-requisite for mental health, and cultural identity depends not only on access to culture and heritage but also on opportunity for cultural expression and cultural endorsement within society's institutions. Māori are confronted by barriers on both scores. Too many are unable to have meaningful contact with their own language, customs, or inheritance, while too few institutions in modern New Zealand are geared towards the expression of Māori values, let alone language. Ethnic identity has assumed increasing importance in the broad mental health field, not only in relationship to positive health and development but also as a key determinant of successful counselling outcomes. The sharing of cultural heritage, a sense of social relatedness, and symbolic ties define ethnic identity. A person does not belong to an ethnic group by choice; rather birth determines eligibility and emotional and symbolic ties strengthen the attachment.[87] Ethnic identity can be divided into an external ethnic identity (observable social and cultural behaviours such as language, participation in ethnic functions, observance of ethnic traditions) and internal ethnic identity (knowledge of values and history, moral sense of obligation, and affective attachment to the group).[88]

Table 2.2 A Māori Identity

Identity Determinants	*Identity Markers*
Self-identification	ethnic affiliation tribal affiliation
Access to cultural resources	Māori language knowledge and skills tikanga Māori knowledge and skills marae participation
Access to Māori physical resources	Māori land fisheries wāhi tapu tribal estates
Access to Māori social resources	whānau friends and associates Māori educational institutions Māori services tribal services

Source: Te Hoe Nuku Roa

A measure of identity based on both external and internal ethnic identity characteristics has been developed to describe Māori identity.[89] But unlike most other identity measures it goes beyond affiliation, knowledge and behaviour to include actual access to the institutions and resources of the group. The underlying premise is that identity means little if it depends only on an abstract sense of belonging with little opportunity to share the group's cultural, social and economic resources. Table 2.2 outlines the components of a Māori identity measure.

Secure, positive, notional and compromised identities reflect different levels of access to cultural and physical resources.[90] A secure identity demands more than a superficial knowledge of tribal tradition. It depends on easy access to the Māori world—especially Māori language, the extended family network and customary land. In contrast, a person with a positive identity expresses high levels of personal commitment to being Māori but does not have ready access to language, land or other resources. A notional identity suggests a Māori affiliation but an absence of access to any Māori institutions, while a person whose identity is described as compromised might have good access to the Māori world (cultural and physical) but little desire for affiliation with Māori.

In a current longitudinal study, known as Te Hoe Nuku Roa, 700 representative Māori households are being tracked over a twenty-year period (1993–2013) in order to measure their aspirations, achievements, concerns and levels of participation in Māori society and in the wider New Zealand society. There is statistically significant evidence that Māori resources are unevenly distributed, and for many respondents access is virtually unattainable. Even though more than half the respondents are very positive about being Māori and have some access to cultural heritage and Māori resources (positive identities), less than a third actually have a secure identity (are competent Māori speakers and have regular contact with Māori cultural institutions and networks, and shares in Māori land). Since a secure Māori identity appears to be positively correlated with good health, and with better educational outcomes even in the presence of adverse socio-economic conditions, the question of access to resources is an important one.[91]

Fewer than half of all Māori in the study have meaningful access to land, fewer again actually receive a dividend from land and about one-third have little or no contact with a marae.[92] Nor do more than one-quarter possess conversational Māori language skills or even minimal knowledge about whakapapa (genealogy) or tribal history. In other words, the level of alienation of Māori from their own resources is severe even though there are high levels of aspirations for greater participation in the Māori world.

Access to Māori institutions and resources depends on many variables, including the availability of information, personal confidence, economic factors and place of residence. A secure identity is not necessarily the privilege of rural Māori. Many urban Māori are confident Māori language speakers, have good access to marae, to Māori land and to whānau.[93] On the other hand, Māori in rural situations often demonstrate disadvantage in terms of access to both cultural and physical resources. The debate about urban and rural Māori is important and it has major implications, but it is more urgent to understand how Māori who are alienated from their own resources, no matter where they live, can gain access and as a result develop a secure identity.

In response to colonisation and attempts at assimilation, Māori identities were often crushed or reconfigured in a fatalistic light. Many Māori rejected their own cultural and social underpinnings of identity and either tried to imitate Pākehā New Zealanders or played out second-class roles as carefree, unambitious and inoffensive labourers. Urbanisation decided the issue for many post–World War II city migrants. No longer exposed to tribal homes,[94] a loss of 'culture, traditions and language' gave way to 'alcohol drugs and crime'.[95] Negative identities were assumed. They were part of the colonised experience and created mental health disadvantage. Indeed, throughout the Fourth World negative identities accompanied by deculturation have been recognised as causes of mental ill health, including alcohol misuse, suicide, aggression, and offending.[96] More recently, indigenous peoples have come to regard the establishment of a positive cultural identity as a key to better mental health[97] and have developed a range of therapies that focus on cultural reawakening.[98] Underlying them all, and it is evident also in Māori centred therapies, is the belief that strengthening cultural identity can improve mental health.

Identity confusion has also been described as a source of anxiety and asocial conduct. Caught somewhere between the values, beliefs, and practices of a parent culture and the demands and expectations of another majority culture, a secure identity can give way to a confused identity. Opting out is one way of reducing the consequent anxiety. The assumption of a strong but negative identity is another. Sometimes the assumed identity can have the characteristics of totalism—the rigid adherence to a set of values or beliefs which serve to reduce anxiety and identity confusion, but at the expense of openness and wholeness.[99] Psychological boundaries become fixed and intolerant of other views, and the new-found identity feeds on the inclusion of some and the total exclusion of others. A Rastafarian identity made sense to groups of disaffected Māori youth on the east coast of the North Island during the 1980s. Not only was there a rejection of Māori identity but there was also an antipathy to those who did not accept Rasta ways or who openly opposed them. The movement, which had the hallmarks of totalism, was born out of separation from traditional lands, often a loss of language, and usually unsatisfactory relationships with family and community. Drug use may have reduced the sense of alienation, but the group's heightened sense of mission arose from the incorporation of a rigid identity based on Afro-Caribbean culture; it was an identity that could only be maintained by denying reality and constructing boundaries to avoid perceived threats from conservative Māori elements.

There is also debate about whether cultural identity for Māori has validity only if it is expressed as a tribal identity. John Rangihau described the notion of a Māori identity as one that was invented by Pākehā as part of a colonising experience. Reminding others of his tribal roots, 'Tuhoetanga rather than Māoritanga' seemed to strike a more meaningful note for him.[100] Certainly, prior to colonisation, there was no sense of a universal Māori identity. But it became apparent during the High Court case concerning the allocation of fishing quota to tribes in 1998 that many Māori saw themselves as Māori, not as members of a tribe or a hapū.[101] For some the tribal option was so removed from day-to-day experience that, at best, it would have been an intellectual exercise lacking any practical meaning. It is also true that the significance of a Māori identity achieved greater importance as Māori people became a minority in New Zealand, and as urbanisation brought together groups of Māori who could relate to common values and experiences, even though their tribal paths had been quite different. Pride in national Māori sporting teams or in the achievements of Māori individuals stems to a large extent from the ease with which Māori can identify with other Māori people. The tribal identity is one dimension; but there is an equal and growing sense of a Māori identity.[102]

Apart from the impact of colonisation and then urbanisation, Māori identity is also affected by influences and trends originating from beyond New Zealand's shores. Globalisation, for example, is creating a new environment within which individuals are able to participate in a worldwide forum. While the global market—the advancement of multinational corporations and the subsequent Westernisation of the world—is sometimes seen as the main objective of globalisation, direct individual participation in the global stage is also possible through new technologies and sophisticated communication networks. Like others, Māori as individuals can join the world through education, trading, professional and business interaction, the internet, or simply by watching overseas television programmes. They become part of a global network. Being a Māori or a tribal member is not necessarily rendered less significant, but neither does it provide a total sense of being. With globalisation there is an expansion of identity to incorporate a transcultural affinity with music, or fashion, or sport, or travel, or religion, or drugs, or expectations of a better life.

Two personal responses to globalisation may occur. In the first, identity as a Māori remains, but it is now complemented by an identity as a citizen of the world. Any serious confusion is avoided by contextualisation so that, as required, the global identity can lead to a sense of inclusion with peers across the globe, while a Māori identity can reinforce a link with a particular past and offer emotional and psychological security in day-to-day realities. In the second response confusion is avoided by rejection of one identity or the other. A Māori identity is abandoned in favour of an identity that is seen to be more portable and less localised. Alternatively, any semblance of a global identity is cast aside and a Māori identity is embraced with fundamentalist fervour. Both responses defy reality and as a consequence reduce coping ability.

By itself a Māori identity is not an insurance against poor mental health, nor does it offer a passport to good health. An identity that confines human experience to a culturally safe environment reduces anxiety and enhances confidence in that environment, but creates maladaptive coping behaviours and rigidities that are out of place in a changing world. On the other hand, a secure cultural identity derived from ready access to Māori cultural, social, and physical resources can provide a strong foundation for health, the more so if it can allow interaction with the other identities that contemporary Māori must incorporate.

MANA AKE: UNIQUENESS

Foundations for health take into account the wider social, economic, historical and cultural circumstances that ultimately impact on Māori lives. But there are other factors which, because they are unique to individuals, lie within the person rather than without. Poor health, including poor mental health, cannot be entirely understood by reference to external causative factors and past experiences. There is another dimension, sometimes described as endogenous, or genetic, or biological, or hereditary—or unique. No matter how adequate the social, economic, cultural and emotional environments, poor health may nonetheless result. Innate factors cannot always be compensated by external socio-cultural factors; nor, however, are they totally unaffected by them. In effect there is a constant interchange between inner and outer energies; health is the locus of multiple interactive pathways.

In her model of health, known as te wheke (the octopus), Rangimarie Pere identified uniqueness, mana ake, as a key component.[103] Individuals cannot be simply understood as the sum total of external forces acting on an inherited substrate. While whakapapa, descent from ancestors, will determine to some extent the genetic and temperamental qualities inherited, the unique combination of genes that endows every child combine to ensure an element of uniqueness. However, inherited genetic material is not the only source of acquired uniqueness. All individuals travel on unique personal journeys, have temperamental and personality characteristics that are not exact replicas of their parents, and are exposed to health risks as a result of their distinctive occupations or interests, or experiences at home and school.

There are not a great number of health problems attributable solely to genetic loading. Insulin dependent diabetes mellitus is one, but for many other so-called genetic disorders the degree of genetic penetrance is more controversial. Alcohol disorders, schizophrenia, bipolar affective disorders, and even some personality disorders may be influenced by genetic inheritance, but the mode of transmission is seldom clear and many other factors come into play. By dismissing a condition as simply 'genetic', opportunities for intervention may be passed over on the basis of a fatalistic concept of disease. In any case, management of the health problem can seldom be premised on altering the genetic make-up; invariably it requires a careful assessment of the many factors which operate on an individual's mind and body, and then the construction of a plan of action that attempts to modify them.

It can also be misleading to draw conclusions about an individual because of ethnicity or cultural affiliation. No two Māori journeys are the same. Although there are common histories, commonly held cultural views, and similar socio-economic living conditions, Māori as a people are diverse[104] and it is dangerous to conclude that any condition can be explained entirely on the basis of being Māori. This does not mean that being Māori is irrelevant; but it does sound a note of caution about seeking explanations derived from cultural or socio-economic stereotypes.

It is unethical to insist that all Māori in hospitals or attending clinics should be managed in the same way, but by the same token it is equally unacceptable that a Māori who has a health problem should be treated as if being Māori was of no consequence. It always is, though not in a way that can be presumed.

Notes

1 Whakatau Mauri refers to establishing a sound foundation for spirit and vitality.

2 Stephen J. Kunitz, (1994), *Disease and Social Diversity*, Oxford University Press, New York, pp. 44–55.

3 Wen-Shing Tseng, John F. McDermott, (1981), *Culture, Mind and Therapy*, Brunner/Mazel, New York, pp. 16–25.

4 American Psychiatric Association, (1994), *Diagnostic and Statistical Manual of Mental Disorders* (4th edn), American Psychiatric Association, Washington DC, p. 281.

5 Ernest Hunter, (1999), 'Considering the Changing Environment of Indigenous Child Development', *Australasian Psychiatry*, vol. 7, no. 3, pp. 137–140.

6 Alex Cohen, (1999), *The Mental Health of Indigenous Peoples: An International Overview*, Nations for Mental Health, Department of Mental Health, World Health Organisation, Geneva, pp. 7–10.

7 Ministry of Health, (1997a), *Mental Health Promotion for Younger and Older Adults: The Public Health Issues*, Ministry of Health, Wellington, pp. 16–35.

8 M. H. Durie, (1985a), 'Māori Health Institutions', *Community Mental Health in New Zealand*, vol. 2, no. 1, pp. 63–69.

9 Elizabeth Murchie, (1984), *Rapuora: Health and Māori Women*, Māori Womens Welfare League, Wellington, pp. 40–41.
10 Heaven and earth.
11 Ministry of Health, (1998f), *Whāia te Whanaungatanga: Oranga Whānau The Wellbeing of Whānau*, Ministry of Health, Wellington, pp. 5–6.
12 Te Puni Kokiri, (1995b), *Omangia te Oma Roa: Māori Participation in Physical Leisure*, Ministry of Māori Development, Wellington, pp. 9–10.
13 Royal Commission on Social Policy, (1988), *The April Report*, Report of the Royal Commission on Social Policy, vol. II, pp. 63–69.
14 Ministry of Health, (1997a), pp. 22–25.
15 Kevin White, (1994), 'Social Construction of Medicine and Health,' in John Spicer, Andrew Trlin, Jo Ann Walton (eds), *Social Dimensions of Health and Disease: New Zealand Perspectives*, Dunmore Press, Palmerston North, p. 248.
16 Mental Health Commission, (1999a), *Housing and Mental Health: A discussion Paper*, Mental Health Commission, Wellington.
17 Alistair Woodward, Ichiro Kawachi, (1998), *Why Should We Reduce Health Inequalities?*, paper prepared for the National Health Committee, Wellington School of Medicine, Wellington, pp. 9–10.
18 National Health Committee, (1998c), *The Social, Cultural and Economic Determinants of Health in New Zealand: Action to Improve Health*, National Advisory Committee on Health and Disability, Wellington, p. 8.
19 Judith Davey, (1998), *Tracking Social Change in New Zealand: From Birth to Death IV*, Institute of Policy Studies, Victoria University of Wellington, pp. 1–7.
20 Peter Crampton, Peter Davis, (1998), 'Measuring Deprivation and Socio-economic Status: Why and How?', *The New Zealand Public Health Report*, vol. 5, no.11/12, pp. 81–84.
21 Philippa Howden-Chapman, Fiona Cram, (1998), *Social, Economic and Cultural Determinants of Health*, paper prepared for the National Health Committee, National Committee on Health and Disability, Wellington, pp. 16–17.
22 Ministry of Health, (1999b), *Taking the Pulse: The 1996/97 New Zealand Health Survey*, Ministry of Health, Wellington, pp. 163–165.
23 Paparangi Reid, presentation to National Health Committee, 21 March 2000.
24 A. Woodward, P. Crampton, P. Howden-Chapman, C. Salmon, (2000), 'Poverty – Still a Health Hazard', editorial, *The New Zealand Medical Journal*, vol. 113, no. 1105, pp. 67–68.
25 Te Puni Kokiri, (1998b), 'Trends in Māori Employment, Income and Expenditure', *Whakapakari: Hunga Mahi*, no. 2, Ministry of Māori Development, Wellington.
26 Te Puni Kokiri, (1998b), pp. 34–35.

27 Te Puni Kokiri, (1998e), *Review of the Ministry of Housing Service Delivery to Māori*, Ministry of Māori Development, Wellington.
28 Te Puni Kokiri, (1998c), *Progress Towards Closing Social and Economic Gaps Between Māori and Non-Māori*, a report to the Minister of Māori Affairs, Ministry of Māori Development, Wellington.
29 Te Puni Kokiri, Minitanga mo Ngā Wāhine, (1999), *Māori Women in Focus Titiro hāngai ka mārama*, Ministries of Māori Development and Womens Affairs, Wellington.
30 Te Puni Kokiri, (2000), *Progress Towards Closing Social and Economic Gaps Between Māori and Non-Māori*, a report to the Minister of Māori Affairs, May 2000, Ministry of Māori Development, Wellington.
31 National Health Committee (1998c), pp. 58–69.
32 Mental Health Commission, (1999a).
33 National Health Committee (1998c), p. 59.
34 Eru Pomare, Vera Keefe-Ormsby, Clint Ormsby, Neil Pearce, Papārangi Reid, Bridget Robson, Naina Wātene-Haydon, (1995), *Hauora: Māori Standards of Health III*, Eru Pomare Research Centre, Wellington Clinical School, Wellington, pp. 145–150.
35 Te Puni Kokiri, (1993a), *Ngā Ia o te Hinengaro Māori: Trends in Māori Mental Health*, a discussion document, Ministry of Māori Development, Wellington.
36 Public Health Commission, (1995), *He Matariki: A Strategic Plan for Māori Public Health*, Public Health Commission, Wellington, pp. 25–39.
37 L. John Horwood, David M. Fergusson, (1998), *Psychiatric Disorder and Treatment in a Birth Cohort of Young Adults*, Ministry of Health, Wellington, pp. 27–30.
38 Vera Keefe, Clint Ormsby, Wayne Ormsby, Fiona Cram, Papārangi Reid, Bridget Robson, Naina Wātene, (1998), 'Mauri Mahi Mauri Ora Mauri Noho Mauri Mate: Health Effects of Unemployment Portfolio', in Te Pūmanawa Hauora (ed.), *Te Oru Rangahau Māori Research and Development Conference Proceedings*, Te Pūtahi ā Toi, School of Māori Studies, Massey University, 175–183.
39 Lorna Dyall, (1997a), 'Māori', in Pete M. Ellis, Sunny C. D. Collings (eds), *Mental Health in New Zealand From a Public Health Perspective*, Ministry of Health, Wellington, pp. 85–103.
40 Kunitz, (1994), pp. 149–191.
41 Public Health Commission, (1994), *Whakapiki Mauri: Māori Health Advancement*, Public Health Commission, Wellington, pp. 5–7.
42 See chapter 5.
43 John Tamihere, (1997), 'Can You Afford the High Stakes?', in Compulsive Gambling Society (ed.), *Gambling as an Emerging Health Issue for Māori*, Report of a Hui held at the Papakura Marae.

44 John Hannifin, Margaret Gruys, (1999), *Problem Gambling Counselling in New Zealand 1998 National Statistics*, Problem Gambling Committee, Auckland.
45 Compulsive Gambling Society of New Zealand, (1997), *Gambling as an Emerging Health Issue for Māori*, paper prepared for the first National Hui on Gambling for Māori, Papakura Marae.
46 Public Health Group, (1996a), *Cannabis*, Ministry of Health, Wellington, pp. 22–23.
47 New Zealand Government, (1999), *Government Response to Report of the Health Select Committee on the Inquiry into the Mental Health Effects of Cannabis*, presented to the House of Representatives in accordance with Standing Order 251.
48 John Broughton, (1996), *Puffing up a Storm Volume I: Kapai te Torori*, Te Roopu Rangahau Hauora o Ngai Tahu, University of Otago, pp. 36–51.
49 Ministry of Health, (1999b), p. 25.
50 John Broughton, Mark Lawrence, (1993), *Ngā Wahine Māori me te Kai Paipa: Māori Women and Smoking*, Department of Preventive and Social Medicine, University of Otago, p. 109.
51 Ministry of Health, (1999b), p. 25.
52 Papārangi Reid, Robert Pouwhare, (1991), *Te Taonga-mai-Tāwhiti*, Niho Taniwha, Auckland, pp. 41–46.
53 Māori Health Group, (1994), *Kia Whai te Māramatanga: The Effectiveness of Health Messages for Māori*, Ministry of Health, Wellington, pp. 33–34.
54 Ministry of Health, (1999b), p. 79.
55 Te Puni Kokiri, (1998d), *Review of ACC Service Delivery to Māori*, Ministry of Māori Development, Wellington, pp. 26–28.
56 Public Health Commission, *Road Traffic Injuries*, Public Health Commission, Wellington, pp. 10–11.
57 Te Puni Kokiri, (1998d), p. 27.
58 Ministry of Health, (1998a), *Family Violence Guidelines for Health Sector Providers to Develop Practice Protocols*, Ministry of Health, Wellington, pp. 33–38.
59 Public Health Group, (1996b), *Child Abuse Prevention*, Ministry of Health, Wellington, pp. 18–19.
60 National Health Committee, (1998a), *Active For Life: A Call for Action: The Health Benefits of Physical Activity*, National Advisory Committee on Health and Disability, Wellington, p. 19.
61 Ministry of Health, (1999b), p. 47.
62 Te Puni Kokiri, (1995b), pp. 12–14.
63 Public Health Group, (1997), *Diabetes Prevention and Control*, Ministry of Education, Wellington, pp. 20–21.
64 Tahuna Minhinnick, (1994), *Achieving and Maintaining a Smokefree Marae*, pamphlet, Paradigm Productions.

65 National Health Committee, (1999b), *Guidelines for Smoking Cessation*, National Advisory Committee on Health and Disability, Wellington, p. 7.
66 Māori Health Group, (1994), pp. 47–48.
67 'Community empowerment the key to injury prevention', *Ministry of Māori Development Newsletter*, issue no. 51, May 1999, p. 5.
68 Te Puni Kokiri, (1995a), *Health Through the Marae: Ngā Tikanga Hauora o Ngā Marae*, Ministry of Māori Development, Wellington.
69 'Marae programme brings lifestyle changes in Far North', *Kōkiri Paetae*, Te Puni Kokiri, 23, August 1999, p. 6.
70 Hiki Pihema, (1998), 'Training: What's in it for Māori', editorial, *Journal of the New Zealand Dietetic Association*, vol. 52, no. 1, pp. 3–4.
71 Te Puni Kokiri, (1993b), *The Healthy Lifestyle Programme—An Evaluation*, Ministry of Māori Development, Wellington.
72 M. M. Ratima, M. H. Durie, G. R. Allan, A. Gillies, J. A. Waldon, P. S. Morrison, Te K. Kingi, (1995), *Men For Change: Living Without Violence*, Te Pūmanawa Hauora, Māori Studies, Massey University.
73 Muru Walters, (1997), 'Kahui Tane: A Challenge to Māori Male Sexuality', in Philip Culbertson (ed.), *Counselling Issues and South Pacific Communities*, Accent Publications, Auckland, pp. 73–92.
74 Lorna Dyall, (1999), *Māori Action Against Problem Gambling: Tā te Iwi Māori Hei Ārai Atu i ngā Mate Petipeti*, Compulsive Gambling Society of New Zealand, Auckland.
75 Woodward et al., (2000).
76 D. Ian Pool, (1977), *The Māori Population of New Zealand 1769–1971*, Auckland University Press and Oxford University Press, Auckland, p. 55.
77 *New Zealand Herald*, 17 August 1874.
78 Ian Pool, (1991), *Te Iwi Māori: A New Zealand Population Past, Present and Projected*, Auckland University Press, Auckland, pp. 75–103.
79 Waitangi Tribunal, (1986), *Report of the Waitangi Tribunal on the te Reo Māori Claim (Wai II)*, Department of Justice, Wellington.
80 In the 1996 Census, the total Māori population was based on Māori descent, rather than the quantum of 'Māori blood'. Comparisons with earlier times are therefore not always reliable. But the general trends are consistent.
81 In the 1996 Census, of the 579 714 people of Māori descent, only 523 374 identified as Māori.
82 Mason Durie, (1997a), 'Identity, Nationhood and Implications for Practice in New Zealand', *New Zealand Journal of Psychology*, vol. 26, no. 2, pp. 32–38.
83 Mason Durie, (1998c), *Te Mana, Te Kāwanatanga: The Politics of Māori Self Determination*, Oxford University Press, Auckland, pp. 135–138.

84 World Health Organisation, Health and Welfare Canada, Canadian Public Health Association, (1986), *Ottawa Charter for Health Promotion,* World Health Organisation, Health and Welfare Canada, Canadian Public Health Association, Ottawa.

85 Ministerial Advisory Committee on Māori Health, (1992), *Hui Hauora Tane,* Department of Health, Wellington.

86 Law Commission, (1999), *Justice: The Experiences of Māori Women, Te Tikanga o te Ture Te Matauranga o ngā Wāhine Māori e pa ana ki tēnei,* Report 53, Law Commission, Wellington.

87 G. R. Sodowsky, K. K. Kwan, R. Pannu, (1995), 'Ethnic Identity of Asians in the United States', in J. G. Ponterotto, J. M. Casas, L. A. Suzuki, C. M. Alexander, *Handbook of Multicultural Counseling,* Sage Publications, California, pp. 134–143.

88 W. W. Isajiw, (1990), 'Ethnic-identity Retention', in R. Breton, W. W. Isajiw, W. E. Kalbach, J. G. Reitz (eds), *Ethnic Identity and Equality,* University of Toronto Press, Toronto, pp. 34–91.

89 M. H. Durie, (1995b), 'Te Hoe Nuku Roa Framework: A Māori Identity Measure', *Journal of the Polynesian Society,* vol. 104, no. 4, pp. 461–470.

90 Te Hoe Nuku Roa, (1995), *Interconnectedness, a paper prepared for the Ministry of Māori Development,* Department of Māori Studies, Massey University.

91 Te Hoe Nuku Roa, (1997), *Reports of the Manawatu-Whanganui and Gisborne Baseline Studies,* Department of Māori Studies, Massey University.

92 See chapter 3 for a discussion on marae.

93 Whānau affiliation is discussed in chapter 7.

94 Anne Delamere, (1998), 'He Pou Tokomanawa Mo te Whanau—A Centre Post for the Family', in Sik Hung Ng, Ann Weatherall, James H. Liu, Cynthia S. F. Loong (eds), *Ages Ahead: Promoting Inter-generational Relationships,* Victoria University Press, Wellington, pp. 49–54.

95 Rangi Mataamua, (1998), 'Child of the Clan, Rich With Many Grandparents and Parents', in Sik Hung Ng, Ann Weatherall, James H. Liu, Cynthia S. F. Loong (eds), *Ages Ahead: Promoting Inter-generational Relationships,* Victoria University Press, Wellington, pp. 55–60.

96 James B. Waldram, (1997), *The Way of the Pipe: Aboriginal Spirituality and Symbolic Healing,* Broadview Press, Ontario, pp. 61–68.

97 Swinomish Tribal Mental Health Project, (1991), *A Gathering of Wisdoms: Tribal Mental Health, A Cultural Perspective,* Swinomish Tribal Community, Mount Vernon, pp. 103-106.

98 Eduardo Duran, Bonnie Duran, (1995), *Native American Postcolonial Psychology,* State University of New York Press, Albany, pp. 85–91.

99 Erik H. Erikson, (1964), *Insight and Responsibility*, W. W. Norton & Co., New York, pp. 91–94.

100 John Rangihau, (1975), 'Being Māori', in M. King (ed.), *Te Ao Hurihuri: The World Moves On*, Hicks Smith and Sons, Wellington, pp. 221–233.

101 High Court of New Zealand, (1998), CP 395/93, Auckland Registry.

102 Waitangi Tribunal, (1998), *Te Whānau o Waipereira Report (Wai 414)*, Waitangi Tribunal, Wellington.

103 Rose Rangimarie Pere, (1984), 'Te Oranga o te Whānau: The Octopus as a Symbol', in Komiti Whakahaere (ed.), *Hui Whakaoranga Māori Health Planning Workshop*, Department of Health, Wellington (no page numbers).

104 M. H. Durie, (1995d), *Ngā Matatini Māori: Diverse Māori Realities*, Paper prepared for the Ministry of Health, Wellington.

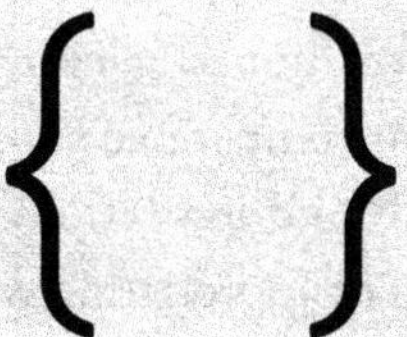

Introducing Communication and Development

Susan Shaw, Ailsa Haxell and Terry Weblemoe

CHAPTER OVERVIEW

This chapter covers the following topics:

+ Learning about people and communication
+ Models and elements of communication
+ Communication and human development
+ The organisation of this book.

KEY TERMS

Intention
Meaningful
Engagement
Meaning

Good communication is at the very centre of professional behaviour and the provision of appropriate support and care. The judgment of appropriate and good communication rests with the person receiving it, and usually reflects their perspective on what they think matters. While ideas of what information is relevant and important may vary between apparently similar people in comparable situations, the concept and importance of being treated individually and respectfully changes little. Approaching people with the genuine **intention** of appreciating what they need and how they may be helped requires a personal acceptance that people are unique and deserve quality and thoughtful attention. There is no substitute for a genuine interest and desire to interact with others in a **meaningful** way. Social interaction and therefore communication is a fundamental human reality and is inescapably important.

Intention A deliberate attempt to behave in a certain way.

Meaningful A sense of significance, relevance, purpose or importance.

Learning about people and communication

It has long been accepted that people working in the health care and disability support sector need to have an appreciation of human development and communication. Traditionally these two subjects are taught in isolation and students (and practitioners) struggle to apply what they have learnt. We believe that putting these elements together enables students to make connections about how to interact effectively and appropriately with colleagues and those they support. Sound interpersonal **engagement** is at the core of good practice and appreciating the perspectives of others. The knowledge and skill to interact with those around us in meaningful ways is of the greatest importance.

Engagement Being genuinely involved.

In addition to placing communication and human development alongside one another, there are other departures from traditional approaches in this book. Generally books about human development focus on theoretical perspectives, while those about communication include fine details about 'micro skills'. Within this book contributors have taken a range of approaches to presenting their chapters. Some have emphasised theoretical perspectives, while others have highlighted the essence of engagement by providing insights into the process of interacting with others. This varied presentation is deliberate, and we hope that it models a range of approaches to considering and presenting information.

The broad range of communication mediums covered within these pages is another departure from other publications for students within these fields of study. People of all ages are using electronic media to communicate and to access information. At the same time, electronic tools are becoming indispensible in the management and delivery of health care and disability support services. However, it is also important to appreciate the **meaning** of communication in terms of art and creativity, and for that reason Chapter 24 considers art, music and poetry.

Meaning The significance of the message and its delivery and context.

While there are groups of practitioners with roles that involve direct communication with patients or service users, this book is designed to consider communication across the spectrum of service development and delivery. The need for accurate, relevant and appropriate communication is as important for scientists in laboratories as it is for receptionists taking calls from patients and clinical staff discussing bad news with families. The way in which people within all of these roles communicate among themselves is also of great significance. Organisational, professional, cultural and personal understandings and approaches to communication all impact on the quality of services and experience of those interacting with them (Leonard, Graham & Bonacum, 2004).

Communication is embedded in context and culture. In both Aotearoa New Zealand and Australia there are many cultural considerations of particular significance within the health and disability support sector. The details of how to manage particular situations can be found within organisational procedures and processes. Information within this book puts the need for these details into perspective and provides a foundation from which to consider culturally appropriate communication.

Models and elements of communication

There is a great deal of information published about how to communicate with people in different situations, and this includes suggested principles and elements that are enshrined in consensus statements (see, for example, Makoul, 2001). It is our belief that, while there are particular essential elements, practitioners are best served by having a broad appreciation of communication contexts and developing a range of skills that become a repertoire suited to them, their roles and their environments. We do not promote recipe-based approaches to communication as they de-personalise all of those involved and diminish the importance of judgment, reflection and reciprocity.

The teaching of communication skills often relies on borrowed theories or practices from fields such as communication, counselling and business. This book differs from many other health-care communication texts in that it focuses more on the application and adjustment of communication skills than on the presentation of communication models and theories. It is intended as a supporting text for communication skills that are taught and assessed through the actual process of interpersonal communication.

We value and acknowledge the concept of 'helping skills' as discussed by John Heron (2001). To be supporting and enabling—creating more rather than less freedom—provides a way of working in health services not bounded by professional borders. The skills are both facilitative and authoritative, and are chosen primarily for their clarity, simplicity and balance. Heron's six skills for helping clients involve being:

+ supportive
+ informative
+ empathic (cathartic)
+ catalytic
+ prescriptive
+ able to confront with sensitivity.

Communication and human development

The basic premise of this book is that sound communication and a good appreciation of human development are essential to the provision of high-quality health care and disability support services, in their broadest sense. While approaches to communication vary to some degree across the lifespan, we do not believe that there are specific formulae for communicating with individuals according to their age. The use of language needs to accommodate knowledge, connections and connotations that people may have, but this does not mean that there is one procedure for chatting to a 3-year-old and a different guideline for explaining a diagnosis to a 13-year-old. While we present information about lifespan stages and communication, we do not condone reductionistic analyses of communication or approaches to people.

The organisation of this book

One of the challenges for us in developing this book has been how to organise it to enable easy access to information, while demonstrating the integrated nature of communication and development. The book is divided into three parts. The chapters in Part 1 (Communication and Lifespan Development) relate to specific stages of human development. Part 2 (Communication and Human Engagement) includes chapters on how people communicate and the challenges they experience in day-to-day life, as well as within the health care and disability systems. Importantly, this section includes chapters about touch and creative elements of communication, which are often overlooked in communication courses. Part 3 (Professional Communication) considers communication within the context of professional practice, acknowledging the need for it to be responsive and useful for practitioners as well as patients or service users.

CASE STUDY 1.1

A 10-year-old boy, teeth and girls

At the time that the concept of this book was being considered, a particular clinical example came to our attention that clearly illustrated our interest linking communication with lifespan development.

Tom, a bright and sociable 10-year-old boy, attended a dental hygiene clinic and was interested in the whole experience. At the end of the appointment, the clinicians wished him well and one of them casually said to him, 'The girls will think you are great now'.

A week later, Tom confided to his mum that there was something he thought she should know. He went on to 'confess' that he had only made cursory attempts to clean his teeth in the past few days.

His mother was surprised and a bit perplexed given that he appeared to be interested in his teeth and the dental hygiene messages. She asked him why, and he responded that he didn't want girls to think he was great.

While this was rather entertaining for the adults involved at the time, Tom taught us a good lesson: communication needs to be both considered and relevant. We need to be mindful enough to appreciate that 10-year-old boys may not actually want to be noticed by girls!

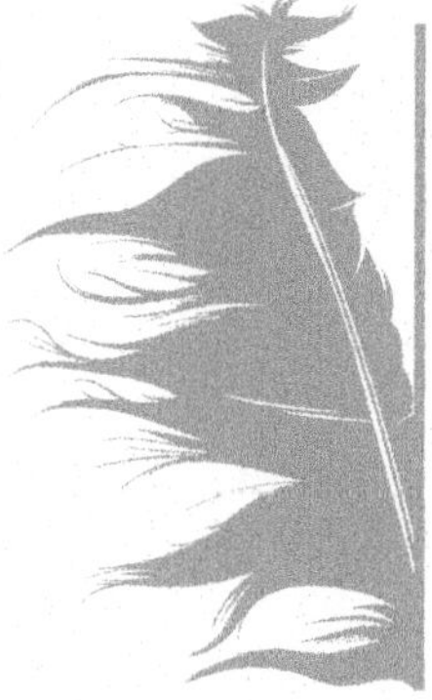

{ SUMMARY }

Good communication is central in the provision of support and care. The intention of working with people in supportive and enabling ways is shared across health disciplines and roles. Such ways of working are about being adaptive to the uniqueness of each situation. The intention here is to engender a mindfulness that integrates knowledge of communication with an appreciation of lifespan development.

REFLECTION POINTS

1.1 Intention (motivation, message, meaning, emotion)

Valuing people as unique and deserving of quality and thoughtful attention underpins all interactions in the health-care sector.

1.2 Reception (received message, response, feedback)

Who might be the best judge of appropriate and effective communications?

1.3 Perception (style, manner, impression, analysis)

Reflecting on your own life, what were some of the moments you remember about interacting with health practitioners? How did you want to be treated?

QUESTIONS FOR REVIEW

1 What basic intentions underpin effective communications?
2 In the case study above, what was the impact of a lack of consideration for the realities of being a 10-year-old boy?

REFERENCES

Heron, J. (2001). *Helping the client: A creative practical guide* (5th edn). London, England: Sage.

Leonard, M., Graham, S. & Bonacum, D. (2004). The human factor: The critical importance of effective teamwork and communication in providing safe care. *Quality and Safety in Health Care, 4*(13), 185–90.

Makoul, G. (2001). Essential elements of communication in medical encounters: The Kalamazoo Consensus Statement. *Academic Medicine, 76*(4), 390–3.

WEBSITES

Building Relationships and Eliminating Disparities: www.urmc.rochester.edu/fammed/research/center_comm_health.cfm

Health Literacy www.healthnavigator.org.nz/centre-for-clinical-excellence/health-literacy

The Electronic Health Record in New Zealand: www.hinz.org.nz/journal/2004/03/The-Electronic-Health-Record-in-New-Zealand---Part-2/893

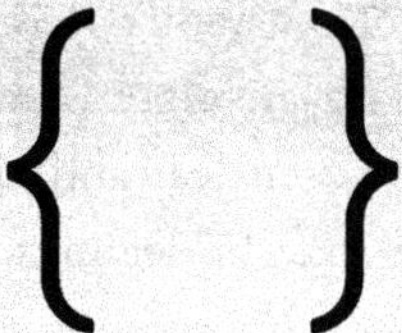

The Antenatal Journey

Andrea Gilkison

CHAPTER OVERVIEW

This chapter covers the following topics:

+ Transition to motherhood
+ The narrative of pregnancy
+ Listening to women's narratives

KEY TERMS

Pregnancy
Maternity care
Childbearing
Conception
Trimester
Antenatal
Narrative

Pregnancy
Carrying a child from conception to birth.

Pregnancy is an extraordinary yet common life event that has a great impact on the lives of the pregnant woman, the father of the baby and extended whānau/family and friends. The experience of pregnancy is always accompanied by an emotional response and involves considerable physical, psychological, social, emotional and relationship adjustments.

The discovery of being pregnant—whether it is the first or subsequent pregnancy, planned or unplanned—may lead to an array of emotions. These include pride and excitement alongside uncertainty or even fear and anxiety about what the implications of the pregnancy might be. There may be feelings of surprise at becoming pregnant, emotional fluctuations, ambivalence and sometimes even denial: 'I can't possibly be pregnant.'

What the impending future might bring and how it will affect their lives are common concerns for parents when they first discover they are pregnant. Concerns may be related to how they will cope with being a mother or a father and how life and relationships might change. Parents' feelings towards the pregnancy can be influenced by many things, including their current relationship, their family situations, study or work situations, plans for the future, financial situations, the timing of the pregnancy, the number of children they already have, and how easy it was to get pregnant. There may be concerns about the mother's health, or that of the unborn baby. The pregnant mother can experience emotions ranging from great joy to despair, depending on her situation, and she may often experience feelings of conflict and confusion about the pregnancy. Over one-third of pregnancies in Aotearoa New Zealand are unplanned (Amin Shokravi, Howden Chapman & Peyman, 2009), so often newly pregnant women will have some unexpected decisions to make when they discover they are pregnant.

After the initial period of discovering that she is pregnant, a woman and those around her have many decisions to make, many of which are guided by the health practitioners she seeks advice from. In Aotearoa New Zealand, midwives are the key health practitioners who work with women throughout their childbearing experience, but many other health practitioners may also be involved in different aspects of **maternity care**. Effective communication is vital for all health practitioners who are communicating with women, especially in this period of her life. To communicate effectively requires excellent listening skills so that communication can be meaningful and sensitive. Parents need to be provided with unbiased information which will enable them to make informed choices about their maternity care.

Maternity care
The care of the woman and her child through pregnancy and for a period beyond birth (postnatal).

Transition to motherhood

Childbearing, the period of time from **conception** until after the birth, has been identified in the literature as a major life event that can bring about many challenges for the woman and her family (Darvill, Skirton & Farrand, 2010). Pregnancy has been viewed as a developmental stage with its own developmental tasks. Both the pregnant mother and father deal with significant life changes and major psychological and social adjustment. According to developmental theories, the pregnant woman prepares for her new role through accomplishment of the developmental tasks during her pregnancy to successfully incorporate a maternal identity in her personality. One well-known theory was developed in the 1960s by Reva Rubin. Rubin (1984) identified four maternal phases that a woman goes through as she adapts to her pregnancy and prepares for her role as a mother (see Table 2.1).

Childbearing The process of pregnancy and birth.

Conception The point during the reproductive cycle at which an egg is fertilised.

TABLE 2.1 *Summary of Rubin's (1984) maternal phases in adaptation to pregnancy*

	Trimester 1	*Trimester 2*	*Trimester 3*
1 Seeking safe passage for herself and her child through pregnancy, labour and birth 2 Ensuring the acceptance of the infant by others 3 Seeking acceptance of self in her role as a mother 4 Learning to give of herself	Concentration on mother's well-being Dealing with physical symptoms	• Concerns about the baby and birth • Responsibility to protect the baby • Baby identified as separate to mother	• Bond established between mother and baby • Safe passage of mother and baby • 'Nesting' behaviour

Another theory of the way that women adapt to pregnancy and motherhood has been proposed by Lederman and Weis (2009), whose framework incorporates several psychosocial dimensions:

+ the woman's acceptance of her pregnancy
+ her motivation to take on the role of motherhood
+ her relationship with her husband/partner

+ relationships between the pregnant woman and her own mother
+ preparation for labour
+ self-esteem and sense of control.

In our society, being in control of what happens in our lives is seen as very important (McAra-Couper, 2007). When a woman becomes pregnant there are some things which she will inevitably not be able to control. It is widely believed that a woman has control over when and if she becomes pregnant through the use of contraception ('birth control'), yet one-third of pregnancies are unplanned and a significant number of women cannot get pregnant at the time that they want to. Conception itself is only partially controllable.

Once she is pregnant, many physical and emotional changes occur that a woman cannot control at all. In one study, Darvill, Skirton and Farrand (2010) found that women who had previously regarded themselves as fit and healthy felt that they had lost control over their bodies in the first **trimester** of pregnancy, due to the onslaught of the physical symptoms and body changes that occurred. According to Darvill, Skirton and Farrand (2010), women sometimes feel more vulnerable to physical harm, and their need to protect the foetus also contributes to their lack of control over their circumstances. As the pregnancy progresses into the second and third trimesters, a mother shifts her focus from her own physical symptoms and self-image to the needs of her unborn baby.

Trimester A period of three months within a pregnancy of nine months.

Parratt and Fahy (2011) critique theories of transition to motherhood, such as those of Rubin and Lederman and Weiss, because they propose that such theories reduce women to a prescribed role: that of being a 'predetermined type of mother' (p. 5). Parratt and Fahy posit that 'transition to motherhood' theory is oriented to stages that are presented as if they were unalterably 'true', when, in reality, they have been predetermined according to socially constructed ideals. Theories about adaptation to pregnancy may devalue the joy and meaning that can be inherent in the here-and-now, moment-to-moment lived experience. If we focus on pregnancy as a developmental stage, then some factors that are of central importance to childbearing women—such as 'inner power' and 'inner knowing', or women's intuition—are excluded as 'not real' or 'non-existent' and therefore become invisible.

The narrative of pregnancy

Health practitioners need to be cognisant of the major life change that pregnancy represents for a woman and those around her, whether the pregnancy is planned or unplanned. The importance of good communication in **antenatal** care is well

Antenatal The period of time before birth.

recognised (Levine et al., 2010) and is fundamental to the Aotearoa New Zealand midwifery partnership model (Guilliland & Pairman, 1995). During pregnancy it is an essential part of communication to develop trust, so that the woman feels comfortable to honestly talk about how she is feeling about the pregnancy, which might be ambivalence, coping with physical changes, body image changes and lifestyle changes. She needs to feel that she can trust the health practitioner so that she can disclose medical and social information of a personal nature.

Pregnancy is not an illness. Communication between health practitioners and the pregnant woman and her partner needs to emphasise accessible and appropriate information that will facilitate informed decision-making for pregnancy and birth. Effective communication encompasses a variety of elements that include development of empathy in the health practitioner–woman relationship, shared decision-making and assurance of satisfaction in the outcomes of the encounter (Levine et al., 2010).

One window to a woman's real feelings is the way she tells her **narrative** (or story/history). The women's individual experience, which becomes apparent when a woman tells her narrative, provides an opportunity for health practitioners to learn about being sensitive to women's individual experiences. It is by recognising a woman's point of view through narratives that health practitioners can provide individualised care and genuine guidance. If a health practitioner relies just on *what* a client says, rather than *how* it is said, then an important aspect of what the client is really trying to convey may be missed, and the health practitioner's response may be routine or standardised (Gilkison, 2011).

Narrative An account or story of an experience or journey.

Listening to women's narratives

As practitioners it is important that we *really listen* to what people tell us. When clients tell us about their experiences, the way they tell their narratives are windows to their view of the world. As a health practitioner it is crucial to acknowledge the feelings that women have about their pregnancy and their thoughts about the future. When a woman tells her narrative (or gives her history), she will connect her experience with her feelings: for example, feelings of joy, sadness, aloneness or anger. When a practitioner *really listens* to those feelings, they acknowledge the centrality of affect and subjectivity in human ways of knowing.

Listening to client's narratives is one of the keys to effective communication. *Really* listening reveals much more than simply listening to the words that people use. We need to 'read between the lines' when we take a woman's pregnancy or maternity history. In Case study 2.1, try to 'read between the lines'.

FIGURE 2.1 *Elements of real listening*

Listening requires cognitive, emotional and intentional presence; sometimes called 'mindfulness'. Notice and understand nuances of language, the range of voice, variations of speech, tones and textures, sounds of joy and anger, mixtures of sadness and laughter, the edgy, uncertain words of fear, the myriad facial and body expressions ... the lengthy silences and continuous stream of words and all the ups and downs of ecstasy and misery.

Think about what is *not* said as well as what *is* said. The parts of stories which a person chooses to omit may tell us about the things which they have overlooked, not seen as important, or they may be too painful to talk about.

Look beyond the surface; a range of possible meanings accompanies each word, sentence and text that extends the range of possible experiences; what stands out in every story is what is meaningful to the listener and to the narrator.

Words matter—think about the words the narrator uses. The words chosen indicate attitudes, beliefs and hold hidden meanings. Listen to metaphors: 'the contractions were like waves', or 'the contractions were like hell'. What do these metaphors tell us about the experience?

Be open to the possibility of anything showing up ... Sit back and wait and listen. We have a tendency to see events or experiences as things which we already understand. We may jump to conclusions too quickly if we assume that we understand the problem.

Source: Diekelmann and Diekelmann (2009), Fiumara (1990), Gilkison (2011), Swenson and Sims (2003).

CASE STUDY 2.1

Emma's narrative

I knew inside me that I was pregnant. I had no idea when my period should have come, but felt like it had been ages. I'd been feeling weird and nauseous. Bill and I had had an on-and-off relationship. We had been living together but we would split up then have these passionate 'getting back togethers'. Gosh, I was only 18 and he was 19. Finally I plucked up enough courage to go to the Family Planning Clinic for a pregnancy test. I took along my jar of urine.

It was 30 years ago, but I can still see that nurse's face and hear her voice. Before she did the test she asked me if I hoped it would be positive or negative. I said 'negative' with a lump in my throat. She was out of the room for an eternity. She came back in and showed me the test. 'It shows you are pregnant,' she said. The room spun around me. All I could think of was how I was going to tell my parents. The nurse was talking to me about things like keeping the baby and adoption. I just wanted to get out of there and go and see my friend. On the bus, I was sure everyone was looking at me and knew. When I told my friend, she just said: 'Wow, you're going to have a baby.'

Interpreting the narrative

Emma's narrative includes phrases that are windows to how she is feeling about discovering she is pregnant. She uses the phrase: *finally I plucked up enough courage.* Emma felt she needed courage to go to the Family Planning Clinic. A person needs courage when they are fearful and Emma was fearful of the result of the pregnancy test, even though she suspected it would be positive. When the nurse asked her what she hoped the result of the test would be, Emma said, *'negative' with a lump in my throat.* She was fearful of going to the clinic, she needed *courage* to go there, and then she feared that the pregnancy test would be positive when she hoped it would be negative. Her emotional response gave her a physical feeling of a lump in her throat.

When the nurse took the urine from the room to do the test, Emma felt that the nurse was gone *out of the room for an eternity.* It was probably only a few minutes, but when a person is highly anxious time sometimes goes slowly, and at other times too quickly. When she heard the result was positive, she said *the room spun around me.* The nurse at this stage was talking to Emma about her choices and some decisions she might need to make. Because Emma was so emotionally distraught, she could not hear a word of the discussion, because all she *could think of was how she was going to tell her parents.*

It is not until the final sentence when Emma remembers her friend's words—*Wow, you're going to have a baby*—that there is a sense of the joy about the pregnancy. Emma has been thinking about the things she fears about being pregnant: telling her parents and her relationship with the father of the baby. It takes her friend's words to remind her that she is not just pregnant; she is going to have the joy of having a baby.

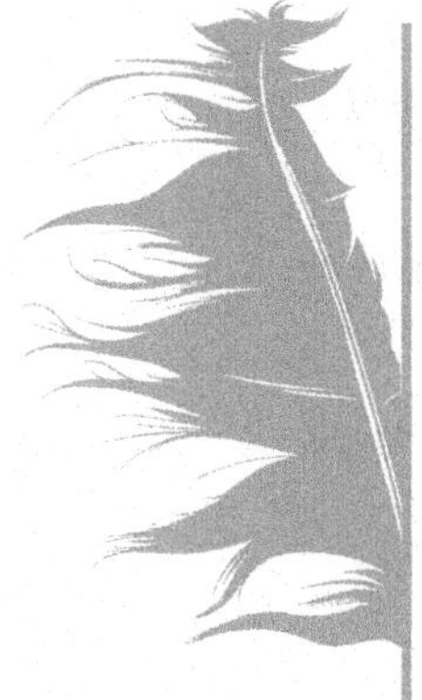

{ SUMMARY }

This chapter has explored some of the developmental theories and concepts that surround adaptation to pregnancy. While developmental theory offers one way of looking at the way a woman might adapt to her pregnancy and the transition to motherhood, some would say that a focus on theory may detract from an understanding of the uniqueness of each woman's individual experience. Women's narratives are windows to their individual experience, and listening to client's narratives is one of the keys to effective communication. If practitioners can learn to *really* listen to narratives—to interpret not only what is said but how it is said—then we can learn a lot about a person's feelings, and in turn provide care that responds to their individual needs. Emma's narrative shows how interpreting the way a narrative was told can uncover what is behind the actual words, and help practitioners to learn how to really listen.

REFLECTION POINTS

2.1 Intention (motivation, message, meaning, emotion)

Listening was described as listening to both what was said and what was not said. What do you think influences what is spoken of and what is not?

2.2 Reception (received message, response, feedback)

Elements of real listening—of listening with 'mindfulness'—involves listening to more than the words or content expressed. What other cues might you listen for?

2.3 Perception (style, manner, impression, analysis)

How might you check if your perception of what was 'not said' is accurate? What risks might this involve?

QUESTIONS FOR REVIEW

1 Do you think the nurse would have had an understanding of how Emma was feeling at the time?
2 What cues might you observe that would show a woman's feelings about coming for a pregnancy test?
3 When you read Emma's narrative, what struck you about the narrative? Were you surprised by anything?
4 What did you notice about the words she used or the way she said things?
5 Were you surprised about the things she did not say in her narrative?
6 How would you handle the situation?
7 How could you provide Emma with the information about her choices?

REFERENCES

Amin Shokravi, F., Howden Chapman, P. & Peyman, N. (2009). A comparison study: Risk factors of unplanned pregnancies in a group of Iranian and New Zealander women. *European Journal of Scientific Research, 26*(1), 108–21.

Darvill, R., Skirton, H. & Farrand, P. (2010). Psychological factors that impact on women's experiences of first-time motherhood: A qualitative study of the transition. *Midwifery, 26*(3), 357–66. DOI:10.1016/j.midw.2008.07.006.

Diekelmann, N. & Diekelmann, J. (2009). *Schooling, learning, teaching: Toward narrative pedagogy.* Bloomington, IN: iUniverse.

Fiumara, G. C. (1990). *The other side of language: A philosophy of listening* (C. Lambert, trans.). New York, NY: Routledge.

Gilkison, A. (2011). *Implementing a narrative-centred curriculum in an undergraduate midwifery programme: A hermeneutic study* (doctoral thesis). AUT University, Auckland.

Guilliland, K. & Pairman, S. (1995). *The midwifery partnership: A model for practice*. [Monograph Series 95/1]. Wellington, NZ: Victoria University Press.

Lederman, R. & Weis, K. (2009). *Psychosocial adaptation to pregnancy: Seven dimensions of maternal role development* (3rd edn). New York, NY: Springer.

Levine, M. D., Marcus, M. D., Kalarchian, M. A., Houck, P. R. & Cheng, Y. (2010). Weight concerns, mood, and postpartum smoking relapse. *American Journal of Preventive Medicine, 39*(4), 345–51. DOI:10.1016/j.amepre.2010.05.023.

McAra-Couper, J. (2007). *What is shaping the practice of health professionals and the understanding of the public in relation to increasing intervention in childbirth?* (doctoral thesis). AUT University, Auckland.

Parratt, J. A. & Fahy, K. M. (2011). A feminist critique of foundational nursing research and theory on transition to motherhood. *Midwifery, 27*(4), 445–51.

Rubin, R. (1984). *Maternal identity and the maternal experience*. New York, NY: Springer.

Swenson, M. & Sims, S. (2003). Listening to learn: Narrative strategies and interpretive practices in clinical education. In N. Diekelmann (ed.), *Teaching practitioners of health care: New pedagogies for the health professions* (vol. 2, pp. 154–93). Madison, WI: University of Wisconsin.

WEBSITES

Choosing an LMC, Kiwi Families: www.kiwifamilies.co.nz/Topics/Pregnancy/Choosing+an+LMC.html
Pregnancy, birth and baby care, Te Ara: www.teara.govt.nz/en/pregnancy-birth-and-baby-care
Your Antenatal Guide, OHBaby!: www.ohbaby.co.nz/pregnancy/your-antenatal-guide

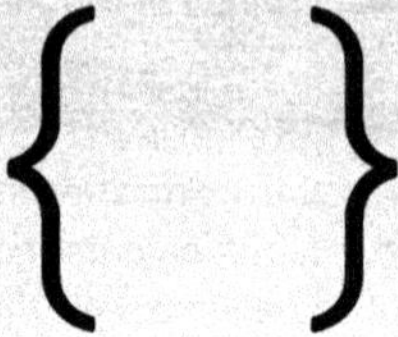

Birth and the Neonate

Annabel Farry and Claire Hotchin

CHAPTER OVERVIEW

This chapter covers the following topics:

+ Birth
+ Supportive communication
+ First communication following birth
+ Early neonatal communication
+ Communicating with babies
+ Practitioners interacting with babies
+ A Māori perspective.

KEY TERMS

Birth
Whānau
Latent phase
Lead Maternity Carer
First stage of labour
Transition
Second stage of labour
Crowning
Behavioural empathy
Sensitive period
Neonatal
Attuned
Post partum

The **birth** of a new family member challenges parents, **whānau** and those supporting them to interact and communicate in new ways that are appropriate to this everyday yet extraordinary event. Comforting communication between a labouring woman and her caregivers helps to create an environment in which she feels safe to become out of control. Losing control is essential to attaining the powerful primal state of birth.

Birth The process of a baby leaving the mother's body.

Whānau Either family and extended family and significant others, or to be born or give birth.

Birth

Birth is an involuntary process that occurs when a complex hormonal combination is released by the hypothalamus and pituitary gland, which are primitive parts of the brain that humans share with all other mammals.

CASE STUDY 3.1

Responses to hormones

Catecholamines (the adrenalines) are vasodilators. Humans respond to fear, whether it is rational or not, by releasing adrenaline. Adrenaline makes mouths dry, eyes widen, sends blood to the skeletal system and leads to a heightened state of awareness.

Oxytocin is responsible for the contraction of the smooth muscle fibres of the uterus and plays a role in creating a sense of calmness and connection.

Endorphins are the body's own opiates. Their levels in the blood stream increase as labour progresses. Without them, labour would be far more painful, and women would therefore be unable to relax enough to allow progress. Endorphins are responsible for the altered state women experience in labour.

Prolactin is involved with initiating and maintaining lactation. It serves multiple roles in mediating care of the offspring, from 'nesting' to the aggressive response mothers have if their offspring are exposed to any threat.

When there are inhibitions in the birth process, they often originate in the 'new brain' or the neocortex. This is the part of the brain responsible for rational thought and decision-making, and is highly developed in humans (Odent, 1999). Women giving birth are not unwell: they are experiencing a normal life event that can be explained in terms of several stages.

Latent phase The period of time prior to labour becoming established.

Lead Maternity Carer The qualified professional identified as providing primary care for a woman during pregnancy, labour and the post-partum period.

First stage of labour The period of time from when contractions become established until the cervix is fully dilated.

The **latent phase** can go on for many hours, sometimes even days, before regular strong contractions begin. The mother is often nervous, and wise communication can play a major role in supporting her. If her fear levels remain high, so will the levels of adrenaline, causing vasoconstriction and a reduction in uterine blood flow and uterine activity (Mander, 1998). A **Lead Maternity Carer** (LMC) can be very effective during this phase by calming both the woman and her support people. She may do this by reminding everyone that labour can take many hours and to look after themselves and each other. It is also useful to promote a sense of 'everydayness' by seeing the woman at home, reassuring her, and encouraging her to go for a walk, have a bath, hold a hot water bottle, enjoy a massage from a support person or just go to sleep.

The **first stage of labour** begins with the onset of regular and strong contractions that dilate the cervix, and finishes when the cervix is fully dilated. The birthing woman has now moved into an altered state of consciousness. She may be loudly vocalising her sensations or quietly breathing through them.

It is at this point where support people declare themselves. Seeing the person they love experiencing pain can cause a number of responses. Some will try to rescue the person from her experience by reminding her of all the pain relief options available. Others will become hyper talkative to cover up their sense of inadequacy. Others may fall asleep. Some may become angry and try to find answers for what they feel is unacceptable. All these responses are due to fear of pain and a lack of awareness about how long a birth can take. A good support person will be able to continue to 'be with' the woman by responding to her but not reacting to her, while continuing to take care of themselves.

Transition The part of labour between the first and second stages.

Transition is the word used to describe the period of time when the woman's body is moving from the first stage to the second stage of labour. Her cervix is almost fully dilated and she is beginning to feel the pressure of her baby on her pelvic floor. As the baby is pushed down the birth canal, past the last centimetre of cervix and onto the muscles of the pelvic floor, women often become overwhelmed and frightened. Women in transition make statements like:

+ 'I've had enough.'
+ 'I can't do this.'
+ 'This is too intense.'
+ 'Please help me.'
+ 'Get me an epidural.'
+ 'How much longer?'

It is at this point that an LMC will use their wisdom to decide what kind of communication is required to help the woman make it through this transition. She may engage all support people to surround the woman with encouraging, loving and strengthening words. She may step in and ask the woman to make direct eye contact with her and breathe with her through each contraction, thus keeping her in the moment and avoiding panic. She may remind her of the physiology of this stage and that the intensity is encouraging as it suggests excellent progress. She may acknowledge the difficulty of this stage of labour and remind her that these sensations are normal and that they will pass. She may use distractions, focusing her mind on a specific task like emptying her bladder. Helping her to the bathroom and back (she will experience contractions along the way) may take her into the next stage.

The **second stage of labour** is from full dilation of the cervix until the baby is completely born. The high state of despair that can occur during transition passes into a very focused bearing down in second stage, when the woman usually gets an overwhelming urge to push during her contractions. Her sounds become more guttural and lower pitch. With each contraction the baby advances and eventually **crowning** occurs.

Second stage of labour The part of labour between full dilation of the cervix and the birth of the baby.

Crowning When the top of the baby's head becomes visible during birth.

Some women manage the second stage of labour and the actual birth of their baby with minimal guidance; they understand instinctively how to gently ease their baby over this threshold, thus minimising the risk of tearing their perineum. Other women need specific guidance at this stage and may later recall not hearing anything but their LMC's voice gently guiding them to 'push or pant'. This intricate three-way communication between the mother, her baby and her health practitioner is, for most women, the period of most intense sensation. This is also when all four hormones are at their peak levels in both the mother and baby's blood stream. Wide eyed with adrenaline, euphoric with endorphins and replete with oxytocin and prolactin, mother and baby make eye contact and an intense bond forms with their mutual gaze.

CASE STUDY 3.2

The importance of support in labour

In 2007, the Cochrane Review of sixteen trials, which involved 13,391 women in eleven countries, concluded that women who experienced continuous one-to-one support during labour:

- were more likely to give birth without using analgesia or anaesthesia
- were more likely to have a spontaneous vaginal birth
- were less likely to report dissatisfaction with their childbirth experiences
- experienced slightly shorter labours.

Common elements of the care provided by these support people include emotional support, information about labour progress and advice regarding coping techniques, comfort measures and advocacy.

The report does not list any adverse effects and states that none are plausible, so it's clear that continuous support during labour provides definite benefits with no attendant risks. It concludes that 'all women should be allowed and encouraged to have support people with them continuously during labour' (Hodnett et al., 2007)

Supportive communication

It would seem obvious that an event of such personal magnitude involving such extreme sensations and of such a fundamentally private nature would require some support from trusted loved ones; however, just two generations ago women were expected to experience labour alone. Women were isolated from loved ones and birth happened to them in an environment over which they had no control. Many routine interventions were imposed unnecessarily and babies were separated from their mothers for long periods between feeds.

In Aotearoa New Zealand many changes have occurred in the last two decades. It is now respected that because the powerful process of labour produces a new family member, family should be central to the event. Often there will be many family members waiting to meet their new sibling, grandchild, niece or nephew. Family are now expected to play a role in the process—if the mother has chosen to have them with her. The LMC often needs to communicate not only with the mother and the father of the baby but also with other significant family members. There may be a language barrier to navigate, in which case the LMC should use a translator (either a professional or a family member) to keep up a healthy dialogue.

During pregnancy the LMC should discuss labour at length. She should listen to what the woman wants for her labour, share information with the woman and spend time helping her make the choices that will form her birth plan. This plan may change, but it begins the process of mutual trust that is essential to a positive birth experience.

Behavioural empathy Actions that demonstrate an understanding or genuine appreciation of the experience of others.

Experienced LMCs often practice a deliberate empathic response termed **behavioural empathy** (Burleson & Holmstrom, 2008) to encourage a woman to feel safe enough to enter into an altered state of consciousness.

Comforting measures should:

+ be highly person-centred; that is, verbal strategies should acknowledge, contextualise and legitimise the feelings of the distressed other
+ involve statements of positive regard, esteem, admiration for the courage or effort shown, understanding the difficulty of the task and confidence that the other will prevail
+ include non-verbal behaviours such as forward body leans, touches and pats, hugs and hand-holding, focused looks and soothing sounds.

During labour some women become completely internal and do not want any encouraging words or touch. They become completely immersed in their sensations, displaying an instinctive need to find a place of safety. Others are fiercely protective of their internal environment during labour. They will respond to disturbance as though it is a threat to their life. They may swear or make commands like 'Don't touch me' or 'Stop talking' or 'Go away'. While this communication may be unthinkable to the woman in a day-to-day context, there is an altered arrangement during labour. Sometimes support people may experience communication from the mother during labour as hurtful. But, more often, it is clear that there is a sacred transformation occurring; the woman's voice is resonant and powerful. The most respectful approach to supporting women during birth is to believe that the woman knows what she needs. Giving birth is a significant event that can have lasting effects on those involved. It has been said that 'birth is not only about making babies. Birth also is about making mothers—strong competent capable mothers, who trust themselves and know their inner strength' (Katz Rothman, 1996, p. 254).

First communication following birth

Universally, one of the first reactions mothers have after the birth of their babies is a desire to look into their baby's eyes. Already familiar with the voices of their parents, the baby gazes back intently. With loving touch and kind words, this gentle welcome to the world tells the baby they are in a safe place. This time, immediately after birth, is a psycho-physiologically **sensitive period**, which floods the baby's senses with the experience (gentle or rough) of being in the world, helping them to stabilise metabolically, and allowing them to initiate breastfeeding.

Sensitive period
A developmental period where particular impressions are most likely to occur and therefore relevant behaviour learnt.

The optimal place for this transition to happen is skin to skin on the mother's chest. Skin-to-skin contact (SSC) involves gently placing the naked baby prone on the mother's bare chest, facilitating interaction through all the senses: touch, smell, sight, hearing and taste. The ideal environment for this to happen is warm, safe, private and uninterrupted.

CASE STUDY 3.3

Early skin-to-skin contact

Skin-to-skin contact (SSC) stabilises and maintains the newborn's heart rate, respiratory rate, blood pressure and blood sugar. A newborn cannot regulate its own temperature; however, a mother in SSC with her infant will increase or decrease her temperature in response to her baby's temperature, in order to maintain the baby's temperature at ideal levels. Babies who experience SSC with their mothers are less likely to cry. Newborn reflexes help the baby who is in SSC move to the breast (stepping reflex), find the nipple (rooting reflex) and begin suckling (sucking and swallow reflex). Breastfeeding, in addition to providing optimal nutrition, fosters early bonding via touch, responsiveness and mutual gazing (Moore, Anderson & Bergman, 2011).

Early neonatal communication

Neonatal Relating to the period of life from birth to 28 days.

Sensory experiences, both negative and positive, from late pregnancy through the **neonatal** period and into the first three years of life, have a direct impact on how a child's brain develops. Nature and nurture work together; both genes and experience are important. A child's early experiences are critical for their brains to form the connections they need to develop. As experiences are repeated, the connections, pathways and networks in a baby's brain strengthen and become permanent (Rowley, 2009).

Responsive tender care from parents or a consistent caregiver creates effective, loving and lasting parents for an infant. Oxytocin is produced by both mothers and babies and increases bonding, setting the scene for the child to develop lasting attachments with others. Being soothed, comforted and responded to allows the baby to feel that they are welcome, loved and wanted. Happiness, joy and responsive care are the experiences that wire the baby's brain to love and trust others. The mother's capacity to create joy, elation, interest and excitement in a baby is key to early healthy development and lifelong physical and mental health.

Neglect, chaotic environments, violence and abuse (lack of attachment) create experiences of persistent stress, danger and fear, and signal the baby to release adrenaline and cortisol (fight or flight hormones). Cortisol in increased amounts over long periods is toxic to neurons, and growing neurons are most sensitive. A prolonged excess of cortisol causes brain dysfunction and destruction. If the stress response is repeatedly triggered, it becomes the template for brain development. The child that experiences persistent stress lives in a constant state of alertness and arousal, watching for signs of danger. A lack of attachment in the first three years correlates to ongoing life problems marked by impulsivity, easy arousal, the unthinking release of aggression and an inability to establish firm trusting relationships with other humans (Perry, 2002).

Communicating with babies

At birth, babies are already communicating in non-verbal ways. All humans are prepared to send and receive messages long before the development of formal language. What on the surface looks like random behaviour is in fact highly organised. Babies communicate about how they experience the world, using all their senses to get to know their family and their environment. Touch is the first sense experienced and perhaps the last to leave as we die. Smell, taste, balance, hearing and vision follow in a sequence that completes development.

CASE STUDY 3.4

How newborns communicate

Eye contact

A newborn's visual abilities are fine-tuned for eye contact. They recognise faces and prefer to look at faces over any other object. A newborn can see best when an object is approximately 20–30 cm away; the distance a mother's face will be if she is cuddling her baby or breastfeeding. At this distance they can imitate facial expressions.

Hearing and understanding

Although babies are not able to understand words when they are born, they are able to discern emotions. Babies are attuned to the emotions of their caregivers as one of their skills to survive. They understand the feelings of caregivers by listening to tone of voice, looking at facial expressions and feeling the pace of their caregivers' breathing. It is not so much what is said, but how it is said that is being absorbed—not literally but emotionally.

Non-verbal communication signs

Babies are responsive to other people and very expressive in their facial movements and gestures. They have a wide range of facial expressions, including bliss, joy, pain, sadness, fear and curiosity. They use their bodies to communicate. Some of these body movements are reflexive and therefore involuntary (for example, babies startle in response to a loud sound and make a tight fist when something is placed in their palm), while others are developmental; for example, turning their head from side to side and raising it from a prone position.

While babies are all individual, there are some generally accepted behavioural signs of what they are communicating. A happy baby is physically relaxed—they may coo, smile and engage in eye contact. When a baby is tired, they may frown, yawn, rub their eyes and become agitated. When hungry, they lick their lips, open and close their mouth, suck their fists or clothing, turn their head from side to side and become restless. Stressed babies fidget, grimace, look away, become agitated, make jerky or thrashing movements and arch their backs. Crying is a late communication sign for tired, hungry and stressed babies. Crying is always a sign of distress and a need for attention. Extended crying is physiologically harmful. It results in hoarseness, reduced oxygen levels, increased heart rate, disturbed digestion and drained energy. It also floods the baby with cortisol, which negatively affects their developing brain (Ludington-Hoe, Cong & Hashemi, 2002).

Despite being born with the capacity for feeling deep emotions, babies are unable to keep themselves in a state of equilibrium, lacking the skills to regulate either the intensity or the duration of those emotions. Without the assistance and responsiveness of a caregiver, babies become overwhelmed by their emotional states, including those of fear, excitement and sadness. When overwhelmed, and separated from their caregiver, they go into a despair–withdrawal response. If their despair (crying) is not answered, they withdraw. Physiologically, they release high levels of cortisol, become cooler, drop their heart rate and become quiet. A quiet and withdrawn baby may not be one that has learnt to be 'good' but one that is experiencing despair (Grille, 2008).

In order to maintain emotional equilibrium, babies require a consistent and committed relationship with one caring person, usually the mother. As the mother tunes into her baby's internal states, her responses produce a response in the baby. One is not independent of the other, and each has a profound effect on the next response. Healthy attachment is simply the development of that **attuned** relationship. Attunement, in the simplest terms, means following baby's cues. When a child looks, reaches, gestures, makes a sound or uses facial expression, this is a non-verbal conversational turn and our response keeps the conversation going. Engaging a baby in meaningful 'give and take' interactions helps their social, emotional and cognitive development.

Attuned The state of being particularly aware of the needs of others.

Babies are equal partners in communication and have their own spontaneous expressions of themselves. Their emotional experience (for example, pain, pleasure, joy or sorrow) is a total body experience. Babies do not pretend or manipulate. What they communicate is emotionally honest and immediate. They cannot plan ahead, have no concept of time and are not equipped to wait. When people respond warmly and promptly to these expressions, they communicate understanding of what the baby is doing, feeling and even thinking. This acknowledges that the baby's feelings are as important as adults'.

Practitioners interacting with babies

Adult communication needs to be adapted to the needs of newborns. Babies thrive on responsiveness, dependability and warmth. When a baby is responded to with tenderness, warmth and love, their body is flooded with pleasurable hormones and their brain forms the connections that they need to develop into a flexible, responsible, empathetic, loving, independent and intelligent member of society.

The early childhood years profoundly affect adult life and in turn affect society as a whole. Health practitioners have a responsibility to share this important information with parents and whānau. Learning to be a parent means learning a new set of skills. Parents and whānau can be supported in the early weeks by enabling mother and baby to be together and maximising their opportunity to bond. Some parents need more help than others to interact responsively with their babies. Teaching and encouraging parents **post partum** how to recognise and respond to their baby's communication cues, how to soothe their baby, and how to interact lovingly and playfully with their baby supports the family from the beginning.

Post partum The period following birth.

Breastfeeding gives the optimal start for a baby's growth, providing exactly what the baby needs for brain growth, as well as providing the sensory pleasure of being held, gazed at and talked with. Parents need support, energy and resources to be able to cope and respond appropriately to babies. Practitioners need to be alert to any potential problems that make it difficult for mothers to cope—for example, depression or living in a violent situation—in order to provide support and early on build parenting skills.

Practitioners also have a responsibility to role model appropriate communication with, and handling of, newborns. When performing procedures on a baby, they need to touch the baby gently, tell them what they are going to do, monitor their response throughout the procedure and stop if necessary. There is never a reason to handle babies in an insensitive mechanical way that disregards their integrity.

A Māori perspective

Pre-colonial Māori surrounded birth with complex rituals and practices that paid respect to the gods of nature (atua) and encouraged the labouring mother to let go, and to give up control over the process to the gods. For many Māori this rich complexity has been lost along with elements of language and culture as a result of colonisation. Within the language, birth is acknowledged as a fundamental part of life. The word 'whenua' means both placenta and land, the word 'hapu' means both pregnant and subtribe, and the term 'whare tangata' means both womb and ancestral meeting house. This meeting house sits at the centre of the marae (sacred open meeting area), which is central to Māori communities. Respect for whenua (both land and placenta), whakapapa (genealogy), tipuna (ancestors) and whanaungatanga (extended family) keep birth in a normal context, while at the same time respecting it as sacred and otherworldly.

Māori who identify as tangata whenua (people of the land) retain a connection to pre-colonial ways of understanding the natural environment. Māori women have been at the forefront in resisting what they see as the encroachment of science into areas of life governed by forces beyond its control. For Māori, the process of birth is one of the most sacred of all such areas of life. Māori women give birth with less intervention than any other ethnicity in Aotearoa (Ministry of Health, 2010). Encouragement during birth is communicated through karakia (prayer), waiata (song), meri meri (massage), calming words and by loving, present physical contact.

One practice that has become almost mainstream is that of returning the whenua (placenta) to the whenua (land). This communicates a deep respect to papatuanuku (mother earth) for the nurturing of this pepe's (baby's) life into Te Ao Marama (the world of light). While many ethnicities practise this ritual, using a tree to mark a spot for their child to visit in years to come, Māori most often bury the whenua in a place with ancestral connections, showing respect for the tipuna who are acknowledged as having a continued place in this child's life.

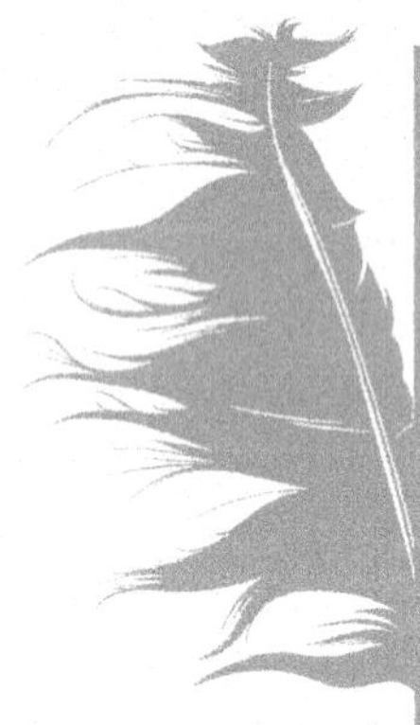

{ SUMMARY }

Continuous support during labour by trusted support people and using comforting communication will encourage the mental relinquishment necessary to achieve physiological labour and birth. Newborns come into this world with the ability to communicate and respond. Consistent, responsive, nurturing, positive, rich experiences in the first three years of life are essential for optimal brain development, resulting in flexible, responsible, empathetic and intelligent members of society. The neonate is an aware, dependent, vulnerable human being who is born with the ability to communicate. Optimal lifelong social, emotional and physical functioning depends upon positive early life experiences in a loving and consistent environment.

REFLECTION POINTS

3.1 Intention (motivation, message, meaning, emotion)

While infants may not understand the meaning of words spoken, they are able to interact. What benefits are there to both mother and baby in sharing skin-to-skin contact at birth?

3.2 Reception (received message, response, feedback)

The newborn infant is described as being born with the ability to communicate. How does a newborn baby convey that it is content?

3.3 Perception (style, manner, impression, analysis)

How might health practitioners role model appropriate communications with a newborn infant?

QUESTIONS FOR REVIEW

1 A 4-week-old baby is brought into the busy health clinic by her mother for a 'Well Child Check'. She is late for her appointment. The baby is crying. The mother is stressed. How would you respond to this mother and baby?

2 You have agreed to be your best friend's support person during her labour. She tells you she is scared of being in pain and out of control. How will you respond?

REFERENCES

Burleson, B. & Holmstrom, A. (2008) Comforting Communication. In W. Donsbach (ed.), *The International Encyclopedia of Communication*. Blackwell Reference Online. Retrieved 12 March 2011 from http://www.communicationencyclopedia.com/public/tocnode?id=g9781405131995_yr2011_chunk_g97814051319958_ss50-1. DOI: 10.1111/b.9781405131995.2008.x.

Grille, R. (2008). *Heart to heart parenting*. Sydney: ABC Books.

Hodnett, E. D., Gates, S., Hofmeyr, G. J. & Sakala, C. (2007). Continuous support for women during childbirth. *Cochrane Database of Systematic Reviews*, issue 3, art. no. CD003766. DOI: 10.1002/14651858.CD003766.pub2.

Katz Rothman, B. (1996). Women, providers and control. *Journal of Obstetric, Gynecologic and Neonatal Nursing, 25*(3), 253–6.

Ludington-Hoe, S. M., Cong, X. & Hashemi, F. (2002). Infant crying: Nature, physiologic consequences, and select interventions. *Neonatal Network, 21*(2), 29–36.

Mander, R. (1998). *Pain in childbearing and its control*. Oxford, UK: Blackwell Science.

Ministry of Health. (2010). *Maternal and newborn information 2003*. Report on Maternity. Wellington, NZ. Retrieved 14 December 2006 from www.nzhis.govt.nz/publications/maternityreport03.pdf.

Moore, E. R., Anderson, G. C. & Bergman, N. (2011). *Early skin-to-skin contact for mothers and their healthy newborn infants*. Retrieved 18 February 2011 from www2.cochrane.org/reviews/en/ab003519.html.

Odent, M. (1999). *The scientification of love*. London, UK: Free Association Books.

Perry, B. D. (2002). Childhood experience and the expression of genetic potential: What childhood neglect tells us about nature and nurture. *Brain and Mind, 3*, 79–100.

Rowley, S. (2009). *The early years—how experience shapes the brain*. Retrieved from http://brainwave.org.nz/wp-content/uploads//2009/10/Chronicle-July-2009-English.pdf.

WEBSITES

Centre for Attachment: www.centreforattachment.com
Liggins Institute: www.liggins.auckland.ac.nz/uoa
The Early Years and Brain Development, Brainwave: http://brainwave.org.nz

READING 11

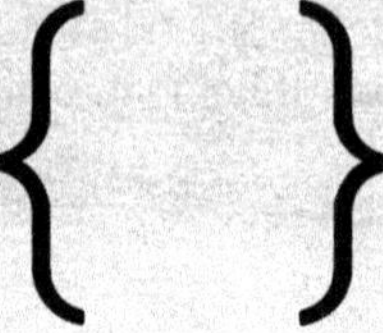

Communicating with Babies and Young Children

Rain Lamdin and Rachel Lamdin Hunter

CHAPTER OVERVIEW

This chapter covers the following topics:

+ Social and cultural contexts of childhood
+ Social context and learning
+ Understanding communicating and language
+ Getting older: 3 years and on
+ Communication through play.

KEY TERMS

Family
Attachment
Vocabulary
Play

Communication with babies and toddlers can be rewarding, puzzling or fraught with anxiety, depending on our understanding of the capabilities and needs of children and babies, and also upon our perception of our abilities or experiences. In this chapter we focus on the developing communication of babies and children, and refer to theories of child development where they are directly relevant to communication. We also consider real-life examples of child-focused practice and communication. Life patterns are established in these early years; therefore communicating respectfully and with an understanding of a baby or young child's development is extremely important. This chapter is written with a predominantly Pakeha perspective, influenced by Western theories. We acknowledge the importance of an awareness of differences in communication styles between and across cultures in ethical health-care practice.

There are three points that underpin our views of communication with babies and children. First, the baby or child is a member of a **family**; they come from, refer to, learn within and explore their worlds as part of that family. Second, non-verbal communication is constant and informative. Finally, whether we are child or adult, we are already and always communicating.

Family A close social grouping of people who are related genetically, emotionally or culturally and who provide basic support for one another.

Social and cultural contexts of childhood

How children are perceived in terms of their dependence or vulnerability affects how adults communicate with them and what they expect in return. It is common for adults to consider people as being children until they are in their teen years. Typically, children between the ages of 12 and 18 months are considered babies, while those under 3 or 4 years are deemed toddlers. In Aotearoa New Zealand, children under 5 years are 'preschoolers'. Most children begin primary school at the age of 5 years; however, 6 years is the legal requirement. Socially and legally, children lack certain rights or responsibilities that adults possess. It is common in Western nations to think of working for money or taking care of family members as being the domain of adults, even though in many parts of the world children are expected to carry out caregiving duties and contribute economically to the family.

'Childhood' was not a clear phenomenon until the late seventeenth or early eighteenth centuries. During medieval times, children may have worked for money, attended school infrequently (if at all, depending on their place within the family or society) and carried their own weapons, along with being accountable for any crimes they may have committed (Aries, 1962). The emergence of developmental theory, in which children were held as developmentally incomplete and thus incompetent (in relation to adults), probably contributed to the positioning of children as dependent, vulnerable beings—a common view held today.

Theories that focus upon child development are inevitably formulated by theorists and researchers who are adults. Accordingly, theories of communication development are told from the perspective of the adult 'looking in' on the child's world. Theorists and researchers need to take care to understand and acknowledge their own beliefs about children and how they see themselves in relation to children. It is also important to acknowledge that various theories about development or communication may inadvertently disempower children, negatively influencing working relationships with them or their advocates.

TABLE 4.1 *Assumptions about children and possible effects on communication*

Commonly held assumptions or stereotypes of young children	*Possible effects on communication in practice with young children*
Children are incomplete humans—not fully developed and 'not there yet' as people.	Their wants and needs are seen as less important and may be over-ridden or disregarded.
Undeveloped verbal skills mean they have poor understanding of what is said or what happens to them.	Adults may not bother to explain our actions, procedures or rationales.
Undeveloped verbal skills mean that children cannot communicate or make their needs known to others.	Adults may not seek to understand or acknowledge the ideas, needs or questions of young children.

CASE STUDY 4.1

Human rights and children

Children's rights have been an international work in progress since 1924, initially through the League of Nations and now the United Nations. Human rights frameworks highlight children as rights-bearing individual citizens, rather than the moral property of adults such as their parents or caregivers. New Zealand and Australia became signatories to the United Nations Convention on the Rights of the Child in 1993 and 1990, respectively. The most recent version (United Nations, 2005) has several Articles that indirectly or directly relate to children and their rights within health care:

- Article 5 highlights the responsibilities of organisations to respond to children within the context of their family.

- Guardians, parents and extended family are responsible for the child and, as such, are integral in the decision-making process during the assessment, treatment and care of children.
- Articles 12 and 13 detail the rights of children to express their views and to seek, receive and impart information. This is not written with specific reference to health care; however, it is clearly relevant when caring for and working with young children.
- Article 24 is specifically written to address the rights of children to the access and attainment of health care, including access to information and education regarding their care.

The enactment of children's rights can be complicated when babies and young children are unable to demand that their rights be met. However, communication in health care is as much the right of a child as is access to health-care treatment. It is the professional responsibility of the health-care practitioner to uphold and advocate for such rights.

Social context and learning

Babies and young children are individuals, and learning how to communicate occurs in the context of their individual surroundings. Early family life is a rich setting for development, providing examples of communication including everyday language, intonation, meanings, mannerisms and values. Most communication in very early life is between babies and their caregivers and family members—those most intimately associated with the baby or young child.

CASE STUDY 4.2

Children, family and society

In 2003, New Zealand Members of Parliament undertook an historic vote overturning Section 59 of the Crimes Act 1961, which had provided a legal defence for parents charged with assault after physically disciplining their children. Redress for parents and caregivers to use 'reasonable force' when disciplining their children meant that parents could legally smack or hit their children, when in other such cases of assault they would be charged and convicted. Exactly what constituted 'reasonable force' was difficult for parents, lawmakers, police and judges to agree upon.

Several high-profile cases, in which parents escaped conviction after assaulting children with hosepipes, riding crops or electrical cords, contributed to growing public unease about the detriment caused to children by such treatment. The rights of society's most vulnerable citizens to live free of fear of such correction contrasted with the rights of parents to 'parent as they saw fit', along with anxiety that children would 'run amok' if not disciplined in particular ways. Implicit within each side of the hotly debated argument were contrasting views on the nature of children. However, both discourses acknowledged the crucial role that parents, caregivers and family play in teaching and shaping children as they grow.

One of the most dominant bodies of knowledge regarding the care of babies and communication arose from the child–caregiver work of John Bowlby (1951), following the Second World War. His work followed research carried out with children who were orphaned or otherwise separated from their parents across a variety of settings. Researchers observed that some indicators of developmental progress were delayed or absent in children who had spent long periods of time in unfamiliar or non-nurturing environments, such as hospitals, refugee camps or orphanages. In particular, the absence of intimate caregiver-type relationships was believed to interrupt the growth, development and health of such children. Such studies were linked with research indicating that adult well-being and mental health were related to childhood experience, primarily before the age of 3 years. Later attempts to restore such developmental input for children were often unsuccessful, promoting the view that children had a prime but limited window of developmental opportunity in their early years.

Bowlby claimed that a primary caregiver—specifically, the child's mother—must be available to respond to a young child's needs in order for them to thrive physically, cognitively and socially, and to avoid what he termed 'maternal deprivation' (Bowlby, 1951). This '**attachment**' bond between mother and child provides a secure social foundation from which children are able to safely explore new surroundings. The concept of attachment still features strongly in many approaches to parenting and understandings of child–parent relationships.

Attachment
Emotional affection and social bonds between people.

It is appropriate to acknowledge that this emphasis on attachment came from a Western perspective of what is 'good' or 'normal' child development. Within this context, growing up and becoming an individual, independent of the family, is highly valued. Children are encouraged to explore their worlds beyond the family and to be self-assured. However, these values are not common across all cultures. The research and analysis that underpins these views also requires some analysis. In Aotearoa New Zealand, for example, early childhood services cannot be compared with war orphanages in terms of stimulation and caring relationships between child and educator/carer (Claiborne & Drewery, 2010). Also, the mother role has been used in arguments for reducing women's place in the workforce, and continues to be an issue for women who are in the position to choose whether they wish to work outside the home.

For health practitioners working with babies and young children, an essential element of communication involves liaising with parents, caregivers and family members of the child. This is an ethical and legal requirement as parents must consent to assessment, investigations and treatment on behalf of their children. Parents need to feel heard, understood and validated in their knowledge of and relationship with their child. Children look to their parent to assess the risk of danger or to provide comfort in novel situations (Bretherton, 1992). Supporting parents to communicate with their child builds strength into the family, as the parent will continue the care and support of the child beyond their contact with the health-care professions and systems. Parents help to shape children's stories and memories of health care and in so doing heighten or allay anxieties.

Understanding communicating and language

A particular level of attention and intimacy is required in order for any baby-initiated messages to be understood. The child–caregiver relationship requires each person to be 'tuned in' to successfully interpret the non-verbal cues and signs that are essential means of communication.

The earliest expression of discomfort, fear or pain is found in crying. A baby may demonstrate particular qualities to their cry, such as a shrill pitch or particularly high volume and some individuals cry more than others. However, there are generally common qualities among certain cries in terms of tone, pitch and volume, indicating messages that are common to all babies at some stage.

TABLE 4.2 *Types of baby cries*

Need or reason for crying	*Type of cry*
Pain or discomfort	Loud, sudden, shrill; silence or long pause between each cry while breath is drawn in for the next cry
Hunger	Begins with an uneven, low-intensity, intermittent grizzle; gradually escalates to continuous wail, increasing in volume and intensity
Fatigue or overtiredness	'Grizzling': monotone of a medium even pitch; seemingly continuous but rises over time in pitch and volume if not attended to
Irritation, frustration or boredom	Can sound most like spoken language—some variances in pitch and volume as if conversing in words
Shock, fear or surprise	Preceded by a quick intake of breath and then a shallow shrill cry, similar but less intense than a pain or discomfort cry; also may have a grizzly, uneven quality

The frequency and duration of crying in young babies, while variable, is mediated by the responsiveness of the parent or caregiver to the baby's needs. When a baby's needs are met there is less need to cry. By the age of 2 months, some babies maintain eye contact with caregivers during feeding and other settled wakeful periods. When a person sustains such eye contact while speaking to the baby, and then pauses, it encourages the baby to 'reply', which models conversation. The baby's responses comprise 'cooing' or 'gurgling'. As the anatomy of the mouth and throat mature, the child's ability to make different sounds improves, resulting in babbling, usually between 4 and 6 months. By 4 months, such sounds may include giggling and laughing.

Even while babies are limited to crying, babbling or smiling, they are able to observe and form rudimentary understandings of what they experience through their senses. Babies communicate, noticing and imitating sounds and facial expressions of other people within the first few months of life, most often from their mother or primary caregiver. Table 4.3 describes common examples of early communication. It should be remembered that there is a wide variation of ages in which each stage is reached, so the milestones mentioned here are approximations.

TABLE 4.3 *Baby communication*

Age (approximate)	Features
6 weeks	First 'social smile'—a response to expressions from other people
3 months	Seeks eye contact with others
	May take turns to coo or gurgle with another person
6–8 months	May follow a pointed finger or look to where someone is referring or pointing
8 months	Notices other's conversations and listens
	Recognises surroundings and can show joy or excitement in response
	May understand simple instructions: 'No!' or 'Show me'
10 months	Can follow simple directions to give or show a toy to another person.
	May wave in response to a wave or direction

CASE STUDY 4.3

The 'nappy-free' baby

Elimination communication (EC) is a form of early communication that is used by some families with young babies. Parents adopting this method of caring for their baby spend time with the baby in close proximity, learning the baby's cues or body language signs preceding a bowel or bladder movement. Such cues include wriggling, sighing, appearing to struggle or even emitting a particular cry. The caregiver responds by holding the baby in a particular squatting position over the toilet or potty and using a chosen cue or sound (such as 'ssss') to signal to the baby that they can release and 'go'. Anecdotal supporters of this method claim that the saving of costs in nappies and the eliminated need for toilet training at age 2 (a challenging time for some families of young children) far outweigh the effort required to tune into and learn the baby's methods of communication. Such methods of toileting are commonplace across several cultures (Sun & Rugolotto, 2004).

In Aotearoa New Zealand, the success of such methods also depends upon the physical proximity of the primary caregiver (usually the mother) to the baby. Families utilising EC in Aotearoa New Zealand might experience some judgment from others not familiar with this philosophy of communication with babies, while families in which both parents have outside commitments (such as work) may find it difficult to be in the requisite proximity to the child in order for the method to be successful.

This example of communication with babies and young children highlights the range of cultural, functional and human elements that impact on communication with children.

Young children understand before they can communicate clearly (Buckley, 2003). Babbling includes a repetitive sound such as 'bababa' or 'nanana', initially using a limited range of consonants that are easy to pronounce. Babbling may occur in response to sounds or voices heard by the baby, or may be self-initiated. Using their voice purposefully may include 'calling' for the parent or caregiver when in another room. During excited or playful times, babies from about 6 months of age may begin to purposefully demonstrate their feelings by kicking, waving their arms, wriggling or turning away. The onset of crawling, usually between 8 and 12 months, enables babies to physically communicate their interest in, say, a family pet or their reluctance to have their nappy changed.

During the second half of the first year, communicative abilities expand to involve people other than the primary caregiver, including family members, other babies and strangers. After initially guarded responses to new people, some babies will actively seek contact with others. A baby may signal a desire for a toy by seeking eye contact with their caregiver and looking from the caregiver to the toy and back again. Reaching out or pointing may accompany the request, as well as babbling (Buckley, 2003, p. 30). Between 8 and 10 months, some babies will develop use of some early 'words', such as 'ohh!' or 'wow!' Even with murmurs rather than exact words, a questioning intonation can be used to express intent or interest, or ask a question such as 'May I have that?' or 'Where has it gone?' Such early sounds are often deemed by parents to be first words. Other early words may include names ('Mama', 'Dada'), consisting of short repetitive syllables that resemble early babbling. Other first words typically include those which have been spoken more commonly in front of or to the child, such as 'no', 'bye' or 'more'.

Approaching their first birthday, babies can begin to understand directions communicated to them by combining several techniques for interpretation, known as non-linguistic strategies (Buckley, 2003). Non-linguistic strategies include noticing facial expressions, gestures or movements used by the other person, and utilising their emerging knowledge of the context and what usually happens next. For example, a toddler picking up a toy bunny off her bedroom floor and showing it to her grandmother might hear 'Ohhh ... give him a cuddle'. Noticing the grandmother clasping her hands to her chest and putting her head to one side, as well as the facial and vocal expression of tenderness, the child may mimic her actions.

While initially understanding a direction in only one context, a child's understanding will grow to encompass a broader range of settings in which, for example, 'Give him (or her) a cuddle' is appropriate, such as when a friend is hurt in play. Over time, the child will rely less upon non-linguistic strategies and more upon verbal content, as knowledge of word meanings increases and the contexts in which the child finds themselves are extended.

CASE STUDY 4.4

Baby sign language

The use of sign language between mother and baby can be developed before oral communication is possible. Here, a mother (and aunt) describes her experiences.

> I watched my nieces communicate with their parents in their own way. It involved their hands, attempts at words and even simple and more meaningful eye contact. One niece and my sister-in-law could go a whole day without using words, such was their shared understanding and the use of eye contact and body language.
>
> With my own son, from a very early age I used very simple signs to indicate things I wanted him to understand. This included holding up one finger and saying, 'I will be back in one minute' if he was awake and I left him. I wanted him to understand that my leaving was temporary. I knew this went against what the developmental psychology theory said, given he was apparently too young to understand that objects exist even when he couldn't see them.
>
> One of the most important things I did early on, which I think helped our communication, was to make a lot of eye contact with him, always respond to him and talk a lot to him. This verbal and non-verbal communication was an effort to reinforce our ability to connect and communicate. While books

promote specific signs, we have developed our own. This wasn't intentional but intuitive, and the result is that my son has created his own signs. His signs are often obvious—licking his finger and closing his mouth to ask for food. When I am not sure what he is asking or talking about, I offer suggestions or ask him to show me and I learn. Now he is at the age of 2 years, we have little frustration with communicating. There are also other factors involved—he is a socially oriented and calm child. The key has been to pay attention to him and respond when he communicates.

Early baby **vocabulary** is also characterised by words that may be incomprehensible to others, but very familiar to family members. The child who wakes from their nap calling for 'Dahdah!' may be calling a pet named Poppy, yet this is only apparent to those in the child's immediate family. Such adopted terms must be translated for others. Some early words also include run-together phrases such as 'mo-more' ('no more'). A single term such as the exclamation 'mang!' may have a multiplicity of meanings, being used to comment on hearing a hammer being used, to complain that the child has just bumped their head or to signal their intent to shut a door. Children also begin to make noises or sounds when handling or identifying objects or toys. Similarly, using actions to accompany early words helps others to interpret meaning; for example, using 'bep-bep' to refer to a car when accompanied by the forward motion of a hand honking a car horn. The content of children's communication at this early stage is focused on the immediate and visible experiences of the child.

Vocabulary The collection of words and symbols that people use to communicate.

Piaget observed the development of his own children and identified stages of sensori-motor and cognitive development (Piaget, 1962). Piaget noticed a change in babies aged between 6 and 12 months in which they began to clearly notice the absence of an object or person after they had disappeared, which he termed 'object permanence'. Slightly older babies would look and then search for the object or person, clearly holding an image of it in their mind. This early mental representation signifies the beginning of symbolic thinking, in which children come to understand that objects, people and events have particular names or representations in language. Such a shift in understanding is believed to lead to rapid increases in understood vocabulary, coinciding with improved motor control of oral muscles (Buckley, 2003). While their own pronunciation remains messy, young children may notice others' pronunciation; for example, a mother using the toddler's term 'blana' for 'banana' may be reprimanded in no uncertain terms by the toddler!

The number of words understood by very young children is far greater than those able to be uttered by the child—a ratio of approximately four to one in children aged between

1 and 2 years. However, the uttered words also increase rapidly during this period. For example, at 13 months a toddler may have an understood vocabulary of about fifty words, but by 18 months the toddler will be able to *express* fifty words (Menyuk, Liebergott & Schultz, 1995). The ability to comprehend increasingly complex instructions or questions begins with simple one- and two-part instructions ('Pick up that letter and give it to Grandma') from about 18 months of age. Children may begin pointing to objects or bringing them to somebody and 'asking' for them to be named; some may attempt to pronounce the word.

Children's initial realisations give way over time to broader concepts of objects as being similar to some others, part of a greater set of objects, and with particular descriptors. For example, a child will learn in several stages (usually between 18 months and 3 years) that:

> 'This is called Molly.'
> 'This is a cat.'
> 'Not all cats are called Molly.'
> 'Molly is a white cat [not a ginger or tabby cat].'
> 'Molly is a cat [part of a large group of animals known as cats] who lives in a house.'

Teaching words or language to very young children can be restricted by their limited capacity to switch attention from one object to another. Caregivers mitigate this by joining the child to explain or use words that are in the child's current area of focus or interest. As children grow, their ability to look up from what they are doing and attend to something different becomes quicker and smoother.

Approaching their second birthday, children may attempt two word phrases, using different intonations to specify their meaning. For example, 'Mum car?' may denote a request to go in the car, while 'Mum car' indicates that the car belongs to Mum. Such early sentences demonstrate telegraphic speech, comprising mostly nouns, verbs and adjectives. Expressive capability in young children is enhanced when caregivers use the child's area of interest to build a conversation, taking turns to speak, waiting for the child to respond and adding to what they have said:

> Hannah (aged 2 and looking at a book): Look!
> Mum (aged 31 and feeling about 90): Oh, look! Maisey!
> Hannah: Maisey ...
> Mum: Maisey's off to a party.
> Hannah: Party ...
> Mum: Wearing her dress.
> Hannah: Party dress.

Getting older: 3 years and on

The size of a child's expressive vocabulary varies according to the type and amount of language to which the child is exposed. Children who are questioned, prompted to join conversations by taking turns to speak, and given positive feedback to what they say demonstrate a larger vocabulary than children from whom less participation is expected (Hart & Risley, 1980). Parents are encouraged to talk to, listen to and read to their children in order to build their understanding. Likewise, health practitioners who give simple, age-appropriate explanations and information to children—as well as time to process information and to ask questions—promote understanding and the capability to communicate.

Around the age of 3, most children begin to add descriptors, such as shapes or colours, to the objects they talk about. This is not always with accuracy. A 3-year-old still needs time to refocus on what the parent or caregiver is directing them to, while a child of 5 may be expected to follow instructions without having to first 'look up' from what she is doing (Buckley, 2003). Such focusing ability is an important skill for children when entering school and working in a busy classroom. Children also grow in their ability to 'repair conversation' (Buckley, 2003) by clarifying or repeating what they have said if not responded to by others, indicating their understanding that they have not been heard or regarded. Similarly, children learn to interrupt with increasing force in order to contribute to a conversation. While talking is often assumed to be the predominant form of communication, children adopt word use later than other communication methods. From the age of approximately 3 years, spoken language becomes the main form of communication for children.

The vocabulary of a 3-year-old is about 1000 words (Claiborne & Drewery, 2010). Some children use different tones of voice when addressing adults or peers, indicating an early understanding of some of the conventions associated with the social positioning of those with whom they communicate. At about this age, children can begin to respond appropriately to questions posed with the beginnings 'why', 'what', 'where' or 'when'. This is often the age when children begin to initiate stories about events, people or phenomena that are familiar or visible to them. Approaching the age of 5, a child will attempt an answer to increasingly complex questions, such as those beginning with 'how' or 'what if'.

Children at the age of 4 and 5 years are increasingly competent at remembering and relating a story as 'news' to interested adults or others. 'Show and tell' in kindergarten and new-entrant school settings is promoted as a way of developing the child's ability to begin, furnish and conclude a verbal account of an event or phenomenon (Claiborne & Drewery, 2010). Children's understanding of basic language concepts relating to time (when, before, during), space (beside, above) or quantity (too much, all, few) precede an emerging ability to understand and cooperate with increasingly specific or detailed instructions (Buckley, 2003).

Conversation provides a rich opportunity to test out children's understanding and interpretation of others' language. Older pre-schoolers attempt to negotiate or to convince others of their point using an increasing variety of questions and arguments, which is sometimes interpreted as challenging behaviour.

Approaching ages 4 and 5, children are likely to be in increasing contact with children of a similar age, and are able to adjust their language and intonation according to whether they are conversing with adults or younger children. Around this time questions directed to adults such as those beginning with 'why?' or 'what?' are as much an expression of the intent to interact with someone as actually seeking to understand a cause or phenomenon (Buckley, 2003). Children also become increasingly able to keep the attention of the other person with frequent questions. With an increased vocabulary, the child is able to name their feelings and this also contributes to their understanding of others' feelings, identified by non-verbal and verbal indicators. Considering this within health-care practice is important. Supporting children's expression of their feelings and thoughts will help to clarify their understanding of what is happening to them and why. We reiterate this as a moral and legal obligation.

CASE STUDY 4.5

Assessing young children

How do we assess babies and young people when we are unable to communicate with them in adult-to-adult ways?

If you apply the principles in this chapter, your first step may be to consider the best way to initially approach the child or baby. Parents convey to the child their acceptance or approval of your work, and have a primary role in giving permission for assessment. They should always be present and informed about what is going to happen. Surprise or distress in a parent will be noticed by the child and mirrored or reacted to accordingly. Caregivers will require explanations and the opportunity to have questions answered before they give their consent for you to work with their baby. Children should be given age-appropriate explanations and be invited to ask questions. Seeking the approval of a very young child may seem difficult, but must be attempted where possible.

Use your assessment skills to direct your communication with the child. Your ability to use your communication knowledge in forming rapport improves your chances of the child being happy, forthcoming and cooperative with you, the stranger.

Always consider how your body language is perceived by the child. For example, eye contact for you may indicate interest or respect, but be received as a threat, especially by children in unfamiliar surroundings such as hospital departments or clinics. Likewise, your height beside a small child can appear frightening, so sitting or crouching to speak to a child should be considered.

Children's experience of one health practitioner is rapidly applied to others. Children who are upset or frightened in the health-care setting may have had fearful experiences with others. Your way of being with the young child frames future experiences with health-care practitioners—another reason to be mindful of your attitude and ways of being with the child and their significant others.

Communication through play

Play Interaction and activity that is relaxed and entertaining.

Engaging in **play** is indicative of understanding and communicative ability in children as they grow older. Play provides an outlet for the expression and regulation of feelings, wishes or fears, and enables children to begin to understand the perspectives of others. When playing, older children practise talking and using their bodies to express themselves (Santrock, 2009). As a form of communication, play can be used by child health practitioners, caregivers and advocates as a means both for understanding and teaching.

Piaget stressed the role of play and the provision of opportunities for the child to internally process anxiety or conflict and to release tension (Piaget, 1962). Children practise different skills and use even solitary play conditions to literally talk to themselves (initially out loud and, later, silently), instructing, reflecting and even praising or berating themselves. Piaget referred to this as 'private speech' or 'inner speech'.

Vygotsky (1962) believed that, over time, inner speech becomes a taken-for-granted process of thinking that supports social and verbal communication. He believed that children who frequently engage in inner speech demonstrate better social communication abilities than those who do not. Piaget's theory of cognitive development is useful because of the concept of object permanence—a child's ability to remember and convey an image in asking for or searching for something is an example of developing communicative ability. Similarly, the work of Vygotsky and Piaget regarding inner speech provides an example of development facilitating communication skills.

Parten classified the ways in which children played, according to the types and levels of social interaction she observed in a study with children aged 2–5 years (Santrock, 2009), as depicted in Table 4.4.

TABLE 4.4 *Young children's play*

Type of play	*Example or explanation*	*Value to communication learning*
Solitary play	Studying a toy or book 'in their own little world'—the child appears uninterested in what is going on around them	Children engage in private speech that contributes to the regulation of emotions
Pretend play	Acting out an event in which children play parts—for example, in a game of 'going to the supermarket' the child may 'be' the mother and request the adult/other children to be the child or checkout assistant; older children will generate stories about less familiar/ unpractised events	Children are enabled to practise other perspectives or roles, such as 'being the mum' or 'telling the children off'
Parallel play	Playing alongside others with little interaction or conversation—children may use same or similar toys beside each other	The child's social development via an emerging awareness of other people is promoted
Associative play	Children focus their attention upon one another and play together with little or no organisation or set games	

As children grow older, their increased interaction with other children provides the challenge of having to share or take turns, negotiate understandings with a limited vocabulary, and respond to other's points of view, with a growing capacity to see a situation from another person's perspective. A final stage in Parten's framework, cooperative play, is generally seen in older children where two or more children will play together, rather than simply alongside one another. The communicative potential in children's play is typified in Parten's work by the continuity of children's communication, aspects of which may be missed or misinterpreted by others, including health practitioners.

There is no single theory of child communication. Theories about children arise over time and depend or reflect the cultural and social perspective of that time. We have drawn upon a variety of perspectives to show the richness of the field, but three areas are key:

+ Children are always members of a family, whether the family is visible or not.
+ Non-verbal communication is continuous and informative, and so always should be looked for.
+ Children and adults alike are always communicating with us, even if we do not realise it. Therefore, we should watch and listen to understand and care for babies and children.

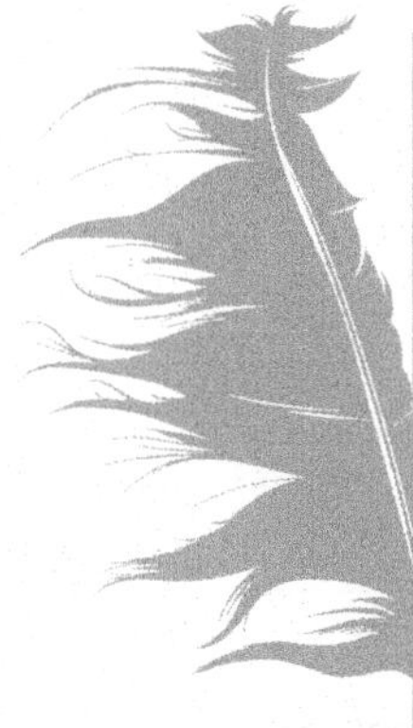

{ SUMMARY }

Babies and children develop certain communication skills over time, and health practitioners must understand and tune into the ways in which babies and young children are already (and always) communicating. Conceptions of children as naive, vulnerable or not fully human might make it easy for adults to disregard or limit communication with them. We have shown that children are entitled to be listened to, regarded and invited to participate in their care by aware and trustworthy professionals. Such attention benefits not only the child but also their family members and caregivers.

Health practitioners should uphold the rights of young children to communicate in ways that are meaningful to the children, and be mindful of less obvious aspects of communication. This requires acute listening and observation. Good communication with this age group requires entering the child's world and attending to the multilayered nature of communication. This includes non-verbal intonations, facial expressions and body movements as ways in which children begin to consciously communicate.

The responses and knowledgeable interpretation of adults encourages children to develop and participate in their world. Health practitioners must comprehend the unfolding of children's understanding and expressive capability, at different ages, to grasp the potential in reciprocal communication that goes far beyond the spoken words upon which many adults have come to rely.

REFLECTION POINTS

4.1 Intention (motivation, message, meaning, emotion)

Observe the children in your world. Who are they with? Who do they relate to? How are they communicating? How do their express fear or the need for reassurance?

4.2 Reception (received message, response, feedback)

In watching children play, how do they make meaning of events and how does this change with age?

4.3 Perception (style, manner, impression, analysis)

What might be the effect of using child rights or human rights frameworks to guide health-care practice with babies and young children?

QUESTIONS FOR REVIEW

1. In what ways do health practitioners enlist the support or guidance of family members to understand the needs or wants of young children?
2. What specific strategies can health practitioners utilise to communicate appropriately with babies and young children?
3. How can you use play to communicate with children?
4. What assumptions do you have about children and communication?

REFERENCES

Aries, P. (1962). *Centuries of childhood: A social history of family life*. New York, NY: Knopf.

Bowlby, J. (1951). *Maternal care and mental health*. Geneva, Switzerland: World Health Organization. Retrieved from http://pages.uoregon.edu/eherman/teaching/texts/Bowlby%20Maternal%20Care%20and%20Mental%20Health.pdf.

Bretherton, I. (1992). The origins of attachment theory: John Bowlby and Mary Ainsworth. *Development Psychology, 28*, 759–75.

Buckley, B. (2003). *Children's communication skills from birth to five years old*. London, UK: Routledge.

Claiborne, L. B. & Drewery, W. (2010). *Human development: Family, place, culture*. Sydney, NSW: McGraw-Hill.

Hart, B. & Risley, T. (1980). In vivo language intervention: Unanticipated general effects. *Journal of Applied Behavior Analysis, 13*(3), 407–32. Retrieved from www.ncbi.nlm.nih.gov/pmc/articles/PMC1308147/pdf/jaba00049-0027.pdf.

Menyuk, P., Liebergott, J. & Schultz, M. (1995). *Early language development in full-term and premature infants*. Hillsdale, NJ: Erlbaum.

Piaget, J. (1962). *Play, dreams and imitation*. London, UK: Routledge.

Santrock, J. (2009). *Lifespan development*. New York, NY: McGraw-Hill.

Sun, M. & Rugolotto, S. (2004). Assisted infant toilet training in a western family setting. *Developmental and Behavioural Pediatrics, 25*(2), 99–101.

United Nations (2005). *The United Nations convention on the rights of the child*. Wellington, NZ: Office of the Children's Commissioner.

Vygotsky, L. (1962). *Thought and language*. Cambridge, MA: MIT Press.

WEBSITES

Attachment Parenting International: www.attachmentparenting.org
Development, kidspot: www.kidspot.co.nz/subsection+26+Toddler-Development.htm
Huggies New Zealand: www.huggies.co.nz

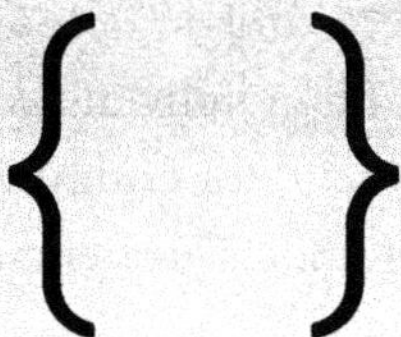

School Age

Anne Grey

CHAPTER OVERVIEW

This chapter covers the following topics:

+ Developmental theories
+ Learning theories
+ Māori perspectives on development
+ Theories of language development
+ Communication with school-age children
+ The influence of communication on children's health care.

KEY TERMS

Holistic
Development
Cognitive
Learning
Nativist perspective
Behaviour

Children of school age are typically between 5 and 11 years of age, who have begun their school years but have not yet entered the adolescent stage. This period is also known as middle childhood. It is a stage of developmental consolidation, because although children are continually learning and developing at this time, there is no rapid development as in the early childhood or the adolescent stages. There are a number of developmental and learning theories, both Western and indigenous, that underpin communication with school-age children. Understanding individual differences among children, and the impact of culture and context, are useful for critically reflecting on communication with school-age children in a way that promotes greater empathy and understanding.

Developmental theories

Holistic An emphasis on the whole person, rather than separate parts.

Development The process of progressive change and growth.

Development is a term that is used to explain the **holistic** growth and change in all aspects of the child's physical, intellectual and social functioning (Brooker & Woodhead, 2010) that occur naturally as a result of the maturational process. Although children's development is a holistic process and each aspect of development is of equal importance to the child (Lindon, 2005), domains of **development** are sometimes artificially separated to enable a deeper understanding of each aspect to be gained. As many of these theories derive from Western thinking and writing, it is important to be aware that these theories can contain 'hidden messages' (Cannella, 1997, p. 59) about children from Western cultures, and sometimes ignore or reflect badly on children from other cultures.

The Western developmental theories explained below outline a general view of the main developmental characteristics of a school-age child, although each theory is specific to a certain domain or aspect of development. To gain this broad perspective, a brief overview is provided on physical development, as well as a discussion on the psychoanalytic theories of Freud and Erikson, and the **cognitive** theories of Piaget, Vygotsky and Bruner.

Cognitive Relating to thought and thinking.

Physical development in school-age children is gradual and regular, and occurs at a much slower rate than in early childhood. Children slowly become taller, heavier and better coordinated. Gross motor skills (such as running and jumping) and fine motor skills (such as writing and drawing) are well developed and continue to improve throughout this period. This enables children throughout the school years to master physical skills such as sports, playing musical instruments, school work and household tasks. Children in developed nations enjoy better health, lower likelihood of childhood illnesses, low risk of infant mortality and increased standards of living, which has enabled many school-age children to participate in sports and cultural activities (Hoffnung et al., 2010). Unfortunately, however, this is often not the case for children in much of the world.

Although psychosocial development is not as readily observable as physical development, there are theories that explain this aspect of development. Psychoanalytic theories form a framework for understanding how the human mind works, and explain how feelings, emotions and imagination contribute to development (Crain, 2005). Sigmund Freud was the first to introduce the notion that behaviour is determined by both the conscious and unconscious mind. Freud proposed that all people need to find a balance between these two drives for well-being to exist. Freud's psychosexual theory focused primarily on sexual development. Freud named the stage of school-age children 'the latency stage', recognising the developmental consolidation that takes place in this period. Because of Freud's emphasis on sexual development, and because his observations were based on a small sample of ill people and were not representative of the general population, today this theory is often negatively critiqued. However, for those working with children, Freud's theory highlights that behaviour and communication may reflect both conscious rational thoughts and unconscious irrational thoughts. To illustrate how these irrational fears may occur, it is useful to reflect on the example of a 7-year-old boy who went to hospital to have his tonsils removed. When the nurse was taking his temperature, he asked if the doctor was going to chop his head off to get out his tonsils (Cook, 1999).

Erik Erikson (1902–1994) built on Freud's theory to construct the psychosocial theory of development. Erikson believed that each individual's identity is the result of interactions with other people and the wider community. He divided the lifespan into eight stages from infancy to old age, with each stage of development involving a crisis or issue that can be resolved either positively or negatively. In most cases, the outcome of each issue would neither be totally negative nor positive, but a combination of both. The crisis or issue that school-age children are involved in is 'industry versus inferiority'. Here, children either develop skills that allow them to feel competent (the positive end of the continuum) or fail to do this and are left with a feeling of incompetence (the negative end of the continuum). In general, throughout this stage the child's sense of competence is developed. It is usual for children to develop a realistic self-image that falls somewhere in the middle of this continuum and involves both positive and negative feelings. For the adult working with school-age children, Erikson's theory emphasises the importance of maintaining a positive environment and interactions to foster a sense of self-worth and competence in children.

Jean Piaget (1896–1980) focused his theory on the cognitive development of children by observing children's thinking and the ways that thinking changed as children matured, and how the maturational process gave rise to **learning**. Piaget believed that children's thinking develops as they interact with their environment by adapting and assimilating new information into their existing knowledge base. He constructed four stages, where each stage is qualitatively different from the stage that precedes it. The stage for school-age children is known as 'the concrete operational stage'.

Learning The process of acquiring skills and knowledge.

Piaget believed that when a child reaches the school age, thinking becomes more logical and organised than previously, but that they still have difficulty in thinking abstractly or reasoning about abstract ideas. This is because Piaget believed that mastery of logical thought developed gradually (Berk, 2008). In recent times, because Piaget emphasised that children's thinking developed in stages, this theory has been critiqued as concentrating more on what children were unable to understand than on their cognitive capabilities. However, it is important to be aware of the limitations to children's understanding. For example, most school-age children can name bones, blood, heart, stomach and lungs when asked about internal anatomy, but cannot explain the location of these organs or what their function is (Rushforth, 1999).

Learning theories

Learning theories refer to the acquisition of knowledge, skills and identity. These theories explain that what is learnt by children is shaped by the relationships that they build, by the cultural values of society, and by the lived daily experiences that form their lives. Moreover, what a child learns is also limited or extended by the economic and social context in which each child lives. In addition, the language a child speaks shapes the child's identity, as well as providing a means of learning (Brooker & Woodhead, 2010).

Vygotsky's sociocultural theory of development provides a different way to understand children's learning and cognitive development. Vygotsky viewed learning and development as a collaborative and social undertaking where children learn from the people who are part of their daily lives, especially those who are more experienced than they are themselves (Wertsch, 1991). Vygotsky believed that language and communication are essential to learning and cognitive development, as it is through language and communication that internal thoughts are expressed. Vygotsky believed each person had a 'zone of proximal development' (what a person can do and understand with help from another person) and a 'zone of actual development' (what a person can do and understand on their own). The process of assisting a person through the zone of proximal development is known as 'scaffolding'. Vygotsky also thought that people, especially children, often talk to themselves in order to guide their own learning. He called this type of communication 'private speech'. Vygotsky explained that each culture had tools that could assist with learning and understanding. In Western cultures these are often books, computers or photos, while in other cultures cultural tools may take the form of legends, songs or dances. Language itself was viewed by Vygotsky as a major cultural tool for learning as language provides the medium for the exchange of ideas between people to build shared meanings about their social, cultural and intellectual experiences (Smidt, 2009). Vygotsky believed that learning individuals are continually extending both their zone of actual development and their zone of proximal development. Vygotsky's sociocultural theory is valuable as it demonstrates the importance of culture and interpersonal relationships for learning, and how individuals learn from participating in a community.

Jerome Bruner, an American psychologist, elaborated on Vygotsky's view of learning. Bruner viewed children as active problem solvers who were motivated to learn quite difficult concepts if those concepts were of interest to them (Smidt, 2009), or had direct meaning for their life, and if those concepts were revisited frequently until understanding was gained. He extended Vygotsky's theory by introducing the term 'scaffolding' to emphasise the role the adult plays to give support, usually in the form of dialogue or communication, to the child's learning and understanding. Bruner also explained learning as being distributed; that is, some learning takes place on an individual basis and some while being part of a social group, and some learning is explicit as a result of direct teaching and some is tacit or absorbed as a result of personal experiences.

Communication involves the processing of information, and the current social environment provides children with an overwhelming amount of information at any one time. The framework that focuses specifically on this aspect of cognitive development is known as the 'information processing' approach. Here the metaphor of a computer is used to explain the human mind. Mental strategies and the flow of information are directed by a central executive area of the working memory (Berk, 2008). In school-age children, information processing becomes more efficient as they are able to pay attention to information for longer periods and can remember and understand complex tasks and topics. They are more selective about the topics they pay attention to, and can switch back and forth between topics as they use various mental strategies more effectively (Hoffnung et al., 2010). This ability to control thought processes is known as metacognition, or the awareness of mental activities and thinking processes (Berk, 2008). This, in turn, leads to greater cognitive self-regulation. The information processing theory is useful to understand communication, as it involves information entering a child's sensory register with mental strategies then employed to enable understanding to take place.

Māori perspectives on development

In Māori culture, theories and concepts of development have been passed down through songs, stories and karakia (waiata, kōrero and karakia) where human development and learning is explained holistically as being a part of the life force (te ira tangata) of the universe (Royal-Tangaere, 1997). From this perspective, each individual, especially each child, is considered to be a taonga, or a gift from the gods. Each individual's learning and development is also connected to the gods as it is believed that the three baskets of knowledge were collected from the heavens by Tane. In order to collect the baskets, Tane climbed Te Ara Poutama, or the stairs that are often depicted in the weaving panels on a marae. Each stair reflects a stage of learning and development that leads onto the next through a learning process of observing, listening and then speaking (titiro, whakarongo, kōrero). Central to the learning process is the concept of tukana-teina, or older sibling–younger sibling, where it is the responsibility of the older or more experienced person to pass on learning to those who are younger or less experienced. As this learning process connects man to the gods, learning is considered a taonga, or a precious gift.

No one aspect of development and learning can be considered in isolation from the others and holism is considered an important principle of human development and learning (Macfarlane, 2007). Moreover, as each individual is connected to the gods, each individual is considered a taonga to be valued and respected (Pere, 1988; 1991). Accepting that there is also a cultural perspective to understanding children's development assists carers to be more empathetic to diversity and difference, and to ensure that communication is culturally sensitive.

Theories of language development

As communication is linked to language, it is important to understand the theories of language development. There is no one theory that gives a clear explanation—several theories explain language development from various perspectives. However, there are particular perspectives from which to consider this. For example, the behaviourist perspective explains language as resulting from environmental learning, while the **nativist perspective** posits that language naturally emerges from the normal process of maturation.

Nativist perspective The view that children build on their innate understanding as they move through developmental processes.

The 'behaviourist' perspective to learning language was outlined by B. F. Skinner. He explained that language occurs through the processes of imitation and reinforcement, whereby children imitate language from those around them and are rewarded, or reinforced, for using these words themselves. It is true that children who are spoken to frequently and who are encouraged to engage in conversations develop strong language skills, but this is no longer thought to be a valid explanation for language development in general. The nativist perspective, outlined by Noam Chomsky, claims that children are born with an innate ability to understand and use language. It is true that children have a remarkable ability to communicate that is not always the result of imitation and reinforcement. For example, children can often make sense of words they have not heard before. Similarly, children who are born deaf, but are surrounded by speaking adults, do not have a sign language to imitate yet invent their own sign systems (Berk, 2008). It can be concluded that children have the ability to acquire language, but this ability requires nurturing if it is to flourish.

In middle childhood, language ability develops significantly, partly as a result of more complex cognitive abilities. By 10 years of age children have a richer vocabulary and are able to choose between words that have a similar meaning but different connotations. This allows children to engage in word play, to tell jokes and to build specialised vocabulary relating to their interests. At this age, children can use language to communicate in different ways, including being able to take another's perspective, empathise with others and to express their own internal fears and emotions in words. This allows children to realise that communication can be a means to understand the world and to resolve conflict, and so language and communication become a means of regulating impulsive emotional **behaviour** (Davies, 2011).

Behaviour
Observable activities, conduct and responses.

The implications of these theories are that although all school-age children should be able to understand communication about health-care treatment, children who are spoken to and read to more often will have a more extensive vocabulary and should be able to understand medical terminology more easily. However, there are many individual differences within this general description of language development in school-age children, so it is important not to stereotype children's language ability.

Communication with school-age children

Communication is a complex rather than a linear process. The importance of culture and context to the communication process must also be recognised as impacting on the meaning, context and purpose of communication, as well as the relationships between those communicating and the influence of the method of communication. Communication also involves a combination of skills that shape the communication process. These skills include language ability (which is influenced by societies and individuals), individual cognitive information processing to find meaning in another person's speech and vocabulary, and the interpretation of the non-verbal components of communication, such as gestures and movements (Vickers, 2006). Skills are needed to communicate effectively, as well as to know which messages are important to communicate (Quality Assurance Report, 1999).

Because of the complexity of communication, and the individual and cultural differences among school-age children, those working with children need strategies for building rapport, explaining, listening and interpreting information. Communication must be respectful of the rights of the child and be conducted collaboratively with the child and family, but should also take account of the child's individuality, age, development, understanding and cultural background, and how circumstances affect the style of communication. Explaining a routine health check to a child may require a different style of communication from explaining about surgery or a serious illness. Health practitioners and the language they use may be unfamiliar to the child, and the environment may contain sights, sounds and smells that are threatening to a child. It is important to consider the child's perspective and to encourage their participation in any communication.

To ensure communication is not threatening to the child, it is first important to build trust between the health care professional and the child by adopting friendly gestures, facial expressions, body language and tone of voice. Carers can get down to the child's level, although not all children make eye contact for individual or cultural reasons. In framing the communication, the professional should explain to the child what has happened, what is happening now, what is going to happen, what this is likely to mean to them, and what is being done to help them (Cook, 1999). It is essential for the carer to explain all key words and phrases in plain language (not medical jargon), ideally in the child's home language, so an interpreter may be needed. If children are given simple, clear information about their illness and the treatment required, they are provided with a meaningful base on which to add new information.

Sometimes it may be necessary for carers to communicate bad news to children. In the past, adults have avoided talking about difficult situations, such as terminal cancer, with children. This has given children an extra psychological burden, and resulted in children losing their sense of competence and control, resulting in depression or excessive fears and fantasies (Beale, Baile & Aaron, 2005). Evidence suggests that terminally ill children as young as 3 years are aware of a diagnosis and prognosis without being told by an adult, and that the avoidance of discussions about death can lead them to feel abandoned (Levetown & the Committee on Bioethics, 2008). It is now thought children should be given honest, accurate information about illnesses and the treatment this entails. In these cases, professionals must be aware that the child needs to know, what the child already knows, how and when the information is best given, and what support the child may need afterwards (Cook,1999).

The following '6 Es' strategy is a guide to difficult communication:

+ Establish open communication with the child and the family.
+ Engage the child at an appropriate time.
+ Explore what the child already knows about the illness and what else they would like to know.
+ Explain medical information in answer to the child's questions, rather than presuming what they want or need to know.
+ Empathise with the child's emotional reactions. The child may be upset and expressing these feelings is necessary before a constructive discussion can take place. In this case, the carer can empathise ('I can see that you've been really worried about this'), validate ('We've been wondering why you've been upset') and clarify ('Can you tell me what

you've been thinking?). Children may prefer to express their feelings in a drawing or through play rather than verbally.

+ Encourage children by reassuring them that they will be listened to and supported. If necessary, explain that although there is no cure for the illness, life still continues. It is not helpful to give the child false hope or reassurance by saying, for example, 'Don't worry—everything will be all right!' (Beale, Baile & Aaron, 2005).

When communicating with children, the information given by the carer addresses two needs. These are the cognitive need to know and understand the information, and the affective/emotional need to feel supported and understood (Levetown & the Committee on Bioethics, 2008). By enhancing awareness of communication strategies when explaining treatment and listening to children's questions and expressions of anxiety, carers can improve the psychological well-being of children.

The influence of communication on children's health care

Several studies demonstrate effective communication is associated with quality of care, which in turn results in better health outcomes. Paediatric health care is improved when children are recognised as having their own cognitive and emotional needs, are respected and are regarded as intelligent, capable and cooperative (Levetown & the Committee on Bioethics, 2008). Studies indicate children have often been passive recipients of health care, and have been given little opportunity to share decision-making with health practitioners. Indeed, it is more usual for health practitioners to ask parents about their child's health than it is to ask the children themselves. Studies show that children over the age of 7 years give a more accurate description of their health, including the pain they experience, than their parents. For practitioners, it is very difficult to accurately assess the extent and nature of pain without description from the child. Some children may not have the vocabulary to adequately describe their pain in words, but may be able to indicate the severity of it by pointing to a face from a continuum of smiles to grimaces. In pain management, it has been shown that patients who control their own pain-relief treatment experience greater pain relief. Children as young as 4 years have been successfully taught to do this. By being listened to, given accurate information about why they are experiencing pain, and by being taught to administer their own pain relief, children experience less negative outcomes as a result of the pain (Levetown & the Committee on Bioethics, 2008).

Asthma among children is common, and studies in the USA have revealed the incidence of children with asthma was greater for children from lower socio-economic backgrounds or ethnic minorities. These children experienced a poorer quality of care than other children because of more barriers to communicating effectively about asthma symptoms, treatment, medication and self-management (Diette & Rand, 2007). The practitioners also experienced difficulties with these children and families because effective communication often took more time than was allocated. Health-care professionals tended to dominate conversations more and listen less to these children and their families. Communication was not child-centred and there were also cultural differences in how symptoms were described. In some cases these factors resulted in the severity of the asthma not being correctly assessed and lower rates of prescription of medication.

Although these children and their families were less able to read information about health, to follow written instructions and to calculate correct doses of medication, the study found when time was taken to explain guidelines for treatment in a one-on-one situation, asthma patients were able to administer their treatment successfully at home. Improved communication was shown to support increased positive health outcomes, while enabling the child to take responsibility for their own health and well-being.

Recently, in accordance with the United Nations Convention on the Rights of the Child, surveys on children's opinions on the quality of their hospital experiences were completed in the USA, Switzerland and Finland. In these surveys communication was noted as both the best and worst aspect of children's hospital experiences. In the USA, 120 children aged 4–20 years were surveyed. They reported they valued relationships with staff and appreciated if nursing staff, doctors and other medical staff listened to them, but confusing communication and not being told about medical procedures were reported as the worst features. These children listed better communication as one suggestion for improvement (Lindeke, Nakai & Johnson, 2006).

In Switzerland, 136 children aged 6–12 years were surveyed on hospital experiences to better understand their priorities. This survey indicated that children do not necessarily have the same priorities and opinions as their parents. The children reported a high satisfaction rate with the nurses (90 per cent), but attitude and relationships were more important to these children than the technical aspect of care. The children appreciated, for example, that nurses took good care of them and explained things to them. The older children commented on their need to feel recognised and reassured, and be able to act on their own behalf. This survey clearly shows children appreciated being asked their opinions on the quality of care they received. This study concluded that children recovered faster if they were prepared for their hospital stay, had explanations about treatment and were supported by being listened to (Chappius et al., 2011).

The study in Finland surveyed 388 children aged 7–11 years about their best and worst experiences of hospitalisation. The children reported that people were one of the best experiences and that the best nurses were pleasant, friendly and nice, and took care of them. Here children described their worst experience as having an unidentified person doing something to them. This study concluded that good communication between nurses, children and their families is linked to increased understanding of treatment and illness (Pelander & Leino-Kilpi, 2010).

These studies all suggest that for hospital environments and treatment to be more child-centred, children's viewpoints need to be heard and children need to be allowed to participate in their own health care. If this happens, children are likely to be less stressed and the treatment more effective.

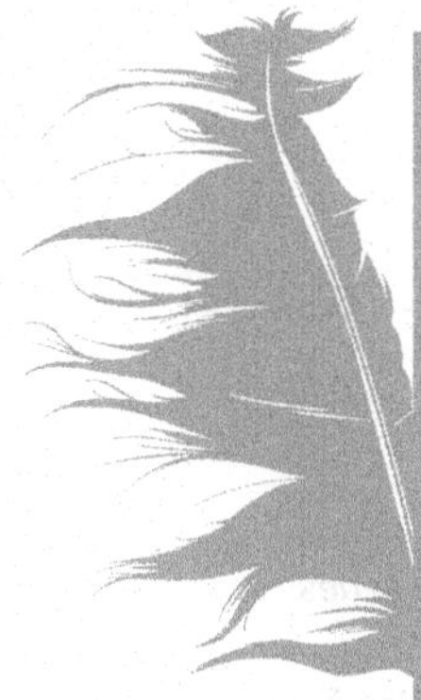

{ SUMMARY }

By communicating with children in a respectful manner, professionals can positively reinforce children's sense of competence (Erikson's theory). School-age children's thinking and understanding is logical when connected to concrete experiences (Piaget's theory), but is influenced by culture and context (Vygotsky's theory). Children in the school age can process information more efficiently (information processing theory) to make sense of their world (Bruner's theory), and are able to understand quite complex concepts if an adult assists their understanding (scaffolding).

Māori views on child development need special consideration as each child is considered holistically as a special gift from the gods and cannot be viewed in isolation from the family or whānau.

Communication with children is both verbal and non-verbal. Although communication transmits information from one person to another, the way the information is interpreted and understood is influenced by individual, cultural and contextual differences.

Health-care professionals working with children need a range of strategies. Information should be as honest and accurate as possible. Children should be allowed to express their feelings and have these listened to.

REFLECTION POINTS

5.1 Intention (motivation, message, meaning, emotion)

When engaging with children, how might you ask open-ended questions that would scaffold a child's ability to describe their symptoms?

5.2 Reception (received message, response, feedback)

Informed consent in Aotearoa New Zealand is less about age and more about the ability to understand, given the cognitive abilities of a person.How would you know that a child has really understood what you have been telling them without asking a simple yes or no question?

5.3 Perception (style, manner, impression, analysis)

Identify communication skills that children value in their health-care providers. Are these the same or different from ones that you value in a health-care provider?

QUESTIONS FOR REVIEW

1 How is communication affected by social/emotional, cognitive and cultural influences? Use a mind map to illustrate the relationships.
2 What are five strategies you could use to make communication with school-age children more effective?

REFERENCES

Beale, E., Baile, W. & Aaron, J. (2005, May). Silence is not golden: Communicating with children dying of cancer. *Journal of Clinical Oncology, 23*(15), 3629–31.

Berk, L. (2008). *Infants and children*. Boston, MA: Pearson Education Inc.

Brooker, L. & Woodhead, M. (2010). Culture and learning. In M. Woodhead & J. Oats (eds), *The series: Early childhood in focus (No.6)*. The Hague, Netherlands: Bernard Van Leer Foundation.

Cannella, G. (1997). *Deconstructing early childhood education: Social justice and revolution*. New York, NY: Peter Lang.

Chappuis, M., Vannay-Bouchiche, C., Flückiger, M., Monnier, M., Cathieni, F. & Piot-Ziegler, C. (2011). Children's experience regarding the quality of their hospital stay: The development of an assessment questionnaire for children. *Journal of Nursing Care Quality, 26*(1), 78–87.

Cook, P. (1999). Will it hurt? Children in medical settings. In P. Milner & B. Carolin, *Time to listen to children: Personal and professional communication*. London, UK: Routledge.

Crain, W. (2005). *Theories of development: Concepts and applications* (5th edn). Upper Saddle River, NJ: Pearson Prentice Hall.

Davies, D. (2011). *Child development: A practitioner's guide* (3rd edn). New York, NY: The Guilford Press.

Diette, G. & Rand, C. (2007). The contributing role of health-care communication to health disparities for minority patients with asthma. *Chest, 2007, 132*, 802–9.

Hoffnung, M., Hoffnung, R., Seifert, K., Smith, R., Hine, A., Ward, L. & Quinn, A. (2010). *Lifespan development*. Brisbane: John Wiley & Sons.

Levetown, M. & the Committee on Bioethics. (2008). *Pediatrics, 2008, 121*, 1441–50.

Lindeke, L., Nakai, M. & Johnson, L. (2006). Capturing children's voices for quality improvement. *The American Journal of Maternal/Child Nursing, 31*(5), 290–5.

Lindon, J. (2005). *Understanding child development: Linking theory and practice*. London, UK: Hodder Arnold.

Macfarlane, A. H. (2007). The value of Māori ecologies in the study of human development. In L. Bird & W. Drewery (eds). *Human development in Aotearoa: A journey through life*. Boston, MA: McGraw-Hill.

Pelander, T. & Leino-Kilpi, H. (2010). Children's best and worst experiences during hospitalisation. *Scandinavian Journal of Caring Sciences, 24*(4), 726–33.

Pere, R. R. (1988). Te wheke: Whaia te maramatangame aroha. In S. Middleton (ed.), *Women and Education in Aotearoa*. Wellington, NZ: Allen & Unwin.

Pere, R. R. (1991). *Te wheke: A celebration of infinite wisdom*. Gisborne, NZ: Akoako Global Publishing.

Quality Assurance Report. (1999). *Improving interpersonal communication between health care providers and patients*. Bethesda, MD: Center for Human Services.

Royal-Tangaere, A. (1997). Māori human development learning theory. In P. Te Whaiti, M. McCarthy & A. Durie (eds), *Mai i rangiatea: Māori well-being and development*. Auckland, NZ: University Press with Bridget Williams Books.

Rushforth, H. (1999). Practitioner review: Communicating with hospitalised children: Review and application of research pertaining to children's understanding of health and illness. *Journal of Child Psychology and Psychiatry, 40*(5), 683–91.

Smidt, S. (2009). *Introducing Vygotsky: A guide for practitioners and students in early years education*. London, UK: Routledge.

Vickers, P. (2006). Communicating with children and families. In I. Peate & L. Whiting (eds), *Caring for children and families*. London, UK: John Wiley & Sons, Ltd.

Wertsch, J. (1991). *Voices of the mind: A sociocultural approach to mediated action*. Cambridge, MA: Harvard University Press.

WEBSITES

Bristol Royal Infirmary Enquiry, Leadership in the NHS: www.bristol-inquiry.org.uk/final_report/report/sec2chap29_13.htm

Improving services for children in hospital, Healthcare Commission: www.cqc.org.uk/_db/_documents/children_improving_services_Tagged.pdf

READING 13

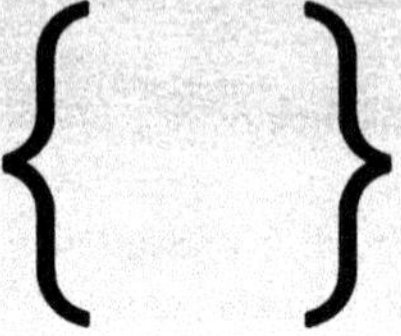

Teens

Gabrielle Le Geyt, Jayne Mercier, Morgyn Hartdegen, Amber Davies and Ailsa Haxell

CHAPTER OVERVIEW

This chapter covers the following topics:

+ The adolescent brain
+ Psychosocial development
+ Physical development
+ Communicating with teenagers

KEY TERMS

Adolescence
Identity
Role
Neurological
Impulsivity
Risk
Resilience

Between childhood and adulthood comes **adolescence**. Transitions in and out of this developmental stage are gradual, usually beginning at age 11 or 12 years, continuing through the teenage years and completing in the early to mid twenties (Turkstra & Byom, 2010). Adolescent communication is frequently stereotyped as comprising slammed doors, grunts and (on good days) monosyllabic responses. However, to gain an understanding of teenage communications, it is useful to consider the major developmental changes occurring in adolescence and how these influence teenage minds and behaviours. This chapter examines some of these processes and their influence on communication, and outlines some ways to enhance communication with this age group.

Adolescence A developmental phase between childhood and maturity.

Adolescence is characterised by considerable physical, intellectual, emotional and psychosocial changes, which allow the young person to attain a sense of independence from parents or guardians and develop their own unique **identity**. There are many processes that support development during this stage, including family, peer affiliation, knowledge seeking and **role** experimentation. Changing biological processes also have a great influence during this stage of life; the adolescent brain continues to develop and mature, which creates advanced cognitive processing and reasoning, and contributes to the emergence of new patterns of behaviour.

Identity The sense of self and individual character that a person has in relation to others.

Role A socially accepted way of behaving and carrying specific responsibilities.

The adolescent brain

Until recently, it was believed that the major 'wiring' of the human brain was achieved during the first three to four years of life, following a dramatic increase in grey matter volume, and that by the age of 10 to 12 years the brain was fully mature. Advancements in neuroimaging techniques have now revealed otherwise. Current research supports the understanding that brain development is not complete until the late teens or early twenties, with the adolescent brain undergoing a great deal of neural restructuring following a second wave of grey matter overproduction in preadolescence (Crone, 2009; Turkstra & Byom, 2010).

The continuing maturation of the adolescent brain underlies advances in cognitive processing, social competence and emotional capacity in teens. The refinement of connections between different brain regions during adolescence is reflected in changes in the way information is processed and communicated. In pre-teens, problem-solving using logical processes is limited to 'concrete operations'; that is, problems that relate to real events and objects (Piaget, 1926). In Piaget's theory of development, teenagers achieve formal operational thought: an accomplishment that allows individuals to consider abstract problems logically and systematically. Thoughtful hypothesis testing also becomes possible; therefore teenagers become increasingly adept at contemplating moral and ethical issues and applying hypothetical reasoning. These skills can be nurtured by facilitating debates, and by encouraging teens to consider multiple perspectives.

Neurological Involving the nervous system.

These **neurological** changes may also provide an insight into a number of teenage characteristics that have in the past resulted in adolescence being discussed as a period of 'storm and stress' (see, for example, the oft-cited writings of G. Stanley Hall, 1904). Physical developments occur in the frontal lobe and the limbic system, regions of the brain that are responsible for self-control, judgment and emotional regulation. In a normally functioning adult brain, these regions plan and coordinate behaviour in a way that takes into account consequences and motivational goals, while regulating and modifying emotional urges to fit into socially acceptable norms. The teenage brain, however, is still developing this ability, which may explain the prevalence of spontaneous actions, poor decision-making, risk-taking behaviour and emotional outbursts in teens. Changes also occur in the way pleasure and reward is processed in the brain—as Steinberg (2005) explains, 'rewarding things feel more rewarding' for teens. Experimenting with drugs and alcohol, for example, is more common in young people than for other age groups. According to New Zealand's Ministry of Health (2010), 30 per cent of 16–24-year-olds reported drug use within the last year, compared with only 16 per cent of New Zealanders aged 16–64. There are many factors explaining the appeal of drugs to young people, including resistance to authority, testing boundaries, peer group affiliation and their use as a coping mechanism. This risk-taking behaviour also correlates with the changing prefrontal regions in the brain that regulate **impulsivity** and decision-making, making biological influences a possible contributing factor. Because of the changing nature of brain structures, drug taking in teenagers can result in long-term consequences; the adolescent brain is not yet fully mature, therefore young people have an enhanced vulnerability to addiction resulting from substance misuse.

Impulsivity The tendency to act without prior analysis.

Communication patterns in adolescence that reflect brain developments may include seemingly irrational outbursts and high-level emotional responses that do not seem to reflect the gravity of a situation. However, due to the advance in cognitive processes, young people may also start to engage in debates and question the decisions and rationale of those around them, including friends, family and teachers, demonstrating an increased ability to negotiate and develop logical arguments. Over time, an increased ability to judge different social situations and adapt their communication accordingly will emerge.

As the ability to consider abstract and moral dilemmas grows, young people may also explore different philosophies, religions and subcultures, and openly reject the values of family. These explorations may be commonly expressed through art, poetry, music or other creative media. These explorations are also heavily influenced by peers, as outlined below.

Psychosocial development

Psychosocial development refers to the development of the self with particular reference to the social context. Psychosocial processes become particularly important during this developmental stage, with adolescents experimenting with different roles, establishing a sense of identity, and achieving a greater social awareness and ability to communicate efficiently in different social situations. As young people start to experience a sense of independence from their parents or guardians, peers become an increasingly important and defining feature of their lives. The importance of identity formation during adolescence was recognised by psychologist Erik Erikson (1968), who discussed this developmental stage as being characterised by a 'crisis' of identity versus role confusion, where the adolescent tries out a number of ways to express their personality and values. If negotiated successfully, the adolescent will eventually develop a stable identity, separate from their family, that can function in wider society. If not negotiated successfully, a firm sense of adult self will not emerge, leading to an over-reliance on the opinions and approval of others (Erikson, 1968).

Newman and Newman's (2003) revisions of Erikson's stages of psychosocial development contemplate an additional stage of adolescence, with early adolescence (12–18 years) concentrating on group identity versus alienation, where the acceptance of the group is paramount and is achieved through looking, thinking and acting the same as one's peers. Newman posits that 'identity versus role confusion' occurs from 19 to 22 years of age.

Understanding the processes involved in achieving identity within a group can provide insight into the different levels of adolescent communication and behaviour. Peer pressure, for example, may encourage behaviours or responses that reinforce the group identity. Loyalty to the group may limit communications on certain levels, and there may be an element of in-group, out-group dialogue. To the outside observer, this may result in what appear to be radical changes in personality as the adolescent conforms to these group norms, or a number of peer group changes as the adolescent also questions whether group norms fit his or her developing identity. Alongside neurological development, peer processes and role experimentation may also play a part in spontaneous actions involving **risk**, and the testing of boundaries. Substance use, for example, may reflect the increased importance of peer affiliation and intergroup processes. Group affiliation can also be communicated non-verbally through choice of clothes, music and activities.

Risk The possibility of injury, loss or death.

As peer affiliation becomes more important, adolescent communication may be characterised by increased time spent sending text messages and interacting on social networking sites. A corresponding decrease in communication with family and other adults may also occur as the adolescent strives to become independent. Those around the young person may observe this in the form of a greater need for privacy, boundary testing and rejection of family norms and values. Further friction is created when parental boundaries directly impinge on the ability to conform to group norms; for example, disallowing body piercings and imposing curfews. Although communication with parents tends to reduce during the teenage years, external approval remains important in the process of identity formation. Teens may, therefore, demonstrate heightened sensitivity to the evaluations and opinions of others and react strongly to criticism and comments that challenge their sense of self (Steinberg, 2005).

The preference for peer communication can also be seen in young people's interactions in help-seeking settings, where research shows that many young people do not access formal support due to fear of lack of confidentiality or not wanting to make a fuss, and prefer to use peers as a source of wisdom (Watson et al., 2003).

However, it is important to note that this withdrawal from adults may not emerge in isolation within the adolescent. Predominant stereotypes of adolescents are negative, with teenagers frequently cast as lazy, selfish and, at worst, criminals (Giroux, 2009; Cohen, 1972), which potentially makes it difficult for adolescents to engage with and place trust in an adult world.

When given an opportunity to be heard, what young people ask for is acceptance: 'Just accept us as we are more' (McCreanor, Watson & Denny, 2006), and to be heard on their own terms (Haxell, 2008).

CASE STUDY 6.1

Feeling misunderstood

A 17-year-old female enters counselling with depressive symptoms, truancy, suicidal ideation and harming behaviours, and regular drug and alcohol use. Family relationships are strained and the young woman relies solely on her same-sex partner as a confidant and support. She feels generally mistrusting of adults, while fear of reprimand for her behaviour (truancy and drug and alcohol use) and uncertainty about confidentiality also prevent her from seeking support from those around her.

To assert her identity she reveals her sexual identity to her family, which increases her sense of feeling misunderstood. This revelation also disconnects her from her peer group, although risk-taking behaviours provide a level of peer affiliation. She continues to feel disconnected and isolated, both at home and at school.

In counselling, the confidentiality policy is explained. The counsellor communicates with empathy in a calm and reassuring manner, without judging or reprimanding the young woman's behaviour. The counsellor also works with the client in a holistic way, focusing primarily on her strengths rather than solely on her risk. This increases the young woman's sense of self-efficacy and encourages her to engage more in activities she enjoys, such as drama and singing. This allows her to connect with a pro-social peer group and have her sense of identity affirmed.

Moments of irrational thinking are sensitively challenged, particularly the idea that ending her life is the only way to change her situation. Through talking, role-play, music, song writing and poetry, the young woman learns more abstract ways to view her situation and manage her seemingly extreme reactions to situations, as well as identifying and being able to express internal feelings.

Physical development

Alongside significant neurological and psychosocial changes, adolescents are also undergoing massive physical development during puberty and subsequent sexual maturation. Changing hormones mean adolescents experience an increase in sexual drives (Udry, 1988), along with an increase in thinking about sexual behaviours and a change in the meaning of them within the individual and from society (Steinberg, 1999).

According to Brooks-Gunn and Paikoff (1993), there are four main developmental challenges of adolescence with regards to sexuality:

+ accepting one's body is changing
+ accepting feelings of sexual arousal
+ understanding that sexual activity is voluntary
+ ensuring that all sex is safe sex.

As with all developmental processes during adolescence, this does not occur in isolation and is influenced by both neurological and psychosocial development. As discussed earlier, changes in the pleasure and reward processes in the brain may influence decisions to have sex. Ultimately, physical changes will be communicated in the adolescent engaging in sexual activities. Youth 07 data notes that 38 per cent of young males and 35 per cent of young females who participated in the survey have had sexual intercourse (Adolescent Health Research Group, 2008). However, Erikson (1968) suggests that the ability to develop intimacy in relationships does not occur until the ages of 18–24 years, when the young person can express feelings, wishes, needs, goals and fears. In this way adolescents may experience physical readiness for sexual relationships before the ability to communicate about and negotiate sexual relationships is fully developed. This may be evidenced by the mediation of peers in intimate relationships, and risk taking in sexual practice.

Continuing development of identity may also result in the questioning and testing of sexual identity, with the Youth 07 survey indicating that about one in twenty New Zealand secondary school students identify an attraction to the same sex or to both sexes (Rossen et al., 2009). The physical changes in the body at this time can also lead to young people feeling self-conscious about their bodies and an increased need for physical privacy. This is often communicated non-verbally through increased hiding of the body; for example, discomfort with getting changed in front of parents or peers where previously there was no issue. Respecting a young person's need for physical privacy is therefore very important at this time.

CASE STUDY 6.2

Teen issues in textspeak

Youthline provides a free live text counselling service for young people. Below are some generic examples of the types of communications received from youth, demonstrating the key developmental concepts they experience.

Developing abstract thinking skills

YP: im grounded. My mum h8s me and i h8 her.

YL: that sux, howcome ur grounded.

YP: its just cos I was late home the otha nite, and its totally unfair, cos i was helping my friend

YL: does ur mum kno the reason why u were late

YP: no she just went mental at me and grounded me

YL: Thats tuff aye? wn u haven't had a chance 2 explain ur story.

YP: yeah, my friend is goin thru some real serious stuff

YL: Do u reckon ur mum wld think differently if she knew why

YP: maybe. shes prob still gonna be angry

YL: Any idea why she mite be angry

YP: She was prob worried about me cos i didn't tell her i was with my frnd.

Impulsivity

I don't see how its eva gonna change and its pointless tlking 2 u. I may as well just not be here

Importance of friends

I am seeing this guy and i really lyk him but my frenz think he is a dik. Not sure if I should dump him.

all my frenz r callin me emo and im not I just like different music from them

Concerns about confidentiality and trust

R u guys gonna tell ne1 what I txt u?

How will I know if i get to tlk 2 the same person next tym?

Sexual identity and development

My gf wants 2 hav sex and im not sure if I want 2. How do u know n ur ready?

ive been lookin at my friends body when we r getting changed for phys ed class. Does that mean im gay?

Communicating with teenagers

The huge developmental, physical, social and emotional changes occurring during adolescence have an impact on how young people engage with those around them; equally, successful communication with teenagers involves both an understanding and an appreciation of a young person's development. The frustrations that an adult might feel at a teenager's seemingly irrational or thoughtless decisions can be balanced with an understanding of the changing underlying processes. The knowledge that teenagers may experience increased impulsivity and heightened emotional arousal should guide responses when communicating in difficult situations with teens. A calm, reassuring approach is more likely to lower arousal and encourage reasoning than a confrontational stance, which may challenge the young person's sense of self and provoke defensive retaliation.

While many adults feel uncertain around teenagers, from a young person's perspective adults can appear to have a lot of power to make decisions about their life or curb developing independence. Communications with adults or professionals in regard to personal issues, therefore, may be subject to a period of wariness or testing to establish trust. This will possibly involve questions from the young person, silence or even acting out behaviours, such as being overly rude and saying things aimed at shocking the adult to check out their response. Appreciating that when young people are pushing limits and boundaries they may also be testing care and acceptance may help adults get through what can feel like periods of rejection.

This can be a very vulnerable and private time for some adolescents as they try on different identities to see which ones fit. They can easily feel shamed and withdraw if their expressions are met with disdain or dismissal. To permit sincere communications with teens, adults need to take time to build rapport and be curious about the young person's emerging individual identity. Sometimes it can be difficult to explain how one feels, and being asked this outright may result in the young person becoming conscious of being put on the spot in having to explain themselves. An alternative way of exploring what's important in the life of a young person is through showing an interest in the individual's culture and their motivations. An entry point into difficult subjects can be had, for example, by asking if there are song lyrics that express how they feel.

Young people's sensitivity to how they might be perceived by adults is accompanied by their developing ability to analyse situations, which means that teens are fairly adept in judging when someone is not being genuine. Genuineness is about communicating on the level of the young person, but without using language that is unfamiliar to the communicator or that they do not feel comfortable using; for example, slang. A teenager will know when people are trying too hard and this will decrease rapport. This also means the communicator asking when they do not understand the young person's way of talking, rather than pretending that they know—which is disempowering—or adopting the unhelpful attitude that there is a 'generation gap' and 'teenagers speak a different language'. Being genuine may also involve letting the young person know some personal information such as likes and dislikes. Even with established rapport and genuine communication, adults may still need to be the one to raise sensitive topics, such as sex, and speak directly and plainly about the subject. Discomfort on the part of the adult is likely to make the young person uncomfortable and disinclined to engage in conversation.

Theories of psychosocial development emphasise role and identity formation. It is important, therefore, to consider whether communications support positive or negative identity formation when working with teens. By concentrating on faults and failures, a problem-focused approach risks reinforcing the problem as being an inherent part of the young person's identity. Think back to Hall's portrayal of adolescence as a time of 'storm and stress'. This idea of young people in a permanent state of turmoil suggests that conflict with parents is inevitable and risks leading to disengagement. A more constructive form of communication takes a strengths-based approach. A strengths orientation encourages the young person to recognise their competencies and strengths, and supports these as part of their identity (McLaren, 2002). Positive approaches like this have the potential to encourage connectedness and supportive relationships; this approach is also understood to foster **resilience** in teens (Youth Mentoring Network, 2011), or the ability to bounce back from difficult situations. Regular and positive communication with teens can also support positive role identification by providing pro-social role models (for example, youth workers and mentors).

Resilience The ability to recover from stress or injury.

Holding a strengths-based approach does not mean that communicating with a young person solely involves providing positive affirmation. A strengths-based approach with youth involves encouraging the positive things they are doing while sensitively challenging risk-taking or anti-social behaviours (Ministry of Youth Development, 2007). Adults who have realistically high expectations of young people's behaviour and a firm belief in what they can achieve will support the young person to have equally high expectations of themselves. Young people may enter relationships with a deficit approach. They may experience a limited sense of self or lack hope for their future. In this way, a key task for the strengths-based practitioner is to assist the young person to find their strengths and remain focused on the young person's potential—despite personal and contextual challenges—and, often, holding hope for the future before the young person can see this for themselves. Aronowitz (2005) referred to this process as 'envisioning the future' (p. 205), which in turn builds resilience.

CASE STUDY 6.3

A strength-based approach in health promotion

Working with young people inside of a strengths-based approach challenges service providers to consider young people not only as recipients of a service, but also as central to the provision of that service.

In providing an online discussion board, young people can post a question and have it answered by others who may have worked through the issues for themselves.

Topic: What's it like going to family planning clinic?

I've made an appointment with family planning as I want to start using contraception, but I'm terrified that someone will see me going in. I feel like there will be a big red arrow hanging over my head. Everyone will know I'm having sex.

And what happens when you go in? It's all a bit nerve-racking for a shy person (well, the shyness is currently in remission). I'm ok talking about this stuff with my boyfriend but talking about sex with anyone else makes me squirm.

Any advice?

Posted by Sarah

Re: What's it like going to family planning clinic?

Hey Sarah—i know it seems scary—i've been there! but trust me, the people that work at family planning are really used to people like us (or like I used to be) (i dont think ANYTHING would surprise them). I found them really supportive.
They talked with me and my friend bout lots of options. Did you know u can take a friend? or the boyfriend if you want. They don't mind at all, they figure they are helping twice as many people in one go!

Don't worry about people seeing you go in, yeah they may see you go in, but if the clinic is on a floor in a bigger building, no one will know where you are going, and even if they do bother to stop and think about it (and i doubt they would—most ppl are too wrapped up in there own stuff), they probably wouldnt care.

Pay it forward; if you discover its OK … tell someone else or post on here

Posted by Ellie

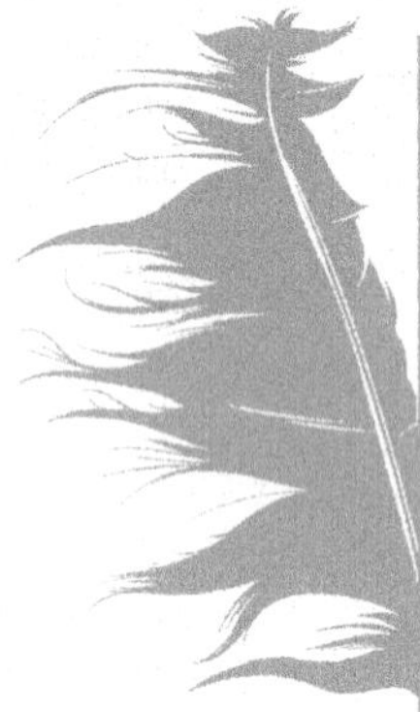

{ SUMMARY }

Developmentally, a young person is coming in to their own. They are learning about who they are, how they relate to others and how they want to be in the world. When working with young people it is important to establish a trusting and accepting environment that encourages the person to reflect on possibilities, rather than simply telling them what they should be doing. In other words, the focus should be on creating more rather than less, of working with strengths rather than deficits, and of growing resilience rather than failure.

REFLECTION POINTS

6.1 Intention (motivation, message, meaning, emotion)

Think about what it is like when someone focuses on your strengths rather than your weaknesses. What impact does this have on how hopeful you feel about the things you can accomplish?

6.2 Reception (received message, response, feedback)

How might establishing boundaries and limits also demonstrate caring?

6.3 Perception (style, manner, impression, analysis)

Establishing trust, being genuine and having a positive regard for a young person's strengths are all part of building rapport. What behaviours demonstrate these attributes?

QUESTIONS FOR REVIEW

1 What are the developmental tasks for adolescence?
2 How is resilience fostered in young people?
3 What is involved when taking a strengths-based approach in working with young people?

REFERENCES

Adolescent Health Research Group. (2008). *Youth'07: The health and wellbeing of secondary school students in New Zealand. Initial findings*. Auckland, NZ: University of Auckland.

Aronowitz, T. (2005). The role of 'envisioning the future' in the development of resilience among at-risk youth. *Public Health Nursing, 22*, 200–8.

Brooks-Gunn, J. & Paikoff, R. L. (1993). 'Sex is a gamble, kissing is a game': Adolescent sexuality and health promotion. In S. G. Millstein, A. C. Petersen & E. O. Nightingale (eds), *Promoting the health of adolescents: New directions for the twenty-first century* (pp. 180–208). New York, NY: Oxford University Press.

Cohen, S. (1972). *Folk devils and moral panics: The creation of the mods and rockers*. London, UK: MacGibbon and Kee.

Crone, E. A. (2009). Executive functions in adolescence: Inferences from brain and behavior. *Developmental Science, 12*(6), 825–30.

Erikson, E. (1968). *Identity, youth and crisis*. New York, NY: Norton.

Giroux, H. A. (2009). *Youth in a suspect society. Democracy or disposability*. New York, NY: Palgrave MacMillan.

Hall, G. S. (1904). *Adolescence: Its psychology and its relation to physiology, anthropology, sociology, sex, crime, religion, and education* (vols. I & II). Englewood Cliffs, NJ: Prentice-Hall.

Haxell, A. (2008). Cn I jus txt, coz I don wan 2b heard: Mobile technologies and youth counselling. Paper presented at the Ascilite. Hello! Where are you in the landscape of educational technology? Retrieved from www.ascilite.org.au/conferences/melbourne08/procs/haxell.pdf.

McCreanor, T., Watson, P. D. & Denny, S. J. (2006). 'Just accept us as we are more': Experiences of young Pakeha with their families in Aotearoa New Zealand. *Social Policy Journal of New Zealand, 27*, 156–70.

McLaren, K. (2002). *Building strength*. Ministry of Youth Affairs. Available from www.youthaffairs.govt.nz.

Ministry of Health (2010). *Drug use in New Zealand: Key results of the 2007/08 New Zealand Alcohol and Drug Use Survey*. Wellington, NZ: Author.

Ministry of Youth Development. (2007). *Youth development strategy Aotearoa: Action for child and youth development*. Wellington, NZ: Author.

Newman, B. & Newman, P. (2003). *Development through life* (8th edn). Pacific Grove, CA: Brooks/Cole.

Piaget, J. (1926). *The language and thought of the child*. New York, NY: Meridian Books.

Rossen, F. V., Lucassen, M. F. G., Denny, S. & Robinson, E. (2009). *Youth'07: The health and wellbeing of secondary school students in New Zealand: Results for young people attracted to the same sex or both sexes*. Auckland, NZ: The University of Auckland.

Steinberg, L. (1999). *Adolescence* (5th edn). New York, NY: McGraw-Hill.

Steinberg, L. (2005). Cognitive and affective development in adolescence. *Trends in Cognitive Sciences, 9*(2), 69–74.

Turkstra, L. S. & Byom, L. J. (2010, December 21). *Executive functions and communication in adolescents*. Rockville, MD: The ASHA Leader.

Udry, J. R. (1988). Biological predispositions and social control in adolescent sexual behavior. *American Sociological Review, 53*, 709–22.

Watson, P. D., Clark, T. C., Denny, S. J., Fa'alau, F., Ameratunga, S. N., Robinson, E. M. et al. (2003). A health profile of New Zealand youth who attend secondary school. *New Zealand Medical Journal, 116*(1171), 1–9.

Youth Mentoring Network (2011). *Panui whakamarama: How to assist your mentee to build resilience*. Retrieved 13 January 2011 from www.youthmentoring.org.nz.

WEBSITES

Information for Teenagers; Child, Youth & Family: www.cyf.govt.nz/info-for-teenagers
New Zealand Aotearoa Adolescent Health and Development: www.nzaahd.org.nz
Youthline: www.youthline.co.nz

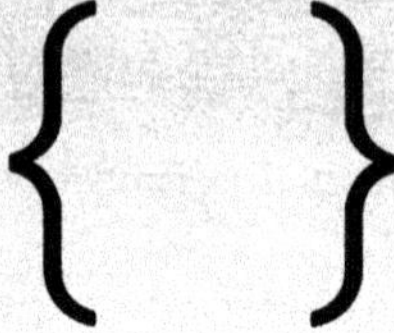

Early Adulthood

Charles Mpofu and Ailsa Haxell

CHAPTER OVERVIEW

This chapter covers the following topics:

+ Physical development
+ Risks
+ Cognitive development
+ Social development
+ Emotional adjustment.

KEY TERMS

Risky behaviour
Post-formal thought
Epistemic thinking
Dualistic thinking
Relativistic thinking
Fluid intelligence
Crystal intelligence
Reproductive technologies
Emotional intelligence

The early adulthood period is presented here as the ages 18 to 40 years. Although developmental psychologists tend to give an age range of 20 to 40 years, the age range adopted here takes into account the context of Aotearoa New Zealand where at age 18 young people assume various legal and social obligations that are associated with entry into adulthood. Individuals at this stage of their life are likely to be at the peak of their physical and cognitive capacities and focused on career advancement and intimacy.

Physical development

Physical development is perhaps the most noticeable aspect of development in human beings. It is about changes in the structures and physiological features of the human body. In terms of physical functioning, young adults are considered to be at the peak of their strength and energy in the middle adult years. Most body functions are fully developed by the time a person is in their mid-twenties. The peak of physical health and fitness occurs on average at approximately age 30 and the vast majority of young adults have no chronic conditions or impairments (Thies & Travers, 2009).

Brain development is an aspect of physical development that has implications for cognitive development during this period. The frontal lobe, which is responsible for reasoning, continues to develop in early adulthood. Knowledge about frontal lobe development is particularly important in terms of judgment and planning, intellectual capacities and problem-solving.

Risks

Within this age group, injuries are a major reason for medical visits. In Aotearoa New Zealand the most significant causes of death among young people are motor vehicle accidents and suicide. Among young adults aged between 25 and 44 years, unintentional and intentional injury (40 per cent combined) is the major contributor to mortality (Ministry of Health, 2001).

Motor vehicle accidents are one of the most common reasons for mortality among young New Zealanders (Fergusson, Swain-Campbell & Horwood, 2003). Drivers aged 20 to 24 are over-represented in traffic accidents and the same trend has been reported in Australia (Fergusson, Swain-Campbell & Horwood, 2003). It is important to note that there is a gender imbalance in this over-representation in favour of males, and this has been attributed to their tendency to engage in **risky behaviour** (Ministry of Health, 2001).

Risky behaviour Actions that may lead to injury or death.

Cognitive development

Post-formal thought Cognitive processes that emphasise relativism and the non-absolute nature of information.

Epistemic thinking Reflecting on how one arrives at facts, beliefs and ideas.

Dualistic thinking A tendency to see things as binary opposites; for example, as black and white, good or bad, or right or wrong. In addition, such ways of seeing assume that these are permanent states and are independent of one's own thinking.

This aspect of development is about changes in thinking, reasoning, memory and other intellectual capacities.

Advancing beyond what Piaget had labelled 'formal operational thinking' is a concept loosely referred to as **post-formal thought**. One of the distinguishing features of adults is the movement away from models of thinking where facts, beliefs and ideas are acquired, and towards a model of thinking that is personally considered and involves justifiable conclusions. This is a stage that Perry (1998) describes as **epistemic thinking**: a time of reflection on how people arrive at their beliefs. This marks a shift from **dualistic thinking**—where such beliefs might be described as true or false, right or wrong, or good or bad—to appreciating that beliefs held by others might differ yet still be valid for that person. **Relativistic thinking** involves an acceptance that what is 'true' or 'right' or 'good' varies greatly among people. This thinking is flexible, accepts diverse opinions and leads to an acknowledgment that there may be multiple truths. Pragmatism—doing what is possible given the limitations—also has been identified as a characteristic of adult thought (Shaie, 1978). This is based on the idea that young adults are at a period where they make use of skills previously obtained to achieve career goals, domestic goals and other life goals. This places an emphasis on context and relativity.

CASE STUDY 7.1

Margaret

Margaret is a 22-year-old woman born into a very religious family in Aotearoa New Zealand. Margaret describes herself as single on her Facebook page, but with lots of friends, both male and female. Margaret's friends describe her as a very social person who likes being with others and partying. Her parents are concerned for her, as she has twice called them needing transport home in the middle of the night. In each instance, she was worried about drink driving, as the plan to have a sober driver in the group had failed. Margaret identifies that she finds it hard to say 'no' to her friends, especially if she has been drinking, and that she finds it hard to be as 'good' as she knows her parents would like her to be.

To ensure that Margaret maintained the family's religious values when she was growing up, she was rarely allowed to play with other children. They discouraged her from joining clubs or participating in social events with her peers. Therefore, school and university were the only places when she was around people from different cultures and with other values.

Recently, Margaret attended an entrepreneurship workshop and was inspired to work with a partner to set up a podiatry practice. Margaret is worried about not being able to say 'no' to her business partner about obtaining a loan to establish the practice. Margaret is also reluctant to discuss this aspect of the business with her family.

Labouvie-Vief (1985, 2003) emphasises that young adults need to function in a world that is complex, and where there are multiple options or paths that could be taken. This requires the development of thinking that is unique to the circumstances of such situations. Labouvie-Vief also points to how the emotions play a part in decision-making: that there may be discrepancies between how a person feels about something and the logic of a situation. Such discrepancies become more organised and integrated with maturity and with the increased exposure to decision-making that early adulthood brings. In Case study 7.1 Margaret can be identified as moving towards relativistic thinking modes in considering how she is beginning to make choices; that is, she is just beginning to develop insight into how her emotions are influencing decisions.

Relativistic thinking Considering information according to its relationship with other known facts.

Rather than focusing on the process of decision-making, Horn and Cattell (1967) investigated types of intelligence in adults that they referred to as crystal and fluid intelligence. **Fluid intelligence** can be viewed as the ability to think and reason abstractly, and to solve problems independently of any related previous experience. **Crystal intelligence**, by contrast, relates to the accumulation of knowledge and skills acquired with experience (Horn & Cattell, 1967). Fluid intelligence starts to decline at around 30 years of age, while crystal intelligence continues to increase through middle adulthood. Horn and Cattell argued that this pattern was physiological rather than subject to context or culture. This increasing crystallised intelligence can be explained by the continued exposure to a wealth of experiences and skill acquisition.

Fluid intelligence The in-born ability of an individual to think and reason quickly and responsively.

Crystal intelligence The ability to think and reason based on experience acquired during life.

Social development

In reference to early adult development, Erik Erikson's theory of psychosocial development proposed that the main task is either to flourish in the achievement of intimacy, or to avoid the crisis of isolation as a result of failing to achieve intimacy (Erikson & Erikson, 1997). The outcome of navigating these two opposing forces has a bearing on achieving a mature personality and successful later development. The key issue here is seeking identity through intimacy and adjusting this identity when new relationships are sought. It is important to note that Erikson's concept of intimacy was not limited to relationship partners, but also referred to the capacity to make meaningful and lasting relationships. These include relationships with friends and colleagues, and could even be applied to developing a love for one's work. In Case study 7.1 it can be seen that even though Margaret is not in a long-term intimate relationship, she has friends, has maintained connections with family and is considering commitments towards career advancement.

CASE STUDY 7.2

Maiuu

Maiuu Fafo is a 23-year-old New Zealander whose parents come from Samoa. He was sent to Aotearoa New Zealand at the age of 17 by his grandmother to find a job and to financially support his extended family in Samoa.

Maiuu is very clear that his priorities lie in fulfilling his grandmother's wishes of being a breadwinner for the extended family. He tells his New Zealand-born friend Brian that he is finding it very hard coping with this pressure. Brian tells Maiuu that these issues don't really matter and that he should find a girlfriend. If this girlfriend is good then the next step is to find a flat where he would live with her while they are deciding about marriage and having children. Brian is baffled by Maiuu's response when he says that his family in Samoa will not approve of these ideas. Maiuu is similarly astounded by Brian's apparent selfishness and disrespect for elders.

Maiuu remembers his grandmother told him that if he has problems he should contact other extended family members in Aotearoa New Zealand, but he is not sure they would understand the pressures he is under. In addition, he knows these other members of his family have responsibilities for disciplining him if he misbehaves. He decides not to discuss his concerns with them.

Young adults find themselves making life decisions that are similar across many societies. These commonly involve career development, choosing a partner and establishing a family. However, contemporary New Zealand society is so diverse that within any community or group there will be people from a wide range of backgrounds who live with various expectations about their behaviour, how they use their time and how they plan for the future. Along with these differences are many expectations about the role and influence of family members. Case study 7.2 presents Maiuu as he is entering into adulthood in Aotearoa New Zealand, which is in some ways similar but in other ways quite different from his life in Samoa. He is increasingly aware of these contradictory demands and the inability of his previous methods of problem solving to resolve the stresses he experiences. Trying to meet the expectations of the differing groups that he interacts with creates additional stressors on him as he moves towards adulthood.

Erikson's theory of psychosocial development emphasises entering relationships, establishing long-term commitments, living with a partner and perhaps considering starting a family as key transitions for young adults.

Fertility is at its peak in the early adulthood years. The twenties are said to be the best times for pregnancy and giving birth because foetal and maternal risk increase after the age of 30 (Thies & Travers, 2009). However, women are increasingly participating in the paid workforce. This means that such decisions require balancing many considerations, such as the loss of income and the pressures of establishing careers, in conjunction with studying and perhaps the legacy of some student debt. These issues all contribute to many women deciding to defer when they have children.

In 2008, Statistics New Zealand reported the median age for women giving birth to their first child was 28 years. Advances in **reproductive technologies** have contributed in supporting the possibility for having children later in life; however, this raises further ethical and legal issues in addition to social and physical considerations.

Reproductive technologies The use of medical and surgical techniques to assist with fertility and conception.

Emotional adjustment

Young adults encounter many issues that make demands on their emotional adjustment. These adjustments occur within the context of both personal and professional relationships.

Erikson contributed to the understanding of emotional development during early adulthood when he noted that a strong sense of personal identity is critical to the development of intimate relationships. Erikson also noted that those with a poor sense of self tend to be associated with less committed relationships, and a higher likelihood of suffering emotional isolation and loneliness, which may lead to depression (Erikson & Erikson, 1997). Developing emotional competence and the capacity for clear communications, therefore, is useful in fostering resilience in early adulthood.

To help foster resilience, Goleman (1996) provides a model for enhancing **emotional intelligence**. The focus is on developing:

1. self-awareness—learning how to read one's emotions and recognise their impact while also using 'gut feelings' to inform decisions
2. self-management—controlling one's emotions and impulses as appropriate to changing circumstances

Emotional intelligence Insight into emotional needs and skills of self and others.

3 social awareness—developing awareness of and sensitivity to others' emotions while navigating one's social networks
4 relationship management—having the ability to inspire, influence and develop others while negotiating conflict.

The link between cognitive and emotional development in the form of emotional intelligence has also been researched in relation to its positive impact on learning among Australian adolescents (Downey et al., 2008).

In both case studies introduced in this chapter, it is apparent that the areas of cognitive, emotional and social development are clearly interrelated.

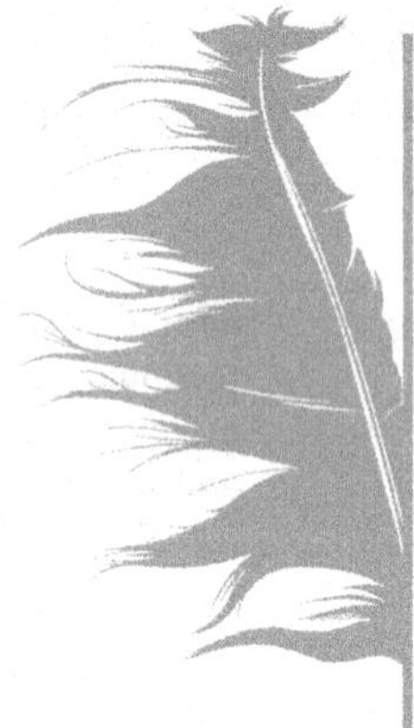

{ SUMMARY }

Early adulthood is a period when individuals begin (and are often expected) to take various social responsibilities, such as seeking an intimate partner, having children and establishing a career. A number of theories can be used to describe and explain physical, psychosocial and cognitive aspects of development in the early adulthood age group. However, concepts must be considered in relation to the wider social environment of the individual. Understanding the experiences of people in relation to their period of life and the wider context in which they live assists in ensuring that communication is appropriate and meaningful.

REFLECTION POINTS

7.1 Intention (motivation, message, meaning, emotion)

Having autonomy is often considered a hallmark of what it is to be an adult. Should autonomy always be respected?

7.2 Reception (received message, response, feedback)

Think about when you have been stressed, anxious, unwell or in pain. How receptive are you to learning at these times? Having educated someone about his or her condition, how would you check if information shared has been understood?

7.3 Perception (style, manner, impression, analysis)

In interactions with practitioners, what expectations do you hold about how you would like to be treated?

QUESTIONS FOR REVIEW

1. What are the dangers of assuming that young adults are at the best years of their health?
2. What conflicts between emotional and cognitive development may people in this age group experience?
3. What part do physical and social development play in risk-taking behaviour?

REFERENCES

Downey, L. A., Mountstephen, J., Lloyd, J., Hansen, K. & Stough, C. (2008). Emotional intelligence and scholastic achievement in Australian adolescents. *Australian Journal of Psychology, 60*(1), 10–17.

Erikson, E. & Erikson, J. M. (1997). *The life cycle completed* (extended version). New York, NY: W. W. Norton.

Fergusson, D. M., Swain-Campbell, N. R. & Horwood, L. J. (2003). Risky driving behaviour in young people: Prevalence, personal characteristics and traffic accidents. *Australian and New Zealand Journal of Public Health, 27*(3), 337–42.

Goleman, D. (1996). *Emotional intelligence: Why it can matter more than IQ*. New York, NY: Bantam Books.

Horn, J. L. & Cattell, R. B. (1967). Age differences in fluid and crystallized intelligence. *Acta Psychologica, 26*, 107–29.

Labouvie-Vief, G. (1985). Intelligence and cognition. In J. E. Birren & K. W. Schaie (eds), *Handbook of the psychology of aging* (2nd edn) (pp. 500–30). New York, NY: Van Nostrand Reinhold.

Labouvie-Vief, G. (2003). Dynamic integration: Affect, cognition, and the self in adulthood. *Current Directions in Psychological Science, 12*, 201–6.

Ministry of Health (2001). *The burden of disease and injury in New Zealand*. Wellington, NZ: Author. Retrieved from www.moh.govt.nz/moh.nsf/pagesmh/952?Open.

Perry, W. G. Jr. (1998). *Forms of intellectual and ethical development in the college years: A schema*. San Francisco, CA: Jossey-Bass.

Shaie, K. W. (1978). Toward a stage theory of adult cognitive development. *Journal of Aging and Human Development, 8*(2), 129–38.

Statistics New Zealand (2008). Births and deaths. March 2008 quarter. Retrieved www.stats.govt.nz/browse_for_stats/population/births/BirthsAndDeaths_HOTPMar08qtr.aspx.

Thies, K. M. & Travers, J. F. (2009). *Growth and development through the lifespan*. London, UK: Jones and Bartlett.

WEBSITES

Births and Deaths: March 2008 quarter, Statistics New Zealand: www.stats.govt.nz/browse_for_stats/population/births/BirthsAndDeaths_HOTPMar08qtr.aspx

Burden of Disease and Injury in New Zealand, Ministry of Health: www.moh.govt.nz/moh.nsf/pagesmh/952?Open

Demographic Trends 2009, Marriage, civil union, and divorce, Statistics New Zealand: www.stats.govt.nz/browse_for_stats/population/estimates_and_projections/demographic-trends-2009/chapter3.aspx

READING 15

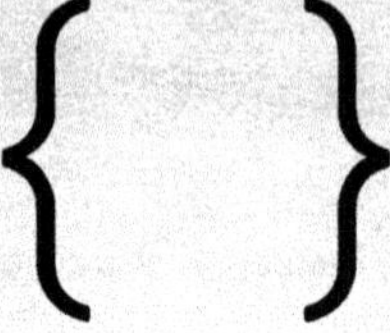

Middle Years

Kirk Reed

CHAPTER OVERVIEW

This chapter covers the following topics:

+ Defining the middle years
+ Roles in the middle years
+ Managing life events.

KEY TERMS

Life roles
Transition
Crisis
Life events

The journey through the middle years can be explored by considering the common developmental tasks as outlined in the work of Erikson (1994) and Havighurst (1972). Another view can be found in the **life roles** that are generally experienced by those in their middle years. Communicating effectively with people at this stage of their life requires a respectful understanding of their perspective, the journey they are on and the issues and challenges they are likely to be experiencing.

Life roles The set of rights, obligations and behaviours associated with various tasks and positions (for example, learner, parent and employee).

Defining the middle years

From a Western lifespan perspective, Erikson (a psychologist) and Havighurst (a physicist and educationalist) identified some developmental tasks that tend to be associated with the middle years. Havighurst (1972) identified that in the middle years, which he described as being from 30 to 60 years, the key tasks include: selecting a mate; starting and rearing a family; managing a home; getting started in an occupation, and reaching and maintaining a successful career; finding a congenial social group; and achieving adult and civic responsibility. He also indentified that the middle years include adjusting to having ageing parents, assisting teenage children to become responsible and happy adults, and accepting and adjusting to the physiological changes of middle age.

Erikson (1994) described middle age as being from 35 to 65 years and called this life stage 'generativity versus self-absorption'. He stated that middle age is when a person tends to be occupied with creative and meaningful work and with the issues that surround family life. One of the significant tasks of the middle years is to perpetuate culture and transmit cultural values through family, while working to establish a stable environment for family and the community. During this stage of life, Erikson identified that significant relationships are within the workplace and family, and that a sense of strength comes through the care of others and the production of something that contributes to the betterment of society. He called this 'generativity', which he described as a response to a sense of fear of inactivity and stagnation. As goals, relationships and family life change, a person may be faced with major life changes—a mid-life crisis—and struggle to find meaning and purpose to life. Erikson argued that if a person did not successfully get through this life stage then they could become self-absorbed and stagnant.

From the work of Havighurst and Erikson, it is clear that there are some common key developmental tasks associated with the middle years, namely: management of a career, negotiating and maintaining a relationship, expanding caring responsibilities, managing a household, adjusting to ageing parents and coping with the physical changes of ageing. At this stage of life there are a range of health issues that are common, which may include: heart disease, stroke, chronic illness, work-related illness, respiratory disease, alcohol and other drug misuse, and depression. In addition, screening for conditions such as breast cancer and prostate cancer, and risk factors associated with chronic heart disease are recommended. These health issues are, of course, different for each individual, but managing and coming to terms with physiological and cognitive changes is an inevitable part of growing older, especially towards the end of the middle years and into older age.

As people enter their middle years with a great many hopes, goals and ambitions, some of these go unrealised as a person settles into the daily round of activities. At around age 40 some adults experience a mid-life **transition** or 'mid-life crisis', where a reassessment of their personal goals and aspirations takes place. Up to this point they may have hung onto their personal story that their life would be a success in every way. There was plenty of time to get a better job, start a family, write a book, take an overseas trip or purchase a fast car. But at some point a person may begin to realise that time is rapidly running out to do all these things. Some adults who go through a mid-life transition do so very well and accept their life as it is. Others refuse to abandon their goals and train for a new job or take a positive step to getting what they set out to. Still others become depressed or turn to alcohol or other drugs as a means of escape when they realise their goals and aspirations may never be achieved.

Transition The journey from one place or position to another.

CASE STUDY 8.1

Kath

Kath is a 42-year-old woman living a long way from her family networks. She is married, and she and her husband own their own home and have a 3½-year-old son. She works full time, gets up at 5:30 am to commute an hour to work and picks her son up from day care at 5.30 pm. Kath has a strong commitment to her career in a large company; she enjoys the challenge of her job but is beginning to realise that when her son goes to school she may have to reduce her hours or resign from her job to manage getting him to and from school. She has a number of friends who live locally, but she does not see them often as she needs the weekends to rest and spend time with her family, and also catch up on household chores. She has few leisure interests outside of her family and home, simply because she does not have enough time in the day. In the past 18 months she has had some health problems and has had her gall bladder removed. Kath is beginning to realise that the health of her parents is beginning to deteriorate, which she finds difficult when she lives so far away from them and cannot be there when they need her.

Roles in the middle years

Depending on a person's life stage, they will take on varying roles. Nine roles were identified by Super (1980). From his perspective as a psychologist he presented explanations that may account for the roles that most people engage in most of the time. These nine roles are: child, student, leisure user, citizen, worker, partner/spouse, homemaker, parent and retiree. In the middle years, and for any particular individual, some of these roles may be absent or insignificant; however, most of these life roles will be present to one extent or another. Super also identified four key areas in which these roles may be acted out: in the home, workplace, school or community. These are all important parts of the environment or context in which people live out their lives, and the environment may significantly influence or impact on a person's roles. For example, an employer may expect their employee to work late or at the weekends to get tasks done, and this may become a routine part of a person's life. This in turn may impact on their leisure time roles and cause conflict with their spouse or partner.

It is important to consider if a person's roles indicate balance. If there are either significant gaps or roles that are too demanding, they may impact on health and well-being. A person in their middle years is likely to have one or more of the roles identified by Super. It is worth considering from the person's perspective what their involvement is in these roles, the meaning the role has and how one role impacts on other roles. Super's roles may be explored in relation to the middle years in the following ways:

+ Child—as life progresses, a person in their middle years may take on more responsibility for caring, looking after and supporting parents, particularly if their parents become frail or need assistance. It is likely that a person in their middle years will still socialise with their parents and have obligations at family events or during holidays or festivals.
+ Student—during the middle years a person may take on the student role and engage in ongoing learning, professional development or higher education. Becoming a student in this stage of life might be linked to career aspirations and advancement, retraining to find a worker role that is more aligned to self-identity, or the need to retrain or upskill because of job loss. The student role is likely to be in conjunction with balancing other life roles; for example, a person might attend an evening course purely for personal interest. It is likely that those in this life stage who engage in higher education will have been successful in this environment in the past, although for some this might be their first time experience, and it may take some time to become familiar and comfortable with the demands of a formal education setting.

+ Leisure user—activities and leisure time may have been curtailed while raising a family and spending more time in the worker role. Leisure time may start to increase in the middle years as children leave home and there is more spare time. It is likely that leisure interests will change in response to a mid-life crisis or decreasing health or physical ability associated with ageing. There may be more time and resources to engage in new leisure activities.
+ Citizen—in the middle years, a person may feel the need to contribute to their local community and give 'something back'. A person may take on civic roles such as city councillor, become a member of a governance group such as a board for a school or non-profit organisation, or join a community group.
+ Worker—this role is likely to be predominant and stable during the middle years, and work commitments and responsibilities may increase due to length of time in the job and promotion. Job loss or redundancy may have a significant impact on a person's sense of identity and self-belief.
+ Partner/spouse—it is likely that a person in the middle years is in a committed relationship or is seeking their second or third long-term committed relationship as a result of the loss of their partner or the dissolution of their marriage or civil partnership. Significant time and energy may be devoted to maintaining the relationship and spending time with their partner.
+ Homemaker—this is likely to be a significant role in the middle years, due to home ownership and management, home renovation, and maintenance of the home environment. These are all likely to take up a considerable amount of time. As a person ages, they may choose to do less around the home or in the garden, and employ someone else to do these tasks while they focus on work or leisure. A person in their middle years may make changes to the physical environment of their home to ensure easy access, downsize the family home or move house in preparation for retirement and/or older age.
+ Parent—during the middle years the role of parent may change as children leave home and 'make their way in the world'. The 'empty nest syndrome' may be experienced where parents mourn the loss of their children as they leave the family home and establish relationships and a home of their own. There may be increased responsibility as a grandparent as a person's children start to create their own family.
+ Retiree—some people in their middle years may take early retirement or may be made redundant. This is a significant change and some might take a long time to deal with the sense of loss. As a result in the change of worker role, a person may reorganise their life to accommodate the loss of the worker role by taking on a part-time job or increasing their leisure interests. Others may begin planning and preparing for retirement, reducing the hours spent in work as they move to the next stage of their life.

Managing life events

While the list above gives a broad and general view of the types of roles a person may have in their middle years, it is by no means comprehensive. As life progresses, a number of events beyond the person's control may take place. This can range from the loss of a partner or spouse or job loss due to the economic climate to deterioration of personal health or a mid-life **crisis**. In order to cope with these **life events** Reese and Smyer (1983) suggest eight factors to consider when working with a person to manage life events. It is important to consider the person in context and work with them to identify the following:

Crisis A significant point of change with potential risks of loss or harm.

Life events Situations or experiences that are significant for the change related to it.

1 Trigger—what set off the event? Was the event expected or anticipated? Was the trigger internal or external to the person?
2 Timing—how did the timing of the event impact on how it was experienced or managed?
3 Control—how much control did the person have over the event, both when it happened and the way it was managed or progressed?
4 Role change—what impact has the event had, or will have, on life roles?
5 Duration—how long did the event last? Was the change permanent or temporary?
6 Previous experience—had the person experienced a similar life event in the past? How has this previous experience impacted on the current event?
7 Concurrent stress—what are the other stressors in the person's life and how have these demands impacted on the current event?
8 Assessment—did the experience have a positive or negative impact? Did this change over time?

While on first appearances this might simply appear to be a list of factors to work through with the person as a means to understand the life events they are experiencing, it is important to make sure that this is done with respect and empathy. Developing a sense of rapport with the person will allow them to feel comfortable and enable them to tell their story in detail. A person in this age group may relate better to someone they connect with their family, rather than a professional. It is therefore important to clarify roles and purpose when talking with them. It may also be useful to adapt language and vocabulary so that it is relevant to their age. Carefully listening to responses will provide cues about how they are going about managing their life event. Be aware that a person may become upset and this must be responded to in a respectful and sincere manner.

CASE STUDY 8.2

Drew

Drew is a 35-year-old gay man living in the inner suburb of a large city. He has a wide circle of friends, who he sees as often as he can, plus a broad range of interests, which include travelling overseas, networking with his friends, jogging, going to the gym, spending time on the net and cooking. He spends most of his weekends with his friends and they often go to bars or clubs. He sees his family from time to time, but this is usually at family events such as birthdays. His father has a long-term illness and lives away from the family home, so his mother lives alone. He tries to support her usually by calling or visiting once a week, but he does not have much time to see her.

He has a successful job and has been studying to update his knowledge. There has been some talk of restructuring at his workplace and he may be made redundant, but he is not too concerned if he loses his job because he feels like a new challenge. He feels like he is well positioned to get a more senior job and that working somewhere else would help him with his career goals. Drew has recently ended a long-term relationship and is looking for someone to settle down with. His general practitioner has warned him that his blood pressure is high; he knows he should do something about this but he is not worried as he knows he is still young and has plenty of time to make those kinds of changes to his lifestyle when he gets older.

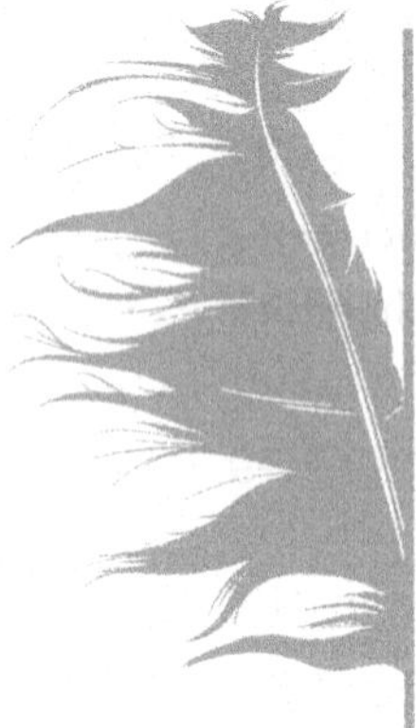

{ SUMMARY }

The middle years are generally considered to be between a person's thirties and retirement and is a time when a person is highly productive and secure, and has a high sense of achievement. Health-care students need to be aware of the roles and responsibilities that are typical in the middle years, but also need to be aware that typical patterns may not apply to every individual's circumstances. These roles and responsibilities can be disrupted due to internal and external factors, such as feeling unsuccessful or having a sense of loss as family leaves home or if the person is made redundant. Having skills and knowledge in understanding a person's life roles and how they manage life events will enable a student to gain an understanding of a person in their context so interventions can be tailored to address the needs of the individual.

REFLECTION POINTS

8.1 Intention (motivation, message, meaning, emotion)

How are the key developmental tasks of the middle years similar to or different from your own life stage?

8.2 Reception (received message, response, feedback)

What would be the ideal role balance for someone in their middle years?

8.3 Perception (style, manner, impression, analysis)

What connections can you make in the case studies of Kath and Drew to the key developmental tasks of Havighurst and Erikson?

QUESTIONS FOR REVIEW

1 Using Super's life roles, can you identify the roles of someone you know who is in their middle years?
2 In what ways does a mid-life transition/crisis resemble an adolescent coming to terms with their identity and place in the world?
3 How would you alter your communication style in order to work with someone that is older than you?

REFERENCES

Erikson, E. H. (1994). *Identity and the life cycle: A reissue*. New York, NY: Norton.

Havighurst, R. J. (1972). *Developmental tasks and education.* New York, NY: Longman.

Reese, H. W. & Smyer, M. A. (1983). The dimensionalisation of life events. In E. J. Callahan & K. A. McCluskey (eds), *Life-span developmental psychology: Non formative life events*. New York, NY: Academic Press.

Super, D. E. (1980). A life-span, life-space approach to career development. *Journal of Vocational Behaviour, 16*, 282–98.

WEBSITES

Agewell: www.agewell.org.nz
Growing Up in New Zealand: www.growingup.co.nz
ThirdAge: www.thirdage.com

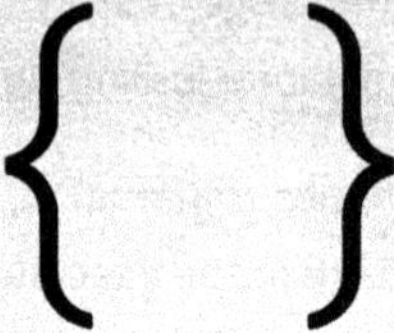

Senior Years

Helen Gaeta and Terry Weblemoe

CHAPTER OVERVIEW

This chapter covers the following topics:

+ Psychosocial theories of ageing
+ The ageing population
+ Socio-environmental theory
+ Communication and ageing.

KEY TERMS

Gerontology
Geriatrics
Activity theory
Disengagement theory
Abandonment theory
Continuity theory
Socio-environmental theory
Ageism
Fluid intelligence
Crystal intelligence

The concept of people in their 'senior years' is commonly reflected in the image of a retired person receiving a state pension. Although this is the case for the current generation of 'seniors', the pension is a fairly modern concept that has its underpinnings in the rise of industrialisation in Europe, especially in Germany. In 1879, Otto von Bismarck, Chancellor of the German Empire, abandoned free-trade policies and adopted protective tariffs on home industries to provide revenue for the German government. The adoption of tariffs proved to be very profitable for German industry, generating an increase in employment opportunities in the urban areas where industry was established. This created an influx of German workers from the countryside to these urban areas. The shift in the working population from agricultural to industrial coincided with the rise of socialism in Europe, a political position that Bismarck opposed. In order to keep the socialist movement at bay, he decided that German workers needed to have a stake in the political affairs of the state of Germany.

The same political influences that were reforming Europe were also impacting on New Zealand. In 1898, the Liberal government led by Richard Seddon, introduced a small means-tested pension to destitute older people over the age of 65 years. Like Bismarck, Seddon was influenced by the plight of the workers, especially the welfare of ex-miners on the West Coast. In 1939, the first New Zealand Labour Prime Minister, Michael Joseph Savage, spearheaded the legislation that was the forerunner of the current 'New Zealand Superannuation Scheme'. This entitled people from 60 years of age to an income- and asset-tested pension, consolidating the notion that 60 years marked the onset of the 'senior years'. Alongside these developments, the fields of **gerontology** and **geriatrics** emerged.

Gerontology The study of social, psychological and biological aspects of ageing.

Geriatrics The study of diseases of ageing.

Psychosocial theories of ageing

Activity theory provides a perspective on ageing that links activity in social roles with life satisfaction (Havighurst et al., 1968, 1969). Optimal ageing involves staying active, maintaining social involvement and finding replacement roles for those activities lost through retirement (Maddox, 1968; Neugarten, 1971). Within this view, failure to age successfully is a failure of motivation on the part of the individual. One of the weaknesses of this perspective is that it makes implicit assumptions about the relationships between people's action and their roles (Gubrium, 1973). Proponents of activity theory assume that people control the types of roles available to them, as well as the activities necessary to the performance of those roles. They assume that people have the capacity to construct and develop appropriate sets of activity goals. However, it is hard to see how this can be so for the elderly who are financially challenged, and the elderly deprived of social support. Another

Activity theory A deterministic approach that sees the older person as responsible for making their own decisions and adjustments to their changing situation.

problem is that it assumes it is better to be active than inactive, and that life satisfaction and activity are positively related. However, research studies have shown there is not a uniform relationship between activity levels and life satisfaction (Lemon, Bengston & Peterson, 1972; Maddox, 1974). Furthermore, it does not take into account that reduced activity is necessary for some elderly because of declining health, and that this does not mean that life satisfaction must decline.

Disengagement theory A belief that ageing involves withdrawal and severing of ties between a person and others in society.

Disengagement theory is an explicit theory based on research conducted by Cumming and Henry (1961). There is a focus on the self and a reduced involvement in organised social structures. Successful ageing is seen as acceptance of, and a desire to, reduce social interactions. The disengagement process is seen as mutually satisfying for the older person and for society. It ensures that society maintains optimal function by preserving social equilibrium and enabling self-reflection for the older person. It provides an orderly transfer of knowledge, capital and power from the older to the younger generation, ensuring that a vacuum is not left when valuable older members of society die. Changes in an older adult's biological and cognitive abilities are not perceived as a threat because the disengagement process prepares one for the anticipated decline that comes with old age. Opponents of the theory claim that it is context-free and biologically homogeneous. Prasad (1964) conducted a study of retired industrial workers and showed that none of the aged men in the study showed any desire to disengage. A number of studies showed that disengagement from employment often worked against an individual's best interest (Glanz, 1983, 1985; Ruffini & Todd, 1979). Furthermore, it was often wasteful or dysfunctional because experienced and productive individuals were being pressured to withdraw or narrow their activities after retirement. Other studies found that when there was disengagement from active life it was usually for health reasons, not ageing per se (Lowenthal, 1968; Mass & Kuypers, 1974).

CASE STUDY 9.1

Disengagement

It was just a sudden decision that I made, but what triggered it was the death of my oldest sister … so I made up my mind then that I was going to put in my resignation right there and then. I was just thinking I needed to spend some time with my grandchildren. But before I left the office I was asked by the office if I would just do a little project part-time for them for three months, so I thought 'yes' … and that was the start of my consultancy. Now I'm gradually weaning myself away from the workforce again, taking a couple of days off a week, and that's something that's much more desirable for my stage of life.

Ministry of Social Development (2009)

Abandonment theory was conceived to explain the increasing loneliness and neglect that characterises old age for some people (Burgess, 1960). It aims to explain inevitable and universal negative features of the ageing process. The view is that older people experience a downwards direction with respect to lifestyle, which is accompanied with increasing levels of abandonment and social isolation.

Abandonment theory The perspective that ageing is linked to decreased social engagement and increased isolation.

It suggests that being old means enduring a degree of social deprivation. Baum and Baum (1980) argue that this view has its origins in industrialisation, which has no use for older people. Knowledge and skills are the modern currency and these change quickly in modern Western civilisations. Thus the services of older people are of little economic value, making them outdated and less 'useful'. Status, therefore, is lost in a culture that prizes youth, beauty and success. Prior to the formalisation of abandonment theory, Barron (1961) suggested that the aged become a 'disprivileged minority group'.

Abandonment theory also implies that financial deprivation, through loss of income, accompanies ageing. Furthermore, old age brings psychological and physical segregation of the elderly, particularly when they live in institutions, retirement villages and nursing homes. These views of the elderly are still prominent today, even though most older people in Aotearoa New Zealand stay in their own homes, with less than 10 per cent in supportive environments. In addition, changing demographics and the high cost of housing is shifting asset wealth from younger to older adults. Thus the older adult is increasingly seen as a valuable consumer, contrary to the notion of financial impoverishment.

CASE STUDY 9.2

Abandonment

When I was looking for a job, I'd just go into these recruitment consultants. It was a joke. They were staffed with young kids. If I did manage to score an interview, I'd know immediately. I was told there is virtually no chance to get a job at my age … just so annoyed by the attitude of 'these kids' that say 'you are not qualified' or 'your skill set is not quite what is required'. Only once, and that was the job I got, I thought, 'I've got a chance here'.

Ministry of Social Development (2009)

Continuity theory was formulated to explain development across the lifespan. Its importance for ageing is that it links the person's past to their present. To this extent, Erikson's (1980) developmental theory of the eight stages of life can be considered a continuity theory. Erikson claims that a person must successfully pass through all prior seven stages to successfully pass through the

Continuity theory The view that ageing is a continuation of the earlier part of life, a component of the natural cycle of life.

eighth stage of life, where synthesis of all prior developmental stages enables the older adult to reflect and accept, with satisfaction, the passage of their life. An individual who achieves this attains what Erikson termed 'ego integrity'. With ego integrity comes wisdom, though Erikson does not expand on what he means by wisdom. An individual who does not achieve 'ego integrity' will experience despair and fear of death.

Continuity theory posits that stability guides psychological development throughout the lifespan. In other words, personality, values, morals, preferences and basic patterns of behaviour are relatively constant through the lifespan, regardless of the life changes an individual experiences (for example, widowhood, illness or loss of income). A major criticism of continuity theory is its deterministic nature. This means there is little, if any, flexibility for change from early behaviours or attitudes as the individual is pre-programmed to age in a particular way. To overcome this inflexibility, new interpretations of continuity have been formulated to encompass evolution and adaptation, reducing the emphasis on stagnation. Newer perspectives still claim that there are basic structures that persist over time (personality traits), but that capacity for change can be incorporated into a person's history. Atchley (1989) states that adults 'employ concepts of their past to conceive of the future, and structure their choices in response to the change brought about by normal ageing' (p. 183). A substantial number of research studies have supported continuity theory (for example, Ross, 1977; Maddox, 1968; Palmore & Kivett, 1977). However, many of these studies have used cross-sectional and short-term designs for data collection. Thus only inferences can be made about the stability of personality over time.

All of these socially based perspectives of ageing have been developed against the backdrop of industrial economies in the Western world. Although most of the research has originated in North America, the underlying principles can be generalised to all Western capitalist industrial models. Activity theory, disengagement theory and abandonment theory are strongly influenced by notions around the usefulness of citizens to economic productivity. During the period in which these perspectives were being developed, only 10 per cent of the New Zealand population was over 65 years old. By contrast, 65 per cent of the population was between 15 and 64 years old. Thus older adults were not needed in the workforce, given there was a plentiful supply of efficient economic units to meet the productivity needs of society. However, the declining birth rate and increasing life expectancy is changing the population demographic. Concomitant with the changing demographic is a shifting perspective of ageing and a need to revise social theories of ageing. The impact of the ageing population is expanded in the next section, followed by a presentation of a newer social theory of ageing that incorporates the changing population demographic and its linkage to recent economic developments.

The ageing population

A common feature of all Western societies is that life expectancy is increasing and birth rates are falling. Consequently, the population is ageing. It is estimated that by 2026, more than 20 per cent of New Zealand's population will be over 65 years, compared with just 12 per cent in 2006. From the late 2040s, this age group will comprise more than 25 per cent of the population (Statistics New Zealand, 2009).

Over the next 50 years or so, the percentage of New Zealanders older than 65 years will approximately double. After this point, the transition from a young society with high mortality rates to an older population with low fertility rates and greater life expectancy will be complete, and a more stable demographic will have been reached (assuming projected fertility rates do not change).

This changing demographic has implications for the labour market that will begin to be felt from 2011, when the baby boomers (those born between 1946 and 1965) begin to turn 65. A shrinking workforce will need to support a larger, more dependent population. In 2000, there were 25 retirees for every 100 workers in Aotearoa New Zealand. If labour force participation rates of the older population stay constant, by 2050 there will be 70 retirees for every 100 workers. This creates a fear that a shrinking working-age population will be obliged to finance the pensions, health care and other services required by a rapidly increasing elderly population, which will lead to higher taxes on a workforce that is already over-burdened with high personal debt.

One approach to managing the impact of the ageing New Zealand population is to maximise the potential of older workers by extending their working lives. For older workers, employment is generally regarded as having positive effects on physical and mental health, as well as providing greater social connectedness and interaction (Ministry of Social Development, 2006), consistent with the perspective expressed in activity theory. According to Statistics New Zealand (2009), 17 per cent of people aged 65 years and over were in the labour force in 2006, up from less than 7 per cent in 1986. This is one of the highest rates of employment for older people in the OECD. Thus the increasing proportion of older adults comprising the population, the need to constrain government spending in support of the ageing population, and the need to retain a skilled workforce are changing the discourse around ageing. Consequently, previous social theories of ageing—that were driven by expansion of the industrial economy where young adults predominated—now need to be revised to accommodate changing Western economies, which are being driven by technological expansion and the need to retain a skilled workforce.

This does not negate some of the perspectives expressed in activity, disengagement or abandonment theories. Instead, it demonstrates how social theories of ageing are very context dependent. A satisfactory theory of ageing needs to take social context into account. A more recent perspective on ageing is to explore the synergies between the older adult and their interactions with their environment.

Socio-environmental theory

Socio-environmental theory An understanding of ageing based on the assumption that the environment of older adults is built on interrelationships between individual and social context.

Socio-environmental theory is predicated on the dynamic interaction between the individual's resources and social resources. The individual context refers to the person's health, financial, intellectual and social support resources, which influence the person's choices and impact on whether they socially withdraw or stay active. The social context refers to the social norms created around the ageing environment and the social resources made available to older adults in the way of housing and local support (Gubrium, 1972). The socio-environmental model states that the life satisfaction of older adults results from the interactions between the social environment available to the older adult and the personal resources of the older person. Furthermore, older adults follow a different ageing trajectory based on different degrees of resources available to them.

The socio-environmental perspective does not dismiss earlier social theories of ageing. Rather, it encompasses them, claiming that abandonment, activity and disengagement theories have both internal and external constructs that vary among individuals. For example, the internal components are a person's tendency to behave in a fixed way towards others and events in the environment. By contrast, the external components are the social expectations of the way older adults should behave. As long as the internal and external constructs are congruent, life satisfaction and high morale will be experienced by the older adult.

This framework proposes that older adults consider the expected social norms of their social situation and accept or reject them based on their personal resources (see Case study 9.3). The environment is defined in terms of physical space, psychological space and economic resources. Furthermore, actions to change social norms can be taken by individuals or by organisations (for example, Grey Power New Zealand, a lobby organisation that promotes the welfare and well-being of citizens aged over 50 years).

The dynamic interaction between individual resource and social environment implies that older adults are heterogeneous with respect to capabilities, resources and motivation. It further implies that ageing individuals can bring about social change by their actions. This reciprocity between individual and social resource sets up a feedback mechanism for the person that enables them to monitor their social effectiveness. For example, a person who experiences abandonment may work to change the social norms that enabled abandonment to occur.

CASE STUDY 9.3

Socio-environmental narrative

Mary is 64 years old and retired. She was a senior manager for a financial company. She is married and her husband continues to hold a senior management position. She has three adult children. Two are married and between them they have five children. The third and youngest is currently living in Italy. Mary and her husband met as students at university. They worked hard at their careers in business and built substantial wealth. Mary worked throughout her pregnancies and returned to work within months of each birth. Mary and her husband could afford to employ home help and childcare to help raise the children and run the home. Mary did not need to retire, but chose to when the firm was about to undergo restructuring. The firm was keen to retain her services, but Mary is interested in literature and theatre, and her career and family never allowed her time to pursue either of these interests satisfactorily. Mary's motivation to retire was to be able to read the books she never had time for, to go to theatre and not feel guilty because she should have been preparing for a meeting in the morning, and to spend time with her grandchildren as they grew up.

Because of Mary's employment history, there was an assumption that she would be bored 'hanging around the house'. It was assumed she would take up voluntary work in community-based activities. She would have plenty of time and she was well qualified to do this. Mary resisted this as it was not what she planned for her retirement. She was made to feel guilty for staying home and reading books when she could be helping in the community. She experienced incongruence between her personal resources and her social environment. This caused her a degree of dissatisfaction and some disengagement from her previous social circles. However, she was able to resolve the incongruence by spending time with her grandchildren and involving herself with their activities; for example, sports clubs and theatre groups. In this way, she was seen as meeting social norms and was able to fulfil her own needs.

The socio-environmental framework is designed to allow flexibility for variations in individual motivations, attitudes and activities among different contexts. An individual may be highly motivated to be active in one social context but not in another. In this model, a person in good health and with sufficient financial resources may still be dissatisfied with their environment; for example, if they are forced to retire from work they enjoy. The key to this model is the degree of congruence or incongruence between personal norms and resources and those of the wider society. The degree of life satisfaction and morale depends on the balance between context-dependent congruence and incongruence (Deci & Ryan, 1987).

Social theory, assumptions and communication

Over the past 200 years, a considerable amount has been written by younger people about older people that objectifies them, minimises their experience and dismisses them from the important issues, such as the ability to compete for rewarding and self-fulfilling employment and to make valuable contributions to society. Some of the above academic arguments have coloured society's attitudes about ageing, retirement and older individuals to the point of considerable society-wide environmental and institutional prejudice, aptly named '**ageism**'. Like institutional racism, those who are not affected by the results of prejudice do not recognise its pervasiveness, while those who are affected are keenly aware and may even adopt the beliefs of their oppressors.

Ageism
Discrimination on the basis of age.

The view that seniors have outlived their usefulness is in direct contrast to the view of the older person as gaining wisdom and possibly to achieving status as a community elder—a view held by many non-Western cultures, as well as our own pre-industrial society. While Erikson may have never defined wisdom, other theorists such as Maslow (1999) have expanded on his concept of generativity as a shift over time from more concrete subsistence-achievement goals to those that are more social or self-actualising.

Experience working with 'seniors' suggests that no one is more aware of these conflicting views than seniors themselves, and that empowerment is key to communicating with seniors. The goal of therapeutic communication is that of respect, empowerment and a 'personal acceptance that people are unique' and deserving of quality and thoughtful attention. Without preconceived ideas of what seniors are or should be like, communicating with them is often a very enlightening and entertaining experience.

The very first consideration when communicating with seniors is that not all individuals age at the same pace, nor do physical, social and psychological aspects deteriorate at the same time. More so than at any other age, it is important to discover and adjust communication and practice to the individual's capabilities, avoiding assumptions based on chronological age.

Communication and ageing

Physical domain

While there is great variation in how people age—based on genetics, environment and behaviour—eventually some deterioration of some senses will occur, while others may remain acute. There may be some physical hearing loss with age, but more frequently there is a deterioration of the ability to distinguish conversations from background noise. This can interfere with clear communication, particularly if the communicator has a soft, high voice, mumbles or gives directions in a noisy room. Consider speaking in a low clear tone, and not necessarily more loudly, and being sure that the receiver of the message can see the face of the person sending the message.

With exposure to the sun's UV rays, the lenses in the eye yellow and become less flexible over time. This can effect colour perception, depth accommodation and the ability to focus on small objects. Even with corrective lenses, this can inhibit reading small print or deter much-loved activities like handicrafts, repair or artwork—even driving for groceries or meeting with friends. When giving written instructions (including, for example, information on drug labels), consider whether the individual will be able to read them, or whether they would like to receive and retain the information in a different way.

Social domain

Everyone is a product of their environment, from their thoughts to the generational periods they have lived through. These events shape the way individuals perceive their world. While it is common today to have a fascination with the 'new', our seniors are often the experts in experiencing and adapting to change. What may seem new to the younger generation may appear to be an 'old concept in a new coat' to someone who has seen many changes. This can create false assumptions in both generations. To be able to communicate meaningfully, it is necessary to always assess and correct assumptions, and to appreciate how older people see their world.

There is some suggestion that as individuals mature, they may shift on an introversion–extroversion continuum of social expression (Myer-Briggs Foundation, n.d.), often moving to a more balanced position. Those that preferred solitary pursuits and achievements may become more social or family oriented, and those who have spent considerable time in the public arena may seek fulfilment of individualistic activities. It is more helpful to discover what retirees want for this and the next stage of life than it is to assume that they are naturally 'disengaged'. The socio-environmental framework can be helpful to remind us that behaviours and attitudes about how seniors should 'act' is strongly influenced by social, cultural, institutional and financial considerations.

Cognitive domain

Raymond Catell (University of Indiana, 2007) informs us about fluid and crystal intelligences. It has been suggested that older adults may have reduced **fluid intelligence**; that is, they are less able to store large amounts of novel information in short-term memory, such as swotting for an examination.

Fluid intelligence
The in-born ability of an individual to think and reason quickly and responsively.

Crystal intelligence The ability to think and reason based on experience acquired during life.

On the other hand, seniors have a larger capacity for practical, **crystal intelligence**, such as making complex financial predictions and decisions based on years of experience. This has considerable impact on understanding how adult learners learn, and this is even more the case with senior adult learners. Because seniors already have considerable understandings from life's experiences, what they often need is the appropriate connections between the new and the old information. A good communicator can discover what the senior already knows and together they can make the connections to new information.

Emotional domain

Once a person has reached 25 years of age, most adults agree that they do not 'feel' any differently as they age. Regardless of our chronological situation, we experience fear, self-doubt, companionship, romantic love, silliness, loneliness and excitement. Often the difference with maturity is in the appropriate control or expression of emotion—or the 'emotional intelligence' (Goleman, 1996). While emotional intelligence is frequently discussed as one of multiple intelligences (Gardner, 2004), it is also a skill in that it needs to be learned and practised. Thus there can be considerably variability, depending on the senior's skills. One individual may be what we might consider inappropriately expressive about their feelings or distress, while another may be stoic to the point of self-harm. It is important to discover and distinguish the internal feelings from the various expressions of feelings in order to support them emotionally.

Emotional support can take many forms of communication, including touch. With our society's glamorisation of physical youth and devaluation of ageing, isolated seniors often speak of not having been touched, cuddled or had their hand held for months at a time. We are already aware of the effect of babies in orphanages being 'untouched'; it is not surprising that adults need touch as well. The willingness to communicate respect, trust, admiration and friendship non-verbally through appropriate touch can often be just as healing as any medical procedure.

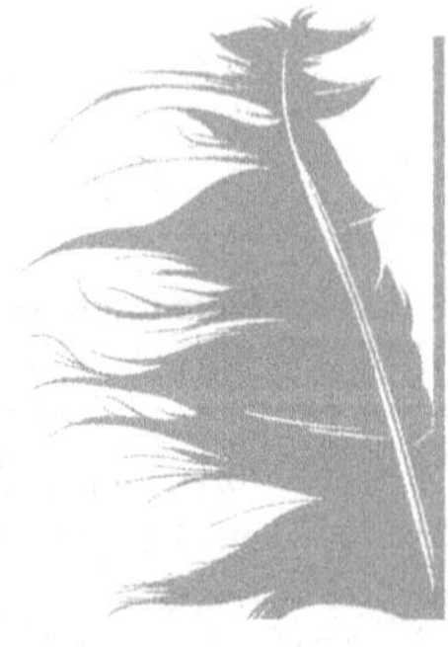

{ SUMMARY }

The notion that the onset of the 'senior years' occurs between the ages of 60 and 65 has its origins in the industrialisation of the Western world. Influential social theories proposed to account for ageing development include activity theory, disengagement theory, continuity theory and abandonment theory. Activity theory is the most popular perspective of successful ageing and is indicative of the current prevailing social view in Aotearoa New Zealand.

However, a demographic change towards an ageing population and economic considerations have caused a shift in the way older adults are perceived. This has given rise to a socio-environmental account of ageing that encompasses a dynamic relationship between individual and social contexts. The degree of congruence or incongruence between these two contexts contributes to the sense of life satisfaction and morale the older adult experiences, which can vary greatly.

When communicating with older people, it is important to show respect, to empower the individual, to acknowledge that people do not age at the same pace, and to take into account varied changes in the physical, social, cognitive and emotional domains.

REFLECTION POINTS

9.1 Intention (motivation, message, meaning, emotion)

Most of the theorists presented in this chapter suggest the elderly relate in particular ways more because of *interpersonal* and societal factors rather than because of *intrapersonal* or internal factors. Do you think that this is specific to this age group?

9.2 Reception (received message, response, feedback)

Reflecting on elderly adults that are known to you, in what ways might either disengagement or abandonment theory explain how this person relates to others?

9.3 Perception (style, manner, impression, analysis)

Assuming communication is a two-way interaction, can abandonment and disengagement occur concurrently? In what ways might you alter this dynamic?

QUESTIONS FOR REVIEW

1 How has Western industrialisation influenced thinking about older adults?
2 How does economic theory impact on attitudes towards older adults?
3 Which of activity, disengagement, abandonment and continuity theory is fundamentally different from the other three and how is it different?
4 What are the problems that socio-environmental perspectives of ageing were designed to overcome?

REFERENCES

Atchley, R. C. (1989). A continuity theory of normal aging. *The Gerontologist*, *29*, 183–90.

Barron, M. I. (1961). *The aging American*. New York, NY: Cornell.

Baum, M. & Baum, R. C. (1980). *Growing old: A societal perspective*. Englewood Cliffs, NJ: Prentice-Hall.

Burgess, E. W. (1960). *Aging in western societies*. Chicago, IL: University of Chicago Press.

Cumming, E. & Henry, W. E. (1961). *Growing old: The process of disengagement*. New York, NY: Basic Books.

Deci, R. I. & Ryan, R. M. (1987). The support of autonomy and the control of behavior. *Journal of Personality and Social Psychology*, *53*, 1024–37.

Erikson, E. H. (1980). *Identity and the life cycle*. New York, NY: Norton.

Gardner, H. (2004). *Frames of mind: The theory of multiple intelligences*. New York, NY: Basic Books.

Glanz, D. (1983). Higher education for retirees: The Israel experience. *Gerontology*, *6*, 32–6.

Glanz, D. (1985). Aging and education in Israel. *Educational Gerontology*, *8*, 101–5.

Goleman, D. (1996). *Emotional intelligence*. London: Bloomsbury.

Gubrium, J. F. (1972). Toward a socio-environmental perspective on aging. *The Gerontologist*, *12*, 281–4.

Gubrium, J. F. (1973). *The myth of the golden years*. Springfield, IL: Thomas.

Havighurst, R. J., Munnichs, J. M. A., Neugarten, B. L. & Thomae, H. (1969). *Adjustment to retirement*. Assen, The Netherlands: Van Gorcum.

Havighurst, R. J., Neugarten, B. L. & Tobin, S. S. (1968). Disengagement and patterns of aging. In B. L. Neugarten (ed.), *Middle age and aging* (pp. 162–72). Chicago, IL: University of Chicago Press.

Lemon, B., Bengston, V. & Peterson, J. (1972). An exploration of the activity theory of aging: Activity types and life satisfaction among in-movers in a retirement community. *Journal of Gerontology*, *27*, 511–23.

Lowenthal, M. F. (1968). Social isolation and mental illness in old age. In B. L. Neugarten (ed.), *Middle age and aging* (pp. 81–99). Chicago, IL: University of Chicago Press.

Maddox, G. L. (1968). Persistence of life-style among the elderly. *Middle age and aging* (pp. 181–3). Chicago, IL: University of Chicago Press.

Maddox, G. L. (1974). Aging and individual differences. A longitudinal analysis of social, psychological and physiological indicators. *Journal of Gerontology*, *29*, 555–63.

Maslow, A. H. (1999). *Towards a psychology of being* (3rd edn). New York, NY: J. Wiley & Sons.

Mass, H. S. & Kuypers, J. A. (1974). *From thirty to seventy*. San Francisco, CA: Jossey-Bass.

Ministry of Social Development. (2006). *To work, or not to work? Findings from a survey of 65-year-old New Zealanders*. Wellington, NZ: Author.

Ministry of Social Development. (2009). *Maturity matters: New choices for older people. Findings from the focus groups and interviews of the Turning 65 Project*. Wellington, NZ: Author.

Myers-Briggs Foundation. (n.d.). *Type in personal growth*. Retrieved from www.myersbriggs.org/type-use-for-everyday-life/type-in-personal-growth.

Neugarten, B. L. (1971). Growing old along with me! The best is yet to be. *Psychology Today*, *5*, 45–8.

Palmore, E. B. & Kivett, V. (1977). Change in life satisfaction. A longitudinal study of persons aged 46–70. *Journal of Gerontology*, *32*, 311–16.

Prasad, S. B. (1964). The retirement postulate of the disengagement theory. *The Gerontologist*, *4*, 20–3.

Ross, J. (1977). *Old people, new lives*. Chicago, IL: University of Chicago Press.

Ruffini, J. L. & Todd, H. F. (1979). A network model for leadership among the elderly. *The Gerontologist, 19*, 158–62.

Statistics New Zealand (2009). *The impact of structural population change* (Structural change and the 65+ population articles). Wellington, NZ: Author.

University of Indiana (2007). *Human intelligence: Biological profiles*. Raymond B. Catell. Retrieved from www.indiana.edu/~intell/rcattell.shtml.

WEBSITES

Ageing and Life Course, World Health Organization: www.who.int/ageing/en

Aotearoa Ageing 2005: A Bibliography of New Zealand Research on Ageing 2001–2005: www.retirement.org.nz/aotearoa-ageing-2005-a-bibliography-new-zealand-research-ageing-2001–2005

Grey Power New Zealand: www.greypower.co.nz

READING 17

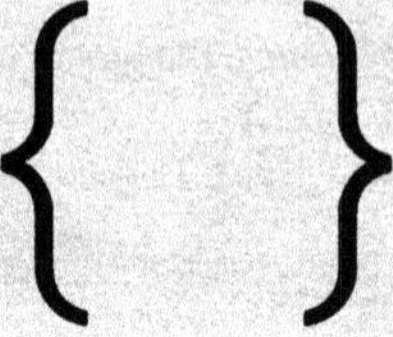

Dying, Grief and Bereavement

Terry Weblemoe

CHAPTER OVERVIEW

This chapter covers the following topics:

+ Cultural considerations
+ How practitioners respond.

KEY TERMS

Grief
Palliative
Hospice
Bereavement
Spiritual

A 'good death' has been defined as the freedom (of patients, families and caregivers) from avoidable distress and suffering that is reflective of clinical, cultural and ethical standards (Institute of Medicine, 1997). Central to the concept of a 'good death' is that a person is allowed to die with dignity, on their own terms, and in a relatively pain-free manner (Dyer, 2006). To die with dignity means that the patient has as much control over their situation and choices as is reasonably possible. It also means that procedures, equipment and situations that cause the individual to experience feelings of a loss of function, respect, dignity or mana are absent or minimised. Inherent in the philosophy is that the individual will have reached some kind of emotional resolution with **grief**, the dying process and end-of-life issues, including how they wish to be remembered.

Canadian physician Balfour Mount is credited with coining the term '**palliative** care'. He based his pioneer Canadian **hospice** movement on the founding work of Cicely Saunders in England and Elisabeth Kübler-Ross in the USA. Cicely Saunders, who founded the modern British hospice movement, envisioned the hospice as a place of care where the communication between hospice workers and families involved respect and dignity, and where residents would be as free from pain as possible (Foster, 2007). Her work as both a nurse and physician at St Joseph's Hospital in London and her subsequent writings developed the fundamental concepts of 'death with dignity', a 'good death' and the idea of hospice as a place of rest and pain relief. In these specialised facilities, patients could receive physical, emotional and spiritual assistance with their end-of-life issues, surrounded by friends, family and health-care workers trained to take care of their special needs. While originally hospice was conceived as a community-based facility, palliative care is now an integral part of many Western societies. They have diversified to serve different needs and communities, such as in-home hospice services or specialised units within hospitals. Australasian paediatric examples include the Royal Children's Hospital in Melbourne and the New Zealand Starship Hospital (Hospice New Zealand, 2005).

Grief The journey of coming to terms with loss.

Palliative Relating to the alleviation of symptoms rather than the cause of them.

Hospice An approach to palliative and end-of-life care that emphasises holism and healing but does not focus on cure.

In studying grief, Kübler-Ross (2009) proposed five distinct stages. These stages are not necessarily a simple progression from one stage to the next, but might also include both jumps across stages and recycling through stages. Of particular importance is that not everyone reaches a stage of acceptance, and some people doubt that ultimate acceptance is ever truly reached. The five Kübler-Ross stages are:

1. denial
2. anger
3. bargaining
4. depression
5. acceptance.

Bereavement The experience of losing a person who was emotionally close.

Bereavement can be defined as the experiencing the loss of a loved one through death (Berk, 2010, p. 659). That experience has both components of intense physical and psychological distress, which we call grief, as well as culturally accepted responses or specific expressions of that pain and loss, which we call mourning. While there are several other theorists who suggest different models of stages of grief and bereavement, the grieving process can be considered to have a number of tasks that need to be addressed or resolved. These tasks include:

1 accepting the reality of loss
2 working through the pain of grief
3 adjusting to life without that person
4 developing a sustaining internal link to the missing individual and rebuilding the mourner's life without them (Worden, 2002).

Cultural considerations

Many individuals—particularly older patients or those from some cultures who have avoided Western hospitals as 'houses of death' (Durie, 1994; Macdonald & Park, 2007)—may have considerable 'worries' about what will happen to them while in medical care. This is true of the South Pacific, which is becoming more multicultural, with patients and staff drawn from a wide range of cultural traditions with varying links to their heritage and beliefs. These contextual issues impact on communication at the most fundamental level. For example, older adults may feel intimidated by staff who are considerably younger than they expect, or they may be concerned about understanding or being understood by staff members with distinct language accents and different cultural backgrounds.

Aotearoa New Zealand is unique in that it has both government-funded Western medical health-care providers and Māori health-care (*Kaupapa Māori*) providers, who differ significantly in the cultural and social aspects of health-care provision. It is interesting to note that many Asian and new immigrant groups in Aotearoa New Zealand have found Māori health-care provision attractive and more suited to their needs. That said, one cannot stereotype about cultural needs, as individual and family preferences can demonstrate both considerable differences and eclectic mixes of cultural influence.

How practitioners respond

Many people are apprehensive about interacting with those facing death. They experience discomfort and anxiety, worrying that they have not received sufficient communication training (Peterson et al., 2010), and that discussing end-of-life issues, or poorly breaking bad news (Taft, 2009), will cause stress. Unfortunately, the silence and lack of adequate communication around these patients can create emotional and **spiritual** harm, and inhibit the patient from receiving adequate information and resolving grief (Kaakinen, 1992), especially in long-term-care facilities.

Spiritual Of belief and understanding beyond physical and cognitive experience.

Within many traditions, communicating with the dying is entrusted to the older, more socially or spiritually experienced members of the group, such as kuia/kaumatua (Māori elders) or counsellors and ministers. Practitioners working in health-care services who do not have this experience or expertise tend to focus on machinery and schedules, and distance themselves professionally and emotionally from communication and spiritual care (Hurtig & Stewin, 1990; Peterson et al., 2010). This avoidance is thought to be rooted in personal unresolved issues of mortality (Peterson et al., 2010). Patients have reported significant psychological and physical suffering resulting from 'stereotypical assumptions and behaviours' within health-care practitioners' interactions that do not recognise their individual situation (Janssen, 2010, p. 251).

New and even long-term professional health-care workers often feel anxiety about communicating with people who are dying and those around them. Research shows that not only do staff feel undertrained in sensitive communication, but also that inadequate communication in general is demonstrably the most common basis for customer complaints within the health-care industry (Health and Disability Commissioner, 2009; Healthcare Commission, 2007). Unfortunately, hard-and-fast rules or guidelines are not very useful in this area, where emotional distress can cloud effective communication for the health-care provider, the patient and their families (Rogers, Karlsen & Addington-Hall, 2000). Typically, personal grief or grief for a loved one is managed in the same way that a particular individual has coped with loss in the past. Their coping strategy is influenced by many different unique and cultural perceptions and learned behaviours. The keys to therapeutic communication for health-care professionals in these situations are:

1 having some resolution with one's own feelings about death and dying, and being comfortable around grief
2 having some skills in principles of 'active listening', 'presencing' or 'qualities of authentic being-with' the dying (Seno, 2010, p. 385)
3 having some familiarity with theories of age-related stages, cultural variations and empathetic abilities to be able to appreciate the world view of another person who may react cognitively and emotionally different from yourself.

CASE STUDY 10.1

'Being with'

During my first year as a nurse in a hospital's 'new graduate programme', I worked in the isolation wards. Working these wards meant that staff cared for the same patients for weeks or months, and often formed close relationships with individuals who would eventually die. In most cases the isolation is intended to keep immuno-compromised patients from contracting common bacteria, viruses and other illnesses from the patient's environment, including from contact with the health-care staff. Isolation meant that everyone had to wash, glove and gown-up to enter the room. This extra effort often meant that staff economised on their trips into a room, therefore patients could feel quite socially isolated.

One of my most poignant memories is of a very athletic, successful-looking American businessman who had been diagnosed with terminal pancreatic cancer. He was in his early forties and had a wife and two young children, about 4 and 6 years old. The patient's wife demanded that ward staff not tell her husband that he was dying. This posed an ethical dilemma for the ward staff because we were concerned about the healthy progress of grieving for this family if there was to be no communication about his prognosis.

Many staff members spent as little time as possible in the room with this man, because it was so awkward to care for him and not to discuss his illness or its outcome. When the family first came to visit, the senior nurses tried to take the wife aside and to convince her to let us communicate with her husband about dying. The wife responded to these attempts by becoming quite loud and hysterical. Her voice could be heard all over the ward, distressing others. She stopped bringing the children to visit, and her own visits became less frequent and more stilted. The whole ward was unhappy and distressed.

One day he turned from the window just as I was about to leave the room, looked me in the eyes and asked: 'Am I going to die?' Caught unprepared and forbidden to answer, all I could think to do was 'be with' him in the moment, and share with him how I sincerely felt. I turned back to face him and quietly tears streaked down my cheeks. I stood silently facing him, unashamed of my tears for as long as he held my gaze. As I watched, understanding solidified on his face. He turned back to the window, and then I left.

He became morose and uncooperative in general and specifically angry and sullen if I entered his room. In the following weeks, he alternated between lying unresponsively in a darkened room with occasional bursts of shouting and anger, including throwing a food tray against the wall. His wife was furious and demanded to discover who had told him and upset him so.

About 10 days before this man died, he turned on the lights in his room, and I could hear him steadily talking to his wife as I worked the other side of the hallway. He spoke lowly and confidently, eventually comforting her as she wept. The next day she brought her two young children in to visit; they had not seen their father for quite a while. I could see, as I passed the room on my other duties, the children sitting on his bed one under each arm, as he soothingly spoke with all of them. After this, the whole family came to visit frequently, and stayed with him as he daily became more and more drowsy.

I visited him again before he died, hoping that he had found his peace. Nothing was spoken out loud. He had always been a strong man and in control of his life, but he again looked me steadily in the face and then slowly smiled.

Individuals in highly emotional and dependent situations often become increasingly sensitive to non-verbal communication (Arnold & Boggs, 1989), particularly attitudes of the people to whom they are increasingly dependent upon. For this reason it is important that health-care professionals working in these areas not be emotionally distant, but be approachable and non-judgmental, have good knowledge of their subject and have good verbal skills (Bailey, 1998).

Active listening (see Chapters 21 and 26) and an emphasis on 'being with' patients and those close to them—rather than 'doing to' or focusing on being busy and occupied with physical tasks—forms the basis for effective and meaningful communication with people experiencing dying, grief and bereavement.

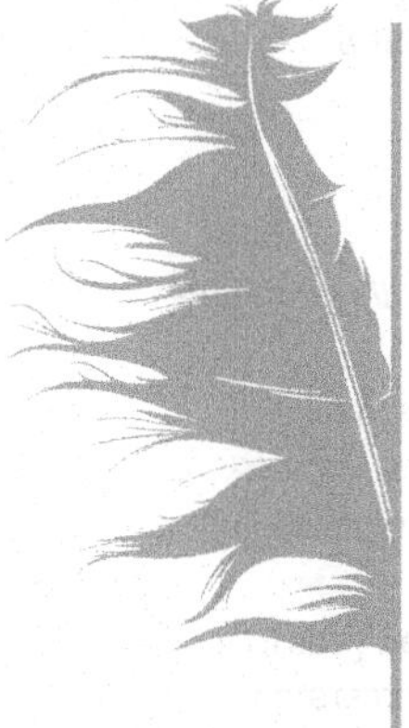

{ SUMMARY }

Communication with patients and families in end-of-life situations is critical and often the most therapeutic tool available to health-care professionals. Therapeutic communication can assist with both bereavement and the grieving process of dying patients, but it needs to be uniquely individualised. The appropriate starting point for such communication is always first gathering information through active listening, then providing appropriate information and a non-judgmental environment for patients to express their fears, wants and needs. Palliative care and hospice principles in recent years have helped 'humanise' the end-of-life within Western medical facilities by offering better pain and anxiety relief, more patient control and choices over the dying, and promoting a better understanding of the grieving process for both the patient and their families.

REFLECTION POINTS

10.1 Intention (motivation, message, meaning, emotion)

What was the intention of the nurse's tears? If 'being with' the patient in the moment produced tears for the nurse, do you think this was appropriate professional communication? Why or why not?

10.2 Reception (received message, response, feedback)

How did the patient respond to the non-verbal communication he was receiving, including avoidance and silence?

10.3 Perception (style, manner, impression, analysis)

Why do you think the patient had to be the initiator of the communication in his family's grieving process? What cultural or environmental factors may have influenced this?

QUESTIONS FOR REVIEW

1 Can you pick out the stages of loss and grieving for the patient, the wife and the nurse in this case study?
2 What would have been Erikson's age-stage related 'tasks' that needed to be resolved for each member of this family in this case study?
3 How might the wife and two young children have been affected had the family not discussed the father's dying?
4 What were some of the non-verbal emotional indicators and behaviours that communicated information in this case study?
5 What were the cultural and political factors that influenced the situation in this case study?
6 Can you think of a way the situation could have been handled differently?

REFERENCES

Arnold, E. & Boggs, K. (1989). *Interpersonal relationships: Professional communication skills for nurses* (2nd edn). Philadelphia, PA: W. B. Saunders Company.

Bailey, K. (1998). Communication issues. Patients' views on nurses' communication skills: A pilot study. *International Journal of Palliative Nursing, 4*(6), 300.

Berk, L. E. (2010). *Development through the lifespan* (international edn). Boston, MA: Pearson/Allyn & Bacon.

Durie, M. (1994). Māori perspectives on health and illness. In J. Spicer, A. Trlin & J. A. Walton (eds), *Social dimensions of health and disease: New Zealand perspectives* (pp. 194–203). Palmerston North, NZ: Dunmore Press Ltd.

Dyer, K. A. (2006). *Definition of a good death or an appropriate death.* Retrieved from http://dying.about.com/od/glossary/g/good_death.htm.

Foster, A. (2007). *Communicating at the end-of-life*. Mahwah, NJ: Lawrence Erlbaum.

Health and Disability Commissioner. (2009). *Other Reports*. Retrieved 14 February 2011 from www.hdc.org.nz.

Healthcare Commission. (2007). *Spotlight on complaints: A report on second-stage complaints about the NHS in England*. Retrieved from www.healthcarecommission.org.uk.

Hospice New Zealand. (2005). *Paediatric palliative care*. Retrieved 14 February 2011 from www.hospice.org.nz.

Hurtig, W. A. & Stewin, L. (1990). The effect of death education and experience on nursing students' attitudes towards death. *Journal of Advanced Nursing, 15*(1), 29–34.

Institute of Medicine. (1997). *Approaching death: Improving care at the end-of-life*. Washington, DC: National Academy Press.

Janssen, A. L. (2010). What can people approaching death teach us about how to care? *Patient Education and Counseling, 81*(2), 251–6.

Kaakinen, J. R. (1992). Living with silence. *The Gerontologist, 32*(2), 258.

Kübler-Ross, E. (2009). *On death and dying* (40th anniversary edn). New York, NY: Simon & Schuster.

Macdonald, J. & Park, J. (2007). The culture of health and illness. In D. Broom, B. Deed, K. Dew, M. Durie, J. Germov, A. Kirkman, J. Macdonald, P. Moon, J. Park, B. S. Turner & S. Walke (eds), *Health in the context of Aotearoa New Zealand* (pp. 155–67). Auckland, NZ: Oxford University Press.

Peterson, J., Johnson, G., Halvorsen, B., Apmann, L., Chang, P.-C., Kershek, S. et al. (2010). What is it so stressful about caring for a dying patient? A qualitative study of nurses' experiences. *International Journal of Palliative Nursing, 16*(4), 181–7.

Rogers, A., Karlsen, S. & Addington-Hall, J. (2000). 'All the services were excellent. It is when the human element comes in that things go wrong': Dissatisfaction with hospital care in the last year of life. *Journal of Advanced Nursing, 31*(4), 768–74.

Seno, V. L. (2010). Being-with dying: Authenticity in end-of-life encounters. *American Journal of Hospice, 27*(6), 377–86. DOI:10.1177/1049909109359628.

Taft, P. (2009). Breaking bad news. *Nursing Standard, 24*(10), 59.

Worden, J. W. (2002). *Grief counseling and grief therapy* (3rd edn). New York, NY: Springer.

WEBSITES

Hospice New Zealand: www.hospice.org.nz

Palliative Care in New Zealand: www.moh.govt.nz/palliativecare

Passing on: learning more about death and dying: www.tpk.govt.nz/en/in-print/kokiri/kokiri-20-2010/passing-on-learning-more-about-death-and-dying

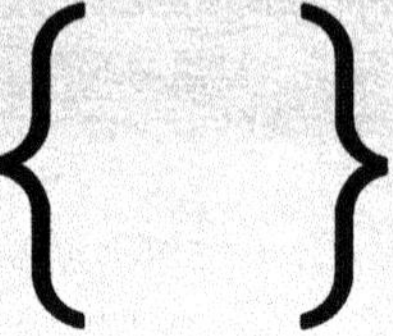

Power Relations

Ruth DeSouza

CHAPTER OVERVIEW

This chapter covers the following topics:

+ Oppression
+ Power
+ Critical social theory
+ Organisational and management theories
+ Social psychological theories
+ Post-structural theories
+ Empowerment.

KEY TERMS

Power
'The state'
Surveillance
Oppression
Critique
Foucauldian
Consumerism

Many practitioners see themselves as apolitical and powerless, particularly with regard to their relationships with the structures of medicine and management. However, in reality practitioners are powerful both as individuals and as members of the groups with which they identify. The structures and cultures within which most health and disability practitioners exist and work are based on beliefs and practices that constrain autonomy. These constraints are at work through a number of mechanisms, such as the market, the infusion of targets and performance measures and quality programmes (Newman & Vidler, 2006). In addition, the changing role of consumers or service users from passive recipients of care in the past to people who may be informed, empowered, articulate and 'demanding' poses a threat to the 'knowledge–power knot' on which professional power rests.

When practitioners view themselves as people who are doing good, they tend to lack awareness of their complicity and embeddedness in relations of **power** that structure inequality. Yet, power is embedded in everyday practices and interactions (Bradbury Jones, Sambrook & Irvine, 2008). Practitioners within the wider health and disability support sector contribute to social regulation through their roles as employees of **the state**. They enact government policies for the benefit of the health of the citizens of the state; so they are both governed and governing. Members of recognised professional groups are provided with a moral authority by their capacity to define problems and pose solutions, and their role in defining and evaluating good or normal behaviour and health practices through **surveillance** of the population and the criteria for interventions on behalf of the state (Gilbert, 2001, p. 201).

Power The exercise of strength or control.

'The state' The politically organised leadership (or government) of groups of people or populations.

Surveillance The act of keeping watch over people and their actions.

These ambivalent relationships with power that are evident among health practitioners require exploration. This can be done by considering the various ways in which power is conceptualised and the micro and macro definitions of empowerment. Some shifts in power have occurred in the last few decades, largely influenced by various social movements. Maternity and mental health are two particular examples of professional practice and service delivery in which power can be recognised and ideas of empowerment can be translated into meaningful engagement between service delivery and those who engage with the service.

Oppression

It can be difficult to understand, but in the process of doing good, people can contribute to **oppression**. For example, medicine has historically dominated health care, but in recent times it has come to be thought about and understood in terms of power and relationships between institutions (and the practitioners

Oppression The unfair or unjust exercising of power over others.

Critique Critical comment, appraisal or evaluation.

within them) and those who seek care and support (Broom, Nicholls & Deed, 2010). This **critique** of power has significantly eroded the traditional position and role of medicine within our society. This desire to rebalance power has challenged assumptions within the professions in relation to personal and professional culture.

For example, there is an assumption that being a member of a group that provides health care and disability support services automatically means individuals are neutral and egalitarian. However, such assumptions have been challenged and the oppressive capacity of these services, systems, institutions and groups has been exposed.

Foucauldian In the spirit of French philosopher Michel Foucault and therefore with an interest in critique of institutions and power.

Young (1990) conceptualises oppression in the **Foucauldian** sense as 'the disadvantage and injustice some people suffer not because a tyrannical power coerces them but because of the everyday practices of a well-intentioned liberal society' (Henderson & Waterstone, 2008). The suggestion is that the actions of many people who are going about their lives contribute to the maintenance and reproduction of oppression, but few of those people (such as health practitioners) would see themselves as agents of oppression (Young, 1990). Oppression, therefore, goes beyond a few people's choices or policies. Its causes are embedded in unquestioned norms, habits and symbols, in the assumptions underlying institutional rules and the collective consequences of following those rules (Young, 1990). It is structural and woven throughout the system. Seeing oppression as the practices of a well-intentioned group removes the focus from individual acts that might repress the actions of others. Instead the focus is on acknowledging that 'powerful norms and hierarchies of both privilege and injustice are built into our everyday practices', which call for structural rather than individual remedies (Young, 1990).

Power

Many practitioners hold empowerment as a central concept to their work with clients, patients and consumers/tangata whai ora. However, in order to empower others, it is important to know what power is. The concept of power has three central themes:

1 Ability—the ability to do something or act in a particular way: capacity, capability, potential, faculty and competence.
2 Control—having the capacity or ability to direct or influence the behaviour of others or the course of events: authority, influence, dominance, mastery, domination, dominion, sway, weight, leverage, clout and teeth.
3 Strength—the physical strength and force exerted by something or someone: powerfulness, might, force, forcefulness, vigour, energy, brawn, muscle, informal punch.

It could be argued that practitioners have all these attributes and are enabled and constrained in their roles and behaviour by the institutions they work for. Practitioners are in positions of political or social authority or control, and have delegated authority (Gilbert, 2001). However, there are different ways of understanding power. Four main theories of power are explored here:

+ critical social theory
+ organisational and management theories
+ social psychological theories
+ post-structural theories.

Critical social theory

Within a critical social theory or liberational framework, power is viewed as a possession and hierarchies are central to the imbalance of power. The group with control has more power and status than other groups in society, which are in a subordinated position. Critical theory is concerned with helping disenfranchised groups in society to overcome this domination. Power is obtained through the surrender of another's power, and empowerment is equated with liberation. In order for this transfer of power to happen, a struggle must occur as powerful people will not readily transfer resources, information or responsibility (Bradbury Jones, Sambrook & Irvine, 2008). Empowerment is collective and is about increasing the power and influence of oppressed groups (Kuokkanen & Leino Kilpi, 2000). However, power is not always repressive and this is a limitation of critical social theory.

Organisational and management theories

Where critical social theory is concerned with oppressed groups, organisational and management theories are concerned with how power is distributed in organisations. Hierarchies also come into play, especially the idea of top-down power (Bradbury Jones, Sambrook & Irvine, 2008). Within this framework, there is an acknowledgement of structural factors and their capacity to empower and disempower, rather than focusing on the individual. According to Kanter (1993), four conditions are necessary for empowerment to occur within organisations, with the degree of empowerment related to how many of the four conditions are present: opportunity for advancement, access to information, access to support and access to resources. Power is then framed as the ability to get things done, and being empowered is having the opportunity to do things. However, the problem with this model and with critical social theory is that power is not only distributed in a top-down manner: it also operates from bottom to top and laterally (Foucault, 1977).

Social psychological theories

Social psychological theories contrast with organisational models of power in that they focus on the psychology or the point of view of the individual, rather than environmental factors. Power is framed as a personal attribute that can be nurtured, and personal growth leads to personal power and therefore empowerment (Bradbury Jones, Sambrook & Irvine, 2008; Masterson & Owen, 2006). However, it does not necessarily follow that individuals are empowered or able to assert their power in any given situation. It may be argued that individualistic empowerment deflects attention from socio-structural disempowerment, as well as social, cultural and structural factors that disempower (Masterson & Owen, 2006). Morrall (1996) challenges individual empowerment, saying that empowering the individual is like treating the symptoms of disempowerment rather than the cause. Other concerns are that an increase in self-confidence might result in an altered perception of power. This would then allow an individual to act or exert influence while power imbalances remain because there has not been an actual transfer of power.

Post-structuralist theories

A post-structural appreciation of power conceptualises it not as a thing (something that is possessed by individuals or organisations) but as a relation: something that is exercised (Foucault, 1977). Consequently, post-structuralism challenges the view that power can be relinquished in order to empower someone else (Bradbury Jones, Sambrook & Irvine, 2008). Michel Foucault (1926–1984) is a key theorist within post-structuralism. Foucault conceptualised power in a number of key ways that differ from the previous three theories: power is always shifting and moving; power is ubiquitous and omnipresent, coming from everywhere and moving in multiple directions and permeating like capillaries into every space and interaction; and power is productive. Within this framework, power is not a logical causal relationship where someone can take over or give up power. Power in this paradigm is about having an influence over thoughts, attitudes and social relationships (Kuokkanen & Leino Kilpi, 2000) and practitioners can be viewed as powerless in some circumstances, and powerful in others (Bradbury Jones, Sambrook & Irvine, 2008).

Empowerment

Empowerment is a central concept in recent approaches to health and health promotion, and acknowledges the importance of people having control or being able to participate in their own life and environment. Notions of 'patient empowerment' and participation in care can be identified throughout recent health-care policy and practice information and documents. Empowerment is almost universally viewed as a good thing. However, empowerment can be misapplied in such a way that a transfer of tasks away from formal care occurs without people and their families being resourced and supported. The risk is that traditional service providers and organisations can absolve themselves of the responsibility for supporting the health and well-being of the population by arguing that people should be taking care of themselves—without transferring the resources to the community for such support. The idea of empowerment can be operationalised in diverse ways in practice and differentially received by clients and families. There might be negative consequences for clients who do not value 'empowerment' as much as they trust professionals. For example, when someone does not want active involvement in certain decisions or tasks, promoting involvement can contribute to negative experiences, dissatisfaction, anxiety, fear and guilt.

CASE STUDY 13.1

Empowerment and recovery

Many people who have experiences of mental illness have been marginalised, experiencing social exclusion and the loss of their dignity, freedom, autonomy and rights. Collective action for empowerment by service users has produced many organisations in Aotearoa New Zealand, including Psychiatric Survivors and Mind and Body. These groups have been at the forefront of de-stigmatisation efforts, contesting negative perceptions of mental illness and exploring new ways of talking about mental health and illness (Masterson & Owen, 2006), particularly recovery. As a result of these efforts, the centrality of service users to New Zealand mental health services has been solidified through both legal and contractual frameworks and culture change, with service users employed within mental health services and playing a part operationally, strategically and nationally.

There is a growing expectation for service-user involvement at all levels of social service delivery, in part due to social and policy changes such as de-institutionalisation and community care.

These have led to a resistance to the supremacy of what has been considered the historically paternalist 'professional knows best' approach, a valuing of people's personal experiences of mental illness, and a growing ownership and pride among consumers. In New Zealand services, consumer participation has had impacts for consumers, health-care professionals and policymakers. Consumers are required to be involved in the planning, implementation and evaluation of service delivery at every level of mental health service provision. Transparent and clear processes that show this in service design and delivery are contractual requirements (Ministry of Health, 1995; Phillips, 2006).

Perhaps the most powerful impact has been on critiquing the normalising judgments of medico-psychiatric discourses that are also widespread in society, where labels of deviance such as 'psychiatric patient', 'schizophrenic' and 'mentally ill' have been accompanied by stigma and caused social exclusion and disadvantage (Masterson & Owen, 2006). The power of medico-psychiatric discourses has placed service users in a sick role, where they have been dependent on the knowledge and resources of professionals. Instead, advocacy, recognition of lay knowledge and personal experience of mental illness have resulted in the creation of alternative discourses, such as the recovery model, which have helped to reduce stigma and the power of health practitioners (Masterson & Owen, 2006).

The recovery model reconceptualises what has been typically called mental illness (Masterson & Owen, 2006), framing it as a natural phenomenon occurring along a spectrum of human experience, rather than long-term dysfunction. Prominent advocates of the recovery model include Deegan (1998), Copeland (1997), Jacobson and Curtis (2000) in the USA, and Campbell (1997), Barker and Buchanan-Barker (2005), and Repper and Perkins (2003) in the UK. In Aotearoa New Zealand, O'Hagan (2001) has developed recovery competencies for mental health workers.

The recovery model provides not only an alternative model but also a critique of professional dominance as seen in mental health policies and practices. Consumers charge that medico-psychiatric discourses obliterate hope, disempowering, stigmatising and removing choice from service users. By contrast, recovery advocates assert that regardless of claims about illness, chronicity and progress that are offered in medico-psychiatric discourses, all service users can achieve recovery. However, it is the individual—rather than services or practitioners—who drives the recovery process and what recovery means to them. Therefore, the recovery project provides a mechanism for empowered action and legitimates the rights of service users, supporting autonomy and self-direction as well the creation of user-run services and reformation of existing mainstream mental health services (Masterson & Owen, 2006). While societal and service 'buy in' is critical (without appropriation and professionalisation), this is not without its challenges. Embracing a recovery perspective requires challenging and transforming some taken-for-granted practices and developing new kinds of relationships with service users. Strategies might include redistributing power in tangible ways (for example, contractually); making professionals dependent on service users for training, education or performance assessment; and renegotiating the professional functions of therapy and carers.

Models and discourses of empowerment

Individual level or micro-level strategies of empowerment include the psychological model and the consumerist model. The psychological model involves developing power from within, by avoiding 'power-over'. Information giving is highly regarded as an essential step towards genuine empowerment (Masterson & Owen, 2006). It is thought that collaborative partnerships between practitioners and service users—founded upon relationships of trust, support, equality, respect, genuineness, empathy and positive regard—facilitate this. However, consumers/clients can be reluctant to challenge decisions made about their care for fear of consequences such as being labelled and experiencing the withdrawal of care or the imposition of punitive care (Masterson & Owen, 2006). Despite the presence of codes of patient rights within nations or organisations, users might be unable to exert them. Professionals might appear to facilitate service user decision-making, but still exert control over their decisions where power might be exercised in terms of limiting the range of decisions and maintaining 'expert' authority.

By contrast, **consumerism** involves delegating or sharing formal power through structural change and where there is a transfer of top-down power within services (Masterson & Owen, 2006). Increasingly in fields such as mental health, policy directives have centralised the role of the consumer and their whānau in terms of being able to shape, participate and evaluate health services. In Aotearoa New Zealand, service users have been taught leadership skills to facilitate their ability to assert themselves in organisations. However, while consumerism can mean service-user participation in decision-making (ostensibly giving them influence

Consumerism
Viewing human interaction with an emphasis on access to goods and services.

and allowing professionals and managers to appear empowering), power is still being retained by professionals and managers who set the terms of engagement, incorporating consumerist ideals into existing power structures without changing them (Masterson & Owen, 2006).

A social or macro perspective of empowerment assumes that large-scale action, to meet people's common needs, changes the social and material circumstances of society. There are two general approaches: socio-structural change and grassroots communal action. Socio-structural change encompasses such strategies as creating equal opportunities through structural change and through legislation, policy, financial and organisational means to ensure the social inclusion of all—regardless of ability, age, gender, race, income, social class, sexual orientation or any other form of difference. Power is evident through the unequal distribution of resources between those who are poor and socially excluded and those who are not. By devolving responsibility to patients and their families, the concept of empowerment achieves the goals of improving perceived control and self-efficacy—which are thought to enhance well-being—while fitting in with neo-liberal political and economic imperatives of efficiency and cost (Funk, Stajduhar & Purkis, 2011).

Consumer involvement in health-care decision-making, planning and policy making (as individual consumers, potential service users, citizens and organised groups) is a feature of the contemporary health-care scene (Coney, 2004). The growing centrality of the consumer is part of many efforts to change health systems so that they are more responsive. However, the advent of 'consumerism' has posed a set of challenges to professional, occupational and organisational power (Newman & Vidler, 2006), not least by threatening the hegemony of the medical model of health, whereby the replacement of the machine model of the body with more holistic models has required more personally tailored responses. This holism has been accompanied by challenges to professional judgment in favour of consumer 'choice' (Newman & Vidler, 2006). Critics of the term argue that 'choice' is inappropriate if a person is an unwilling or involuntary user, or if alternative services are scarce (Newman & Vidler, 2006).

CASE STUDY 13.2

Consumers and birth

The New Zealand midwifery profession has struggled for autonomy in the face of threats from medicine, hospitals and nursing (Stojanovic, 2008). It has shaped itself into an autonomous feminist profession founded on partnership with women (Surtees, 2003), creating a point of difference emphasising 'normal' and 'natural' births and the capability of women to 'naturally' carry and deliver a baby without the surveillance and interventions of physicians in a hospital setting (Macdonald, 2006). Mutually beneficial political lobbying by consumers and midwives in the late 1980s saw legislative changes occur that led to autonomous midwifery practice. Midwives wanted to differentiate their scope of practice from nurses and regain independent practice and autonomy, while maternity consumer activists viewed autonomous midwifery practice as a mechanism for gaining increased control over their own birthing (Pairman, 2006). The subsequent passing of the Nurses Amendment Act in 1990 heralded an era of choice in maternity care for Aotearoa New Zealand, allowing women to choose a caregiver (Lead Maternity Carer or LMC) who would either coordinate or personally provide the care they required from early pregnancy to six weeks post partum (Pairman, 2006). Direct access to government maternity funding means midwives can be self-employed, prescribe some pharmaceuticals, and access pathology and radiology services, hospitals and other birthing facilities. They can also consult with obstetricians or refer women to consultant obstetricians (Davis & Walker, 2010). In 2004, 75.3 per cent of New Zealand women were registered with a midwife to provide lead maternity care, demonstrating a high uptake of midwifery care (Ministry of Health, 2007).

Partnership

The concept of partnership between women and midwives in midwifery practice recognises the centrality of women as consumers in society and to the profession (Freeman, Timperley & Adair, 2004). Partnership was incorporated into the New Zealand College of Midwives' *Handbook for Practice* in 1993 (New Zealand College of Midwives Inc., 1993) and is named as the first of ten standards of midwifery practice: the midwife works in partnership with the woman and the twin forces of feminism and consumerism contributed to this ethic. The women's health movement in the 1970s and the Inquiry into the Treatment of Women for Cervical Cancer at National Women's Hospital (also known as the Cartwright inquiry) in the 1980s identified the omission of informed consent and choices in cervical cancer screening and treatment as evidence of the violation of women's rights (Surtees, 2003). This led to an emphasis on 'accountability, patient-centred care, self-determination and cultural sensitivity in the health service' (Surtees, 2003, p. 30). The centrality of the consumer role became instantiated in roles such as patient or consumer advocates in health services and consumer representation on committees.

The newly formed New Zealand College of Midwives, which had emerged from the New Zealand Nurses Association in August

1988, encouraged consumers as members and representatives in decision-making (Daellenbach & Thorpe, 2007). This partnership was a recognition of the value of the political and public support of midwifery, but also an acknowledgment that there was further collaborative work to be done. The midwifery autonomy regained in 1990 allowed for one-to-one working, and the partnership between the midwife and the woman came to underpin the midwifery model in New Zealand maternity services (Pairman, 2006). Partnership assumed equity between mother and midwife, and acknowledged that both parties were making equally valuable contributions. Midwives brought their knowledge, skills and experience, and the woman brought her knowledge of herself and her family, and her needs and wishes for her pregnancy and birth. Midwives argue that their point of difference from the more hierarchical professional models of medical, nursing and obstetric practice is the shift from authoritative models to partnership and collaboration, where women are empowered (Daellenbach & Thorpe, 2007). However, partnership rests on consumers who are informed and want to be informed (DeSouza, 2006).

Critics from within the midwifery profession challenge the model of partnership on two counts: first, because it assumes a white, middle-class subject; and second, because the relationship between midwives and clients is more akin to individualist contractualism, where individuals contract with each other but do not produce a participatory outcome (Skinner, 1999). Skinner's critique of contractualism contradicts the explicit claim by Guilliland and Pairman (1995) that the concept of partnership originates from their understanding of partnership as it is encapsulated in the Treaty of Waitangi. Instead, Skinnner argues that the Treaty is a contract that only has a contemporary reading of partnership and that the demands for tinorangatiratanga (self-determination), protection and equity remain absent in the midwifery partnership. Skinner (1999) concludes that partnership 'reflects a superficial analysis of society, neglecting to identify the dominant underlying right-wing philosophy of individualism, contractualism and patriarchy. It does not recognise inequalities in power or access to resources and is culturally elitist' (p. 16).

Choice

A second tenet of midwifery is the notion of choice and being an informed consumer. The assumption that choice is empowering is derived from the notion that women can be empowered by being consulted and actively involved in processes that affect them. Informed choice emerged as a women-centred, feminist mode of health-care communication, which provided a contrast to more hierarchical and paternalistic modes associated with biomedical obstetrical contexts (Spoel, 2007). Informed choice became both an ideological principle implicit in midwifery models of care and a rhetorical practice of midwives exchanging information with women in order to facilitate decision-making (Spoel, 2007). This led to the advancement of empowered and choice-making subjects who were no longer passively recipient 'patients' but active 'consumers' of health care (Tully, Daellenbach & Guilliland, 1998, p. 248). This notion of the choice-making subject is arranged around discourses of neo-liberal subjectivity and relies on an individual who is rational and responsible within the discursive culture of midwifery. Choice is also constrained by a tension within contemporary liberalism, where respect for the autonomy and privacy of individuals is posited against the concern for the regulation of social and economic life, and where expert knowledges are a mechanism for regulating the choices of individuals within the limits of government, thereby constraining the choices that are made (Murphy, 2003).

Liberal feminists view increasing choice in childbirth as a mechanism for enhancing women's perception of control, but radical and social feminists argue that choice has led to the illusion of freedom in an oppressive context where the status quo remains unchanged (Leap & Edwards, 2006). Leap and Edwards outline the limitations of the concept of informed choice. First, the person who is doing the informing has a powerful influence on the decisions that are made. Being given information about a limited range of choices is not a guarantee of involvement in decision-making. Ultimately, the health practitioner is a gatekeeper who decides what information is relevant. However, if the mother disagrees with the health practitioner, she needs to have either the resources to find alternative support or the attributes that will allow her to challenge the decision—such as being articulate, assertive and knowledgeable (Leap & Edwards, 2006).

Schmidt's (2008) example of breastfeeding information provided by the Ministry of Health is emblematic of the neo-liberal paradox. Schmidt contends that what appears to be the provision of scientific information about the benefits of breastfeeding and risks of formula feeding frames breastfeeding as the only rational option and appropriate choice for a good modern parent to make. Schmidt contextualises contemporary breastfeeding discourses in the new public health model, where neo-liberal ideals of individual informed choice are advanced in tandem with the narrowing of choices to those that advantage the state, such as those that reduce the costs of health care.

Natural childbirth

The legislative changes of 1990 that paved the way for greater midwifery autonomy in birthing also saw the advancement of natural childbirth as a philosophy that was strongly intertwined with partnership and informed choice. Central to this philosophy is the idea of being close to nature, and of returning women to the rewarding aspects of a labour.

However, natural childbirth discourses reflect class and race biases where control over birth and informed consumer choice are emphasised without the recognition that these require access to cultural and material resources that are available only to privileged women (Brubaker & Dillaway, 2009). The feminist notion of taking control of one's life and body is a very middle-class perspective (Lazarus, 1997). However, evidence is growing that alternative approaches to childbirth do not necessarily guarantee more fair or compassionate treatment, as seen by a growing body of work about the experiences of migrant and refugee birthing women (Bowler, 1993). Therefore, midwifery concepts of partnership, choice and natural childbirth derived from radical feminist critiques of medicalisation have been aligned to middle-class white subjectivity, but have not effectively changed the structures of biomedical dominance.

The emergence of the consumer movement in health occurred in the context of related social movements, including the civil rights, anti-racist and indigenous rights movements, the psychiatric survivors' movement and the women's movement. Groups coalesced around identity politics and demanded a larger say in health particularly in terms of policy, professional regulation and service planning (Coney, 2004). The women's health movement was the forerunner in challenging tenets of modern medicine and predated other consumer movements, such as patient's rights and disability movements. The emphasis on critiquing mainstream health care resulted in scrutiny of who held the power in the health sector: governments, health practitioners, health industries, the pharmaceutical industry, policymakers, researchers and funders.

Alongside these people-led developments came community development and public health approaches that advanced critiques of medical dominance and the desire for community-based primary health-care models. These developments were supported by the Alma Ata Declaration (WHO, 2008) and the Ottawa Charter (WHO, 1986). In particular, indigenous Māori and mental health consumers have articulated the need for community-controlled services.

Public health as a field has broadened its scope from communicable disease to the recognition of the role of social inequalities as determinants of health. With the medical model failing to substantively improve the health of deprived populations, the need for models that address the social determinants of health have led to greater involvement of communities in shaping such services. This has led to the development of new and innovative service delivery models by, for example, Māori, Pacific refugee and Asian communities.

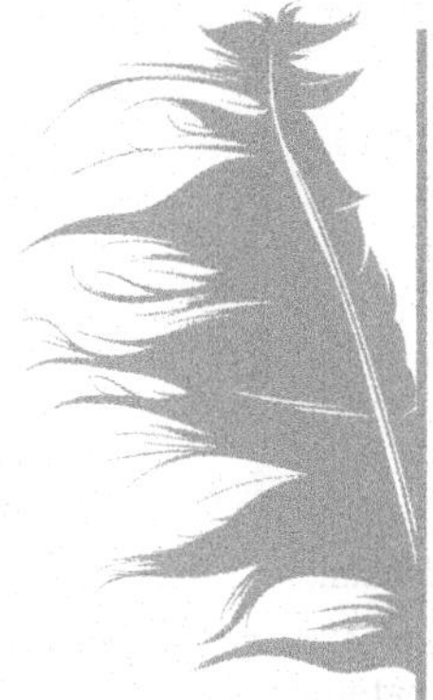

{ SUMMARY}

Power is a complex phenomenon in health care and disability support where many professionals assume that because they are doing good that oppression does not exist. However, the rise of consumer movements demanding the redistribution of power in these contexts has foregrounded the empowerment agenda. Therefore, in order to provide services and support that are empowering, professionals must first understand the part they play in power relations. This chapter has outlined the ways in which power is conceptualised through four main theories: critical social theories, organisational and management theories, social psychology theories and post-structural theories. These theories range from viewing power as a possession to seeing power as a relation. In response to the professional dominance of human experiences, such as having a baby and experiencing mental illness, the empowerment agenda has been advanced in a range of ways. In mental health, the recovery model challenges the dominance of professional knowledge in mental health policy and practice, and demands that service user involvement occurs at all levels of care. Importantly, the consumer drives his or her own process of recovery. In the patriarchal area of maternity services, the use of partnership, choice and natural childbirth are viewed as ways of redistributing power back to women. However, empowerment through the redistribution of responsibility to the consumer and their family can be problematic if the corresponding resources are not made available.

REFLECTION POINTS

13.1 Intention (motivation, message, meaning, emotion)

What motivates the consumer movement in health care and disability support services?

13.2 Reception (received message, response, feedback)

Who has more power when practitioners are giving information to consumers?

13.3 Perception (style, manner, impression, analysis)

Do consumers always understand what practitioners say?

QUESTIONS FOR REVIEW

1 Outline the different models of power and empowerment. Which definitions appeal and why?
2 Is there a risk that practitioners and professions can absolve themselves of responsibility when they emphasise the empowerment of service users?
3 What does being empowered mean to you in a health context?

REFERENCES

Barker, P. J. & Buchanan-Barker, P. (2005). *The Tidal model: A guide for mental health professionals*. London: Routledge.

Bowler, I. (1993). They're not the same as us: Midwives' stereotypes of South Asian descent maternity patients. *Sociology of Health & Illness, 15*(2), 157–78.

Bradbury Jones, C., Sambrook, S. & Irvine, F. (2008). Power and empowerment in nursing: A fourth theoretical approach. *Journal of Advanced Nursing, 62*(2), 258–66.

Broom, B., Nicholls, D. A. & Deed, B. (2010). Approaches to healthcare provision. In S. Shaw & B. Deed (eds), *Health and Environment in Aotearoa/New Zealand* (pp. 60–76). Melbourne, Vic: Oxford University Press.

Brubaker, S. J. & Dillaway, H. E. (2009). Medicalization, natural childbirth and birthing experiences. *Sociology Compass, 3*(1), 31–48.

Campbell, J. (1997). How consumers/survivors are evaluating the quality of psychiatric care. *Evaluation Review, 21*(3), 357.

Coney, S. (2004). *Effective consumer voice and participation for New Zealand: A systematic review of the evidence*. Wellington: New Zealand Guidelines Group (NZGG).

Copeland, M. E. (1997). *WRAP: Wellness Recovery Action Plan*. Brattleboro, VT: Peach Press.

Daellenbach, R. & Thorpe, J. (2007). Independence in practice: A New Zealand case study of midwives in partnership. In L. Reid (ed.), *Midwifery: Freedom to practise? An international exploration of midwifery practice* (pp. 261–81). Philadelphia, PA: Elsevier.

Davis, D. L. & Walker, K. (2010). Case-loading midwifery in New Zealand: Making space for childbirth. *Midwifery, 26*(6), 603–8.

Deegan, P. E. (1988). Recovery: The lived experience of rehabilitation. *Psychosocial Rehabilitation Journal, 11*(4), 11–19.

DeSouza, R. (2006). *New spaces and possibilities: The adjustment to parenthood for new migrant mothers*. Wellington, NZ: Families Commission.

Foucault, M. (1977). *Discipline and punish: The birth of the prison*. London, UK: Allen Lane.

Freeman, L. M., Timperley, H. & Adair, V. (2004). Partnership in midwifery care in New Zealand. *Midwifery, 20*(1), 2–14.

Funk, L. M., Stajduhar, K. I. & Purkis, M. E. (2011). An exploration of empowerment discourse within home care nurses' accounts of practice. *Nursing Inquiry, 18*(1), 66–76.

Gilbert, T. (2001). Reflective practice and clinical supervision: Meticulous rituals of the confessional. *Journal of Advanced Nursing, 36*(2), 199–205.

Guilliland, K. & Pairman, S. (1995). *The midwifery partnership: A model for practice*. Wellington, NZ: Department of Nursing and Midwifery, Victoria University of Wellington.

Henderson, G. L. & Waterstone, M. (2008). *Geographic thought: A praxis perspective*. New York, NY: Routledge.

Jacobson, N. & Curtis, L. (2000). Recovery as policy in mental health services: Strategies emerging from the states. *Psychosocial Rehabilitation Journal, 23*(4), 333–41.

Kanter, R. M. (1993). *Men and women of the corporation*. New York, NY: Basic Books.

Kuokkanen, L. & Leino Kilpi, H. (2000). Power and empowerment in nursing: Three theoretical approaches. *Journal of Advanced Nursing, 31*(1), 235–41.

Lazarus, E. (1997). What do women want?: Issues of choice, control, and class in pregnancy and childbirth. In R. Davis-Floyd & C. F. Sargent (eds), *Childbirth and authoritative knowledge: Cross-cultural perspectives* (pp. 132–58). Berkeley, CA: University of California Press.

Leap, N. & Edwards, N. (2006). The politics of involving women in decision making. In L. Page & R. McCandlish (eds), *The new midwifery: Science and sensitivity in practice* (2nd edn) (pp. 97–121). Philadelphia, PA: Elsevier/Churchill Livingstone.

Macdonald, M. (2006). Gender expectations: Natural bodies and natural births in the new midwifery in Canada. *Medical Anthropology Quarterly, 20*(2), 235–56.

Masterson, S. & Owen, S. (2006). Mental health service user's social and individual empowerment: Using theories of power to elucidate far-reaching strategies. *Journal of Mental Health, 15*(1), 19–34.

Morrall, P. (1996). Clinical sociology and the empowerment of clients. *Mental Health Nursing, 16*, 24–7.

Ministry of Health (1995). *A guide to effective consumer participation in mental health services*. Wellington, NZ: Author.

Ministry of Health (2007). *Notice Pursuant to Section 88 of the New Zealand Public Health and Disability Act 2000*. Wellington, NZ: Author.

Murphy, E. (2003). Expertise and forms of knowledge in the government of families. *Sociological Review, 51*(4), 433–62.

New Zealand College of Midwives Inc. (1993). *Midwives handbook for practice*. Dunedin, NZ: Author.

Newman, J. & Vidler, E. (2006). Discriminating customers, responsible patients, empowered users: Consumerism and the modernisation of health care. *Journal of Social Policy, 35*(2), 193–209.

O'Hagan, M. (2001). *Recovery competencies for New Zealand mental health workers*. Wellington, NZ: Mental Health Commission.

Pairman, S. (2006). Midwifery partnership: Working with women. In L. Page & R. McCandlish (eds), *The new midwifery: Science and sensitivity in practice* (2nd edn) (pp. 73–97). Philadelphia, PA: Elsevier/Churchill Livingstone.

Phillips, R. (2006). Consumer participation in mental health research. *Social Policy Journal of New Zealand, 27*, 171–82.

Repper, J. & Perkins, R. (2003). *Social inclusion and recovery: A model for mental health practice*. London, UK: Bailliere-Tindale.

Schmidt, J. (2008). Gendering in infant feeding discourses: The good mother and the absent father. *New Zealand Sociology, 23*(2), 61–74.

Skinner, J. (1999). Midwifery partnership: Individualism contractualism or feminist praxis? *New Zealand College of Midwives Journal, 21*, 14–17.

Spoel, P. (2007). A feminist rhetorical perspective on informed choice in midwifery. *Rhetor: Journal of the Canadian Society for the Study of Rhetoric, 2*, 1–25.

Stojanovic, J. (2008). Midwifery in New Zealand 1904–1971. *Contemporary Nurse, 30*(2), 156–67.

Surtees, R. J. (2003). *Midwifery as feminist praxis in Aotearoa/New Zealand*. Christchurch, NZ: University of Canterbury.

Tully, L., Daellenbach, R. & Guilliland, K. (1998). Feminism, partnership and midwifery. In R. Du Plessis & L. Alice (eds), *Feminist thought in Aotearoa/New Zealand* (pp. 245–55). Auckland, NZ: OUP.

World Health Organization. (1986). *The Ottawa Charter for Health Promotion*. Retrieved from www.who.int/hpr/NPH/docs/ottawa_charter_hp.pdf.

World Health Organization. (2008). *International conference dedicated to the 30th anniversary of the Alma-Ata declaration on primary health care*. Retrieved from http://www.who.int/mediacentre/events/meetings/alma_ata/en.

Young, I. M. (1990). *Justice and the politics of difference*. Princeton, NJ: Princeton University Press.

WEBSITES

About Mental Health Recovery and WRAP: www.mentalhealthrecovery.com/aboutus.php
Definition of Wellness: www.definitionofwellness.com/dictionary/empowerment-for-health.html
Maternity Services Consumer Council: www.maternity.org.nz

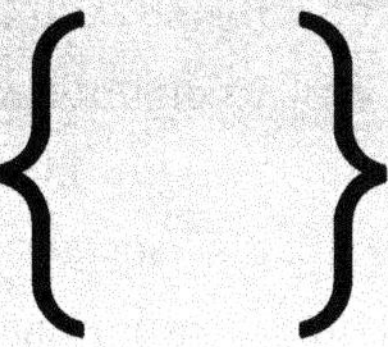

Culture

Denise Wilson, Ray Gates, Junior Sonny Samuela and Terry Weblemoe

CHAPTER OVERVIEW

This chapter covers the following topics:

+ Cultural difference
+ Cultural competence
+ Cultural safety.

KEY TERMS

Cultural difference
Culture
Ethnicity
Race
Colonisation
Assimilation
Cultural domination
Māori
Pacific People
Aboriginal and Torres Strait Islanders
Interpersonal racism
Linguists
Indigenous
Stereotypes
Cultural blindness
Cultural imposition
Institutional racism
Racism
Cultural competence
Cultural awareness
Cultural safety

Cultural difference The variations between groups that relate to their fundamental understandings about themselves, those around them and the communities of which they are a part.

Culture Beliefs, traditions and rituals originating within the family and community into which a person is born and raised, and transmitted from one generation to the next through a common language.

Ethnicity A group of people united by cultural or national heritage but residing in a place different from their place of origin.

Race A group of people who share distinctive characteristics.

Colonisation The movement to a new place by a group of people who maintain strong ties with their place of origin in the process of establishing a settlement.

Assimilation The process of attempting to make all people similar in terms of their beliefs and practices.

Before examining the concepts of **cultural difference**, cultural safety and cultural competence, it is important to understand what **culture** is and what it is not. Culture originates in the family and community in which a person is born and raised, where beliefs, traditions and rituals are transmitted from one generation to the next through a common language. Simply, culture provides a group of people with a shared identity based on beliefs, values and behaviours acceptable to that group, and influences the way its members see the world (Andrews & Boyle, 2007). Everyone has a culture of origin. Health practitioners also have a specific professional culture. Nonetheless, social, technological and global changes influence cultural beliefs, values and practices, which means that culture is dynamic, evolving over time as its members interact with cultural and social groups within and outside of their family or community of origin.

Often the concepts of culture, ethnicity and race are referred to interchangeably, even though they are different concepts. **Ethnicity**, while incorporating aspects of culture, develops within communities, where groups of people share common traits, loyalties and associations. Often people's nationality is used as a de facto term for ethnic identity (in Census polls, for example). It should be noted that this is a crude measure of ethnicity and cannot be used as a reliable indicator of culture, particularly in the case of Asian identity where a great number of nationalities are collapsed within an 'Asian' ethnicity descriptor. **Race**, on the other hand, broadly classifies people based on shared physical characteristics like skin pigmentation, facial features, body build and hair composition. Major race classifications in the Pacific include Polynesian, Melanesian, Micronesian and Caucasian, and are discernible by their physical characteristics. Defining people by race, ethnicity and culture, however, is problematic because identity, globalisation and inter-marriage contribute to identifiable features within the contemporary context.

Cultural difference

Effective communication with others from a different cultural background requires having a critical understanding of a country's history of **colonisation** and immigration. Countries like Australia and Aotearoa New Zealand were colonised by settlers from other countries, which resulted in their indigenous peoples being subjected to a loss of people, land, language and cultural practices through processes of **assimilation** and **cultural domination**. The colonising agenda was for indigenous peoples to conform to the dominant values, beliefs, behaviours and expectations of the settler culture, and the outcome was the cultures, social structures, roles, functions and traditions of the indigenous peoples were eroded. Not only have contemporary indigenous peoples—like **Māori**, **Pacific People**, **Aboriginal and Torres Strait Islanders**—suffered historical traumas, but most also live with significant contemporary socio-economic deprivation. They also experience inequalities in the access and use of health services, and in the quality of these services, which is generally perpetuated by institutional and **interpersonal racism**.

Professionals need to be aware of this in their practice and how it impacts on relationships and communication with indigenous peoples. Culturally determined and valued patterns of engagement and perspectives on communication style provide some insight into communication differences. Patterns of engagement differ in terms of the balances between individualism and collectivism. Pacific People tend to value the group needs, activities and identity (collectivism), whereas Europeans value individual achievement and recognition. In practical terms, this means that working in teams or emphasising the family as a whole may achieve more than emphasising individual efforts and rewards (Ting-Toomey & Chung, 2005). Other values in terms of engagement can be found in the different emphases placed on the roles people have within society. Western Europeans tend to value what a person does, can easily see a role as separate from the individual, and can understand interchangeable roles. For Pacific People, families and the relationships within groups are more important; they tend to define how the individual will work, who they are and how they will relate to each of a large number of people. While Western Europeans are more likely to introduce themselves to a new person by explaining what their role is or what job they do, Pacific People will generally want to know what the individual is like, what kind of person they are and how they are to relate to them (for example, their name, where they are from and who their parents are). Different appreciations of communicative style are also evident between cultural groups in terms of directness and indirectness. Europeans tend to emphasise the importance of verbal communication over non-verbal, the words over the context, and the content of the communication over the way the message makes the recipient feel, while at the same time using verbal softeners such as 'please' and 'thank you' for requests. For Pacific People, non-verbal communication, relationships and context are of greater importance.

Many communities are becoming increasingly culturally diverse due to globalisation and increasing migration. Minority and culturally and linguistically diverse groups are common in Australian and New Zealand communities, so health services and practitioners need to be aware of the challenges people belonging to these groups might face. Communication with those who belong to culturally and linguistically diverse communities requires professionals to work with others, such as interpreters, to ensure

Cultural domination When one cultural group assumes superiority over others.

Māori The indigenous people of Aotearoa New Zealand.

Pacific People People indigenous to the islands of the Pacific region.

Aboriginal and Torres Strait Islanders The indigenous people of what is now known as Australia.

Interpersonal racism When individuals treat others in a prejudiced manner based on judgments about their race.

Linguistics The study of language.

Indigenous The natural or native people of the land; the original inhabitants and carers of the place.

Stereotypes Beliefs held about a particular group that influence the way people respond to and treat people belonging to that group.

Cultural blindness The apparent inability to see cultural differences.

Cultural imposition The deliberate establishment of one set of cultural beliefs over those from other groups.

they provide safe and effective health care and disability support services. However, Mortensen (2010) reported that health practitioners lack the necessary cultural knowledge and skills of the culturally and **linguistically** diverse groups within their communities, which creates a major barrier to experiencing accessible, safe and equitable health services. Effective communication is important, and cultural safety and cultural competence can improve the practice of professionals working in communities that are culturally and linguistically diverse (DeSouza, 2008; Mortensen, 2010).

In situations where professionals lack critical analysis and understanding of contemporary **indigenous**, minority, and culturally and linguistically diverse groups, they risk acting on assumptions, **stereotypes** and faulty information. Often stereotypes are inaccurate, and negatively impact on the quality of health practitioners' communication with patients and service users. Acting on stereotypes or ignoring cultural differences contributes to **cultural blindness** (Johnstone, 2009). Cultural blindness facilitates a platform for **cultural imposition** (Andrews & Boyle, 2007), where professionals believe people should conform to beliefs and values of the dominant cultural group. Cultural imposition is evident in public health services in Aotearoa New Zealand, for example, whereby health practitioners impose the dominant biomedical view of health and illness on health service users.

Health is a socio-cultural construction formed in personal and professional lives (Wilson, 2008). Māori have an eco-spiritual holistic world view, which values collective responsibilities and obligations to whānau (extended family) members. Such a world view is at odds with the biomedical world view that is illness- and disease-oriented, valuing an individualistic perspective. Cultural difference becomes evident when a number of whānau members of a Māori patient in hospital want to visit or be present at a doctor's round, and the doctors and nurses focusing on the individual patient require visitors to adhere to visiting times and leave during the doctor's round. Whānau presence is important for the wairua (spiritual well-being) of a Māori patient.

In Australia and Aotearoa New Zealand there is awareness of cultural diversity, but it tends to be either poorly understood or insufficiently recognised and respected. For example, Aboriginal and Torres Strait Islander people are commonly grouped together and termed 'ATSI' or 'Indigenous'. It has been argued that neither of these terms is appropriate as they ignore unique tribal identities both between and within these groups (Gooda, 2010; Taylor & Guerin, 2010). By failing to recognise, appreciate and manage these differences, many individuals and services—albeit in some cases without intention—reinforce the harm that colonisation, assimilation and institutionalisation has inflicted on Aboriginal and Torres Strait Islander peoples (Ganguly, 2001; Taylor & Guerin, 2010) and Māori (Reid & Robson, 2007).

The continued ignorance of, or blindness to, cultural differences offers explanations for the persistent poor health status of Aboriginal and Torres Strait Islander peoples compared with the rest of the Australian population, and similarly for Māori and Pacific People in Aotearoa New Zealand. This is notably different from the experience of indigenous populations in other countries, where recognition and appreciation of cultural differences has led to improvements in the health of indigenous peoples (Couzos & Thiele, 2007; Ganguly, 2001). Couzos and Thiele (2007) have criticised the Australian Government as failing to meet its international obligations to improve the health of Aboriginal and Torres Strait Islander peoples, based on the belief that there is a continued practice of **institutional racism.**

Institutional racism can be defined as 'the systematic disadvantaging of racial and ethnic minorities through systems or institutions' (Taylor & Guerin, 2010, p. 75). In terms of health, this could include potential barriers to accessing services or care (for example, transportation, service hours and staffing), failure to provide adequate services (for example, lack of interpreters for little- or non-English speaking patients) and failure to provide adequate care due to stereotyping. Jones (2000) identifies **racism** as occurring at three levels: institutional, personally mediated (whereby individuals display discriminatory behaviours or choose not

Institutional racism Racism that is accepted and allowed within an organisational or powerful framework.

Racism Treating people in a discriminatory manner based on their heritage or race.

CASE STUDY 14.1

The dangers of stereotyping

A 56-year-old Aboriginal man presented to a regional hospital's emergency department, shouting, slurring his speech and staggering round the waiting area. Admissions staff had trouble understanding him due to his affected speech and, like many Aboriginal people in the district, his use of a pidgin form of English.

A triage nurse eventually guided him into a preliminary examination room. She knew the local community had a high level of alcohol abuse, and had frequently seen intoxicated community members present to hospital. Although she did not detect any alcohol on the man, she assumed he was drunk and believed all he needed was a couple of hours to 'sleep it off'. She instructed the man to rest on the examination table and said she would return shortly.

The nurse became busy with incoming patients, and was unable to return to the man until several hours later. The man was unresponsive, and on closer examination lacked any vital signs. The emergency was raised but the man was unable to be revived.

It was discovered that the man had been previously diagnosed with type I diabetes and had died from severe hypoglycaemia.

to acknowledge another person's culture) and internalised (when those subject to racist and discriminatory behaviours begin to believe the negative stereotypes imposed on them). Undoubtedly, racism has been linked to poor health outcomes and quality of care, at times resulting in adverse events (Davis et al., 2006; Harris et al., 2006). Blackman (2009) links the impact of racism on communication, stating: 'Perceived racism is a factor that can cripple the opportunity for honest and valuable communication between health care provider and the patient' (p. 213). Further, racism fuels mistrust and does little for the establishment of respectful relationships.

Institutional racism in the health-care system, whether intentional or not, at the very least places minority groups at a disadvantage, and at worst places them in jeopardy. It is important to understand that, in these circumstances, it is the culture of neither the patient nor the practitioner that leads to poor service provision (McMurray & Param, 2008). Rather, it is the failure to recognise and address these differences that leads to poor outcomes. As Fenwick (2006) states: 'If Western health care does not enhance Indigenous health due to the loss of emotional, social, spiritual and political support, it may be considered that the care delivered is culturally unsafe' (p. 220). Making services culturally safe remains an ongoing subject in both the Australian and New Zealand health-care systems.

CASE STUDY 14.2

Culturally appropriate support

It is common for Pacific People to be inaccurately thought of as one homogenous group. AUT University has developed an approach to supporting Pacific students based on the concept of a 'learning village'. The information below is directed at people from non-Pacific backgrounds to assist with interacting with Pacific students.

The setting is important—consider the environment in which information will be shared. Will everyone feel comfortable and culturally safe to speak their mind in that environment, or will they be overheard or feel foolish if they express themselves or their opinions in a way that is different from others? Do not assume how people experience or interpret information. Give them permission and facilitate their communication, especially within groups.

Make proper introductions—Pacific People want to know who they are speaking to, as a person, not just a job title or role. Be human and make an emotional connection with them. Try to put them at ease and spend some time to get the level right. Never trust stereotypes, but discover who they are as individuals.

Discover common ground—it helps if Pacific People can find common ground, such as someone or some place that both know, or even a common purpose. Aotearoa New Zealand and its various cultural groups are quite small. It is always a pleasant surprise to find out who you know in common. Gentle humour that includes them can often put people at ease.

Set the ground rules early—Pacific People need to know how to relate to strangers, what is likely to happen and who is in charge. There are many cultural expectations, in both the medical and the educational field, that Europeans have grown up with and internalised that are never articulated. Spell out what will happen, what is expected of them, what are the consequences and what kind of relationship they can expect.

Show that you truly care and meet them halfway—learn something about their culture and way of seeing the world. Do not just expect them to be culturally competent in your culture but reciprocate. Being interculturally competent does not necessarily mean that someone must know everything about their culture; rather, one should be open and flexible enough to build bridges and solutions between the cultures, and be willing to meet them halfway (Falconer, Watson & Hofner Saphiere, 2006).

Be persistent—keep checking understanding. In practical terms, this can mean such things as defining things as we go, repeatedly checking in with Pacific People that they are following our explanations or seeing if they have a question that we have not yet answered. They need to clearly understand what resources are available to them and exactly how to access them. This may require a step-by-step instruction or a visual demonstration. Do not assume that they necessarily know some of the things that are probably taken for granted in New Zealand culture, but equally do not assume that they do not know—always check, and give them credit for what they do know. Also do not assume that they see the world the same way that you do. Culture influences perception and the assumptions we make about what is going on, so check and check again.

Understand their background—learn something about their culture, their background and why they do what they do. Be interested and ask about their cultural understanding and their experiences, and what makes them comfortable or feel like they can fit in. Check in with Pacific People regularly, giving them permission to tell us when and how they see the world differently, and seeing if we can compromise or find a middle ground. Empower them to express themselves and to negotiate on equal footing.

Give examples they can relate to—the more that we know about their culture, the better we can use the examples and metaphors they already know to explain new concepts. We often forget how much of our illustrations are based on the history and technology of our culture, and therefore do not actually help to clarify meaning across culture. A good example that is culturally neutral, culturally shared or even culturally appropriate is much more facilitative to learning. Remember to be persistent. If one example does not trigger understanding, be willing to try something else or to demonstrate when possible.

Cultural competence

Cultural competence The concept that practitioners have the skills to interact in a culturally appropriate manner.

Cultural awareness A basic understanding that cultural difference exists and requires consideration and appropriate responses.

It has been argued that in order to help break down the barriers that cultural differences can place between patients and health-care practitioners and services, there is a need to establish a level of **cultural competence** (Gruen, Weeramanthri & Bailie, 2002; McMurray & Param, 2008). Many definitions exist regarding cultural 'competence' and it is often confused, or used interchangeably, with **cultural awareness**. In Australia, the provision of cultural awareness training has been incorporated into the curricula of many health and medical courses; however, there is little evidence about whether this translates into competence at the service-provision level. Authors such as Gruen and colleagues (2002), Henry, Houston and Mooney (2004) and Taylor and Guerin (2010) argue that it is not occurring.

Aotearoa New Zealand has adopted the concept of cultural safety, believing health practitioners need to be more than culturally aware. A clear history of this concept is obvious within nursing (Papps & Ramsden, 1996) and more information about it is presented later in this chapter. However, the Health Practitioners Competency Assurance Act 2003 in Aotearoa New Zealand has a focus on health practitioners being competent, and requires registered health practitioners to demonstrate cultural competence. Early versions of cultural competence required health practitioners to 'learn' the cultural practices of people they came into contact with. However, this is problematic as it is not possible to 'know' all cultural practices, given the culturally diverse people health practitioners come into contact with. Wilson (2008) defines cultural competence as the capability to 'articulate and demonstrate culturally appropriate and acceptable health services where clients feel culturally safe' and that these services reflect the professional's 'reflexivity, knowledge and skills, and an ability to work meaningfully with clients to meet their unique health and cultural needs during their health experience' (p. 185). Thus, cultural competence involves:

1 the knowledge, beliefs, attitudes and power dimensions of the professional
2 his or her actions contributing to improving health outcomes and health status of people from different cultural backgrounds
3 the ability to integrate the cultural values, beliefs and practices of clients into their plans of care (Wilson, 2008).

To do this requires a willingness and commitment to provide culturally competent care, and undergo ongoing education (Campinha-Bacote, 2002; Whaley, 2008).

Cultural competence is a progression from cultural awareness. It occurs when a given system (for example, a hospital, health service or collection of health practitioners) is able to identify and use behaviours, attitudes and policies to work effectively despite cultural differences (Nguyen, 2008). The questions in Table 14.1 can be used to guide self-reflection to determine the level of knowledge and skills a practitioner currently possesses, and the further development needed to attain cultural competence.

TABLE 14.1 *A self-reflection activity on cultural competence*

Self-reflection activity
What do I feel about people from other ethnic and cultural groups in my community?
What do I know about the cultural and ethnic world views of the range of people in my community?
What do I think about people from other ethnic and cultural groups in my community?
What interactions have I had with people from different cultural groups?
What stereotypes, prejudices and racism do I have about those from cultural groups different from mine?
What knowledge and skills do I possess to undertake appropriate and safe cultural assessments? What knowledge and skills do I need?
What aspirations do I have to be culturally aware, safe or competent?

A practitioner must not only have a level of awareness of the cultural diversity of their patients, but must also understand how their own cultural background and beliefs can impact upon the practitioner–patient relationship; they should also consider the ways in which they can approach that relationship to achieve a positive outcome for the patient (Nguyen, 2008; Williams, 1999). The aim is not to make the practitioner an 'expert' on the culture of a given patient, but rather to enable the practitioner to recognise and overcome potential barriers to effective service provision. Translating this understanding into the clinical, educational and policy-development systems can facilitate the development of culturally safe services.

Cultural safety

Cultural safety
A concept, closely associated with health practitioners in Aotearoa New Zealand, relating to the expectation that people receiving services should experience security and respect in terms of their cultural identity.

Cultural safety originated from the concerns of Māori nurses (and also Māori students in nursing programmes) about the quality of care patients received and the differences in outcomes compared with others (Ramsden, 2002). Over time, cultural safety has evolved to include cultural groups beyond ethnic groups, such as age, gender, occupation and sexual orientation. While cultural safety is determined by the patient about their experiences of interactions with health practitioners and a health service, there is an onus on health practitioners to undergo a process of critical reflection on their own cultural values, beliefs and traditions, and how this impacts on others. It is also useful to identify and reflect on the power a health practitioner has, which may or not be used to benefit patients. In situations where professionals lack this analysis, they risk acting on stereotypes and faulty information, and inadvertently using their power to disrupt access, use and quality of health services. In the absence of cultural safety, patients have their cultural identity diminished and demeaned, and as a consequence are disempowered during their health experience.

CASE STUDY 14.3

Compromising cultural safety

Matiu is a 40-year-old Māori man who lives with his whānau (his wife, Mihinui, and three school-aged children) in rented accommodation near the local marae. He has not worked for some time as he has serious health conditions associated with having rheumatic fever as a child, including obesity and sleep apnoea. He survives on the sickness benefit and relies on others for transport as he cannot afford the costs associated with having a car. Their home does not have a telephone.

Matiu finds it difficult to keep his health clinic appointments at the hospital, which is a one-hour drive away from his home. This is affecting his wairua (spiritual well-being) as he would really like to get better control of his health, but does not really understand his conditions and the treatments associated with them. When he has tried to ask questions in the past, the health practitioners he has come into contact with either ignore him or use language he cannot understand. In fact, he believes health practitioners only care about his illnesses and not about other things affecting his health. He also believes they trample on his mana, leaving him feeling inferior and worthless by the time he leaves. Matiu would really like to take his wife with him to his appointments to help him understand, but he really does not want to expose her to the disrespectful way in which he gets treated. He has received letters from Mary, the nurse at the health clinic, but he does not understand some of the words used and has decided to ignore them, as the money it costs to pay for petrol for someone to take him to the hospital is better spent on food for his children.

Mary, the registered nurse at the local health services, has given up on Matiu as he consistently does not attend clinic appointments. She has concluded Matiu does not care about himself, and has heard that the whānau are known for not conforming. For example, his tamariki (children) often do not attend school, according to Mary's friend who is a school teacher. Matiu's actions confirm all the things Mary knows about working with Māori—they are lazy, difficult and always late for (or miss) appointments. If they would just do what everyone else does, everything would be fine. To date, Mary has only communicated with Matiu in writing.

This is a situation where Matiu's cultural safety is being compromised as Mary has imposed her own cultural beliefs and values (such as the importance of time-keeping and conforming to expectations) onto Matiu. She has also acted on unvalidated assumptions (such as the hearsay about the school attendance of Matiu's tamariki) and stereotypes. In this situation, Mary would benefit from reflection on her own and her professional cultural beliefs, values and practices, and how this may impact on others she works with from a different culture.

From a cultural perspective, Matiu's whānau are important and a priority, and in his situation of limited resources he has prioritised feeding his children over the costs of transport. He has also decided not to expose his wife to the poor treatment he receives. Having health practitioners who can communicate in a respectful manner—providing Matiu with time to understand the information he is receiving and to ask questions—and acknowledging important cultural beliefs and practices related to his health would pave the way for a different outcome from the one described here.

In addition, cultural safety was grounded in the Treaty of Waitangi, the agreement Māori made with the Crown in 1840. The Treaty of Waitangi outlines the nature of the relationship Māori have with Crown agents, including health practitioners working in publicly funded health services. The Treaty guaranteed Māori the right to self-determination, to equality with other citizens living in Aotearoa New Zealand, and to protection. The principles of the Treaty are translated into health practitioners' practice in three ways: partnership (formation of a meaningful relationship for working *with* the patient and his or her family), participation (involvement of the patient and family in their care) and protection (determining key cultural and spiritual values, beliefs and practices that need to be included into plans of care). A fourth 'P'—power—also should be considered; that is, the power health practitioners possess and the manner in which they use it.

The need to provide culturally safe environments in all services to Aboriginal and Torres Strait Islander peoples has been identified by Australian governments since the late 1960s, and has been recommended in almost every report on Aboriginal and Torres Strait Islander health since the National Aboriginal Health Strategy in 1989 (NATSIHC, 2004). A generally accepted definition of cultural safety, as it applies to Aboriginal and Torres Strait Islander peoples, is 'an environment which is safe for people: where there is no assault, challenge or denial of their identity, of who they are and what they need. It is about shared respect, shared meaning, shared knowledge and experience, of learning together with dignity, and truly listening' (Eckermann et al., 2010, p. 174). Inherent in this definition are elements that can be attributed to basic human rights: identity, recognition, acceptance (or, at the very least, tolerance) and respect.

In the scope of providing health services, cultural safety equates to empowering patients from diverse cultural backgrounds to determine for themselves what sort of care is most appropriate for them (Nguyen, 2008; Peiris, Brown & Cass, 2008). In particular, the power imbalance that commonly exists between practitioner and patient needs to be equalised, so the practitioner can be seen as a resource that the patient can access—or, in broader terms, that health services can be seen as a resource for the community (McMurray & Param, 2008; Peiris et al., 2008).

An example of this has been described by Abbott, Gordon and Davison (2007), where Aboriginal Health Workers (AHWs) are utilised as a means of balancing the relationship between non-Indigenous nurses or doctors and Aboriginal patients. Within this arrangement, the practitioner, AHW and patient are seen as equals who work in partnership to achieve an identified outcome. AHWs often take the role of a 'cultural mentor' for the non-Indigenous practitioner, providing advice and understanding on cultural and other barriers that may limit the implementation of a care plan, and working with both the practitioner and the patient to effectively address and overcome these barriers (Abbott, Gordon & Davison, 2007). Similarly, Māori Community Health Workers are also a useful cultural resource for those working with Māori communities.

CASE STUDY 14.4

Aboriginal Health Workers as cultural mentors

During a 6-month placement at an Aboriginal Community Controlled Health Service in western Sydney, a GP registrar has a patient walk out of the consultation without discussing further details of her complex medical and social problems. He is concerned because the patient is potentially very ill, and confused because he felt that his communication skills were quite good.

He consults the service's AHW about the incident and the issues he encountered during the consultation. They agree that he should videotape some consultations, with full consent from the patients, with the aim of reviewing them together to discuss cross-cultural communication skills in an Aboriginal setting. In the meantime, the AHW contacts the patient involved to ensure appropriate health management can be initiated.

Adapted from Abbott et al. (2007, p. 71)

Facilitating cultural safety in the health service setting requires examination of service provision, not just in terms of what services are available but more importantly in terms of how services are delivered. This has implications at all levels of the organisation, from direct-contact staff (practitioners and administrators) to managers, internal policies and programmes, and even the organisation's infrastructure (Williams, 1999). Many authors, including Wepa (2005), Williams (1999), Nguyen (2008) and, most recently, Taylor and Guerin (2010), have suggested a set of minimum requirements for developing cultural safety principles (see Table 14.2).

TABLE 14.2 *Suggested minimum requirements for cultural safety guidelines*

Individual level
• Undertake a process of critical reflection on personal and professional cultural backgrounds and how these impact on those from differing cultural backgrounds. • Demonstrate a readiness to be culturally safe. • Have a willingness to listen and communicate appropriately with those who belong to indigenous, culturally and linguistically diverse, and minority groups. • Have an understanding and respect for different cultures, knowledge, experiences and obligations. • Avoid practices or attitudes that may diminish or demean an individual's identity or dignity, or disempower an individual. • Minimise the power differential between self and individuals.

(*Continued*)

TABLE 14.2 *Suggested minimum requirements for cultural safety guidelines (cont.)*

Organisational level
• Make a commitment to the practice of cultural safety throughout the organisation that is evident in its organisational policies. • Actively engage with individuals and the community to address appropriate issues. • Provide access to interpreters. • Identify groups and resources within the community to assist. • Recognise and empower community control and ownership. • Achieve clarity and consistency in decision-making.

Health services need to become accountable to the communities within which they provide services, and in so doing facilitate the development of a mutual level of trust and respect (Gruen, Weeramanthri & Bailie, 2002; Vicary & Andrews, 2001). This means recognising the impact that colonisation has had upon the health and well-being of indigenous peoples, and working towards 'decolonising' our health institutions, with the aim of developing reconciliation between indigenous and non-indigenous peoples (Edwards & Taylor, 2008; McMurray & Param, 2008; Sherwood & Edwards, 2006).

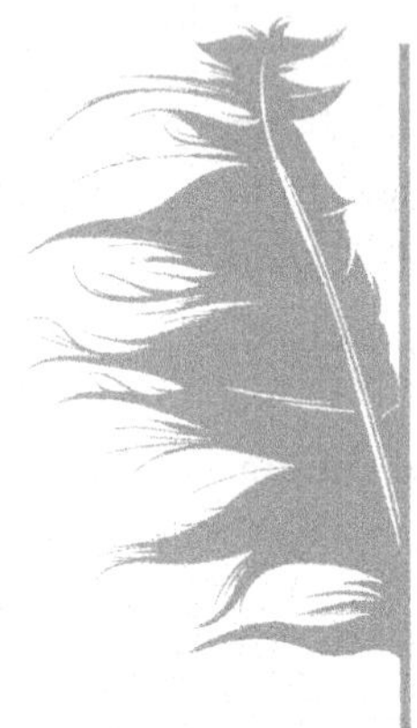

{ SUMMARY }

Cultural differences can present barriers to the effective and safe provision of health-care services to indigenous, culturally and linguistically diverse, and minority groups. There is a professional onus on those working in health services to develop the ability to provide safe and effective services to those who belong to these groups. Developing cultural competence can assist individual practitioners to develop their capability to work effectively with those from another culture, and overcome these barriers. Cultural safety occurs when patients and service users feel their cultural identity is recognised and respected, and their rights to equal health care are observed. Cultural competence facilitates cultural safety when it is practised at both individual and organisational or systemic levels.

REFLECTION POINTS

14.1 Intention (motivation, message, meaning, emotion)

What are some examples of how culture shapes the beginning stages in a therapeutic relationship?

14.2 Reception (received message, response, feedback)

When working with a person from a different cultural background, what cues would indicate how accurately the information you shared was received? How could you ensure the person understood what you were talking about?

14.3 Perception (style, manner, impression, analysis)

Reflect on occasions when communicating with someone from a different cultural background. Knowing what you now know about cultural safety and cultural competence, reflect on the way in which you communicated (that is, your communication style, manner and body language you adopted). How could you check out your communication style, manner and body language?

QUESTIONS FOR REVIEW

1 Consider the outcome in Case study 14.1. What changes would you suggest need to be implemented on the part of both the triage nurse and hospital management to avoid this happening in the future?
2 How would you describe the differences between cultural awareness and cultural safety?
3 How do you evaluate your own cultural competence and cultural safety?
4 Do you think cultural safety is a journey or a destination?

REFERENCES

Abbott, P., Gordon, E. & Davison, J. (2007). Expanding roles of Aboriginal health workers in the primary care setting: Seeking recognition. *Contemporary Nurse*, *26*(1), 66–73.

Andrews, M. M. & Boyle, J. S. (2007). *Transcultural concepts in nursing care* (5th edn). Philadelphia, PA: Lippincott Williams & Wilkins.

Blackman, R. (2009). Knowledge for practice: Challenges in culturally safe nursing practice. *Contemporary Nurse, 32*(1–2), 211–14.

Campinha-Bacote, J. (2002). The process of cultural competence in the delivery of healthcare services: A model of care. *Journal of Transcultural Nursing, 13*(3), 181–4. DOI: 10.1177/10459602013003003.

Couzos, S. & Thiele, D. D. (2007). The international covenant on economic, social and cultural rights and the right to health: Is Australia meeting its obligations to Aboriginal peoples? *Medical Journal of Australia, 186*(10), 522–4.

Davis, P., Lay-Yee, R., Dyall, L., Briant, R., Sporle, A., Brunt, D. et al. (2006). Quality of hospital care for Māori patients in New Zealand: Retrospective cross-sectional assessment. *The Lancet, 367*(9526), 1920–5.

DeSouza, R. (2008). Wellness for all: The possibilities of cultural safety and cultural competence in New Zealand. *Journal of Research in Nursing, 13*(2), 125–35. DOI: 10.1177/1744987108088637.

Eckermann, A., Dowd, T., Chong, E., Nixon, L., Gray, R. & Johnson, S. (2010). *Binaŋ Goonj: Bridging cultures in Aboriginal health* (3rd edn). Sydney, NSW: Elsevier Australia.

Edwards, T. & Taylor, K. (2008). Decolonising cultural awareness. *Australian Nursing Journal, 15*(10), 31–3.

Falconer, T., Watson, B. & Hofner Saphiere, D. (2006). *Cultural detective (NZ): Series facilitator guide* [Registered Training Package]. Retrieved from www.culturaldetective.com.

Fenwick, C. (2006). Assessing pain across the cultural gap: Central Australian Indigenous peoples' pain assessment. *Contemporary Nurse, 22*(2), 218–27.

Ganguly, I. (2001). The third dimension: Cultural awareness for non-English speaking background health professionals. *Australian and New Zealand Journal of Public Health, 25*(2), 109–10.

Gooda, M. (2010). *Social justice report 2010*. Canberra, ACT: Australian Human Right Commission.

Gruen, R. L., Weeramanthri, T. S. & Bailie, R. S. (2002). Outreach and improved access to specialist services for indigenous people in remote Australia: The requirements for sustainability. *Journal of Epidemiology and Community Health, 56*(7), 517–21.

Harris, R., Tobias, M., Jeffreys, M., Waldegrave, K., Karlsen, S. & Nazroo, J. (2006). Racism and health: The relationship between experience of racial discrimination and health in New Zealand. *Social Science & Medicine, 63*(6), 1428–41.

Henry, B. R., Houston, S. & Mooney, G. H. (2004). Institutional racism in Australian healthcare: A plea for decency. *Medical Journal of Australia, 180*, 517–20.

Johnstone, M.-J. (2009). *Bioethics: A nursing perspective*. Sydney, NSW: Elsevier Churchill Livingstone.

Jones, C. P. (2000). Levels of racism: A theoretic framework and a gardener's tale. *American Journal of Public Health, 90*, 1212–15.

McMurray, A. & Param, R. (2008). Culture-specific care for Indigenous people: A primary health care perspective. *Contemporary Nurse, 28*(1–2), 165–72.

Mortensen, A. (2010). Cultural safety: Does the theory work in practice for culturally and linguistically diverse groups? *Nursing Praxis in New Zealand, 26*(3), 6–16.

NATSIHC. (2004). *National Strategic Framework for Aboriginal and Torres Strait Islander Health: Context*. Canberra, ACT: Office for Aboriginal and Torres Strait Islander Health.

Nguyen, H. T. (2008). Patient centred care: Cultural safety in indigenous health. *Australian Family Physician, 31*(12), 990–4.

Papps, E. & Ramsden, I. (1996). Cultural safety in nursing: The New Zealand experience. *International Journal for Quality in Health Care, 8*(5), 491–7.

Peiris, D., Brown, A. & Cass, A. (2008). Addressing inequities in access to quality health care for indigenous people. *Canadian Medical Association Journal, 179*(10), 985–6.

Ramsden, I. M. (2002). *Cultural safety and nursing education in Aotearoa and Te Waipounamu* (PhD thesis). Wellington, NZ: Victoria University of Wellington. Retrieved from http://culturalsafety.massey.ac.nz/thesis.htm.

Reid, P. & Robson, B. (2007). Understanding health inequities. In B. Robson & R. Harris (eds), *Hauora: Māori health standards IV. A study of the years 2000–2005* (pp. 3–10). Wellington, NZ: Te Ropu Rangahau Hauora a Eru Pomare. Retrieved from www.hauora.māori.nz.

Sherwood, J. & Edwards, T. (2006). Decolonisation: A critical step for improving Aboriginal health. *Contemporary Nurse, 22*(2), 178–90.

Taylor, K. & Guerin, P. (2010). *Health care and Indigenous Australians: Cultural safety in practice*. Sydney, NSW: Palgrave MacMillan.

Ting-Toomey, S. & Chung, L. C. (2005). *Understanding intercultural communication*. Los Angeles, CA: Roxbury Publishing.

Vicary, D. & Andrews, H. (2001). A model of therapeutic intervention with Indigenous Australians. *Australian and New Zealand Journal of Public Health, 25*(4), 349–51.

Wepa, D. (2005). *Cultural safety in Aotearoa New Zealand*. Auckland, NZ: Pearson Education New Zealand.

Whaley, A. (2008). Cultural sensitivity and cultural competence: Toward clarity of definitions of cross-cultural counselling and psychotherapy. *Counselling Psychology Quarterly, 21*(3), 215–22.

Williams, R. (1999). Cultural safety—What does it mean for our work practice? *Australian and New Zealand Journal of Public Health, 23*(2), 213–18.

Wilson, D. (2008). The significance of a culturally appropriate health service for indigenous Māori women. *Contemporary Nurse, 28*, 173–88.

WEBSITES

Australian Indigenous HealthInfoNet: www.healthinfonet.ecu.edu.au

Hauora: Māori health standards of health: www.hauora.maori.nz

Tataū Kahukura: Māori Health Chart Book: www.moh.govt.nz/moh.nsf/indexmh/tatau-kahukura-māri-health-chart-book-2010

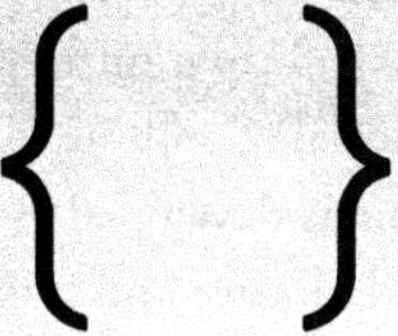

Touch

David Nicholls

CHAPTER OVERVIEW

This chapter covers the following topics:

+ The culture of touch
+ Touch through the lifespan
+ Touch and communication
+ Touch and professional practice
+ Touch and human well-being.

KEY TERMS

Haptic
Integumentary system
Therapeutic touch
Purposeful touch
Inappropriate touch

> ***When we honestly ask ourselves which person in our lives means the most to us, we often find that it is those who, instead of giving advice, solutions, or cures, have chosen rather to share our pain and touch our wounds with a warm and tender hand.***
>
> *Henri Nouwen (1990)*

Of all the senses, touch is probably the most valuable to other people. While hearing, sight, smell and taste provide vital information that enables human function, it is the ability to touch that makes people social. Combine touch with the ability to communicate with words and it is clear how humans developed as higher order beings. Touch allowed people to feel their way out of the dark cave and into the sunlight; to rub sticks together to make fire; to wield tools to provide and prepare food; to build machines and tall buildings; to plough fields; and, importantly, to heal other people's suffering. Touch is the most practical and the noblest of the senses, and is an essential component of modern life.

Touch means much more to us than merely what we can feel with our hands. This is apparent in common references to touch, such as people saying they 'feel for you' when showing sympathy, or that someone 'touched a nerve' in relation to something being painfully true. To 'catch your breath', 'grasp at straws', 'hold that thought' and 'grab a drink' are other examples of touch in everyday language. It is also common to refer to the working of the human mind in terms of tactile language—how people 'feel'.

Touch, therefore, is far more complex than it would first appear, but it is a vital subject for those who aspire to work with others, and particularly those in the professions that use touch as a regular part of their work. Novice practitioners often make the mistake of thinking that tactile, or **haptic**, communication is innate and cannot be taught; that it is a skill that some people are simply born with. While this might be true to some extent, expertise is achieved through months and years of practice, along with the application of skills that certainly can be acquired. Touch is so powerful, rich and complex that students of health must have at least a rudimentary appreciation for its ability to bring relief to people, and they must grasp some of its subtlety and complexity.

Haptic Relating to the sense of touch.

There are several social and theoretical aspects of touch. Culture and history indicate the importance of touch for humans. Across the lifespan, tactile forms of communication take various forms. The complexity inherent in the language of touch is important to understand; its place in professional practice also requires attention.

The culture of touch

People have used touch to hurt and to heal for as long as we have recorded history. From earliest fumblings in the dark world of prehistoric peoples, through the manual labour of the pre-industrial age, to the computer-aided technologies of the twenty-first century, touch has been vital to the identity of humans and has served as a marker of evolution. Touch is now so pervasive and necessary for our civilisation that it is easy to overlook how important it is to human existence, ways of life and standards of living (Calvert, 2002).

Prior to the Industrial Revolution, most Western cultures relied on small-scale manufacture of goods and agriculture for income. By necessity, work was local, with things being made as they were needed and food being harvested in season. With the advent of machinery in factories and on farms, mass-produced commodities began to appear in homes, and food began to be gathered in vast quantities and shipped as refrigerated cargo around the world. Populations subsequently grew in number, size and affluence; birth rates increased and death rates declined.

But while the marvels of modern technology were celebrated, people also began to yearn for a simpler time. As far back as two hundred years ago, writers like Charles Dickens and Thomas Hardy, and painters like John Constable and Jean-François Millet, mourned the loss of a pastoral way of life. Concerns that people were 'out of touch' with nature began to pervade aspects of Victorian culture and led to some seeing technology as the cause of much illness and suffering. In many ways, today's environmental campaigners and advocates for locally grown, organic food are repeating many of the same arguments: expressing a yearning for a simpler time when people made things by hand.

Touch has played a complex and multidimensional role in modern culture, and it is simplistic to say that touch, or touch technologies, are simply good or bad. Take, for example, the current fascination with smartphones and touch technology. It is difficult to imagine the appeal of an iPad or iPhone without the touch-screen, or a computer without a mouse or keyboard. Touch is ubiquitous in modern technology and for many years science writers have written about a future in which haptic technology or haptics play an increasingly important part in our methods of communication. From touch-screens (such as the screens used in the films *Minority Report* and *Quantum of Solace*) to touch-activated communication systems, haptics will offer assistive technologies for people, whether they have difficulties with speech, want to reach a mass audience or simply want to communicate with someone on the other side of the globe.

One of the most interesting aspects of touch in our culture is not the technological innovation coming in the next few years, but the way that touch has influenced our various social histories. Many of the social tensions that now define human civilisation have, in some way or other, involved touch. The sexual revolution in the 1960s broke down traditional stigmas around touch, for example, but these new-found freedoms were soon cut short by epidemics of AIDS, avian flu and SARS that made people more fearful of touching others (this cultural shift is illustrated in the Austin Powers films). HIV/AIDS was such a frightful thing in the 1980s that Princess Diana caused controversy when, in 1987, she publicly touched the hand of an AIDS victim, commenting that people need hugs and that she believed everyone needs to be touched. More confusion and ambivalence in relation to touch are apparent in the ubiquitous nature of cleaning products, in terms of the debate that children's immune systems may not be able to properly develop in sanitised environments.

The sophistication of human society is built on some rather basic physiological functions, not least the prehensile ability, which in anthropological terms means to be able to grasp objects. Many other species 'feel' through their hands and paws, and some have adapted tails (monkeys), claws (cats), noses (elephants) and even lips (horses) that allow them to grasp objects in the absence of human-like hands. But few outside the primates have the ability to move the thumb across the palm to touch the other digits (a function called 'opposition'). The prehensile ability of early humans allowed them to grasp objects, fashion weapons and wield tools, and this vital evolutionary advantage may have even led directly to us walking erect (because animals cannot wield tools in their hands if they rely on four legs to stand and walk). This, in turn, allowed humans to grow in size and brain power, adapt their diet and evolve rapidly. Touch is a tool that has brought us to civilisation.

Touch through the lifespan

The experience of touch (both given and received) is vital for normal child development. A newborn baby first relies on their other senses to find out about the world beyond their grasp. Only when they begin to crawl then walk do they really experience the world of surfaces, materials, textures and temperatures, and then parents and others around them spend inordinate amounts of time teaching them to discriminate between those that are safe and those that are not.

Children learn that not all tactile experiences are good or pleasant. Accidents occur: some will trip and hurt their hands on the gravel, touch a hot pan or trap their fingers in doors. Some will experience physical abuse at the hands of others. Much is learnt and remembered from early tactile experiences and some of it will stay with a person for their whole life.

Adults, too, rely on touch for growth and maturation. Much of our sexuality is inherently derived from touch. The sensuality of the world around us is appreciated in large part from our sense of touch. Indeed, the experience of pain so common in adulthood is thought by many philosophers to be vital to our very existence as humans (see, for example, the work of Friedrich Nietzsche or the writings of Marcel Proust). Touch is also a major form of social engagement for adults who use handshakes, kisses, hand-holding, slaps and punches to communicate to others what words sometimes cannot say.

For the elderly, who are prone to frail skin and illnesses that compromise their **integumentary system**, touch takes on new meaning. An inability to move as

Integumentary system Skin and related structures.

freely and as comfortably as when they were younger often means long periods sitting or lying, and a reliance on others for help with movement. Fragile skin can easily break down and ulcerate, and poor circulation results in very slow healing. A cerebro-vascular accident (or 'stroke') may affect the sensation over half of the body, and heart disease may cause the limbs to swell and the skin stretch until it splits. Arthritis may deform the joints of the hands and make using even simple tools like knives and forks, garden trowels and knitting needles impossible. Touch, therefore, accompanies people through the various stages of life, helping to define their experiences and engagement with the world. This is most clearly seen in the way people use touch to communicate.

Touch and communication

Touch is incredibly complex and multifaceted. Touch cannot be understood simply by knowing the anatomy of the hand, or the cultural history of tools, or the pathology of arthritis. It is not possible to know how important touch is by thinking only of one aspect of its role for individuals and societies. Its role in communication is immeasurably more complex.

While technical skill is hugely important in health-care practice, it is people's ability to communicate that truly makes the difference to people's experience of health care and disability support, and may also determine whether a treatment is effective or not. Given that the vast majority of communication is non-verbal (through gestures, body language and expressions), it is reasonable to assume that touch plays a large part in determining the outcome for those receiving care and support.

However, touch in health care is, in some ways, made more complex by social taboos about what can be touched, when and by whom. Each culture reflects its history and cultural identity in the way that touch is used. In English culture, for example, it is normal to shake hands on meeting someone, while in French culture people exchange kisses. In Māori culture the hongi carries enormous significance as a gesture of welcome. Simple though they are, these gestures betray deep roots that relate directly to collective histories, beliefs and values.

In Western cultures touch has been a problematic issue for many centuries, since certain forms of touch associated with pleasure and sensuality were considered sinful by the early Christian church. The Christian attitude towards 'sins of the flesh' led to a purge against early forms of massage in Western Europe. All forms of **therapeutic touch** were considered blasphemous and many of the handwritten texts of Greek and Roman physicians and healers were burned. Had it not been for the intervention of Persian scholars like Ibn Sīnā (or more fully, Abū Alī al-usayn ibn Abd Allāh ibn Sīnā, 980–1037), who translated these texts into Arabic, the works

Therapeutic touch Touch that is deliberate and intended to help and heal, and is understood accordingly.

of Celsus and Galen would almost certainly have been lost, along with much of what is now known about these therapies.

The height of our Western society's anxieties about touch came in Victorian England towards the end of the nineteenth century. This period coincided with the birth of modern medicine, nursing, midwifery and physiotherapy, and these professions (and others that have followed) had to negotiate how society could give them licence to touch people while not causing offence. One of the ways this was achieved was through clearly defined ethical codes of conduct and the technical teaching of **purposeful touch**.

Purposeful touch
Touch that has a meaningful and honourable intent.

Purposeful touch defines the intent of the giver, and says less about the experience of the receiver. It is not the casual contact between two friends or the unintentional brush against another person on a bus, but the deliberate, thoughtful and often highly technical contact between a skilled practitioner and a client or patient. Importantly, it may require one of the parties to touch the other in a way that would not normally be socially acceptable. Taking blood, inserting urinary catheters, bathing people in bed and replacing hip joints, for example, all require forms of intimate contact that would be totally unacceptable were they to take place in the cinema or at the mall. But in hospital or at the local clinic, under the care of a qualified health practitioner, it is possible to encroach upon people's personal space in the most intimate manner. Given this ability, it is vital that consideration be given not only to the technical aspects of touch, but also to how that touch will be perceived.

Touch is an intimate connection between two people who in all probability have different histories, beliefs and values. Each experience of touch is unique, because the second after being touched change may take place, and the touch no longer exists. There is an aphorism that states: 'You cannot dip your toe in the same place in the river twice.' It means that every encounter in life is specific to that exact moment in time, and this is true of those occasions when people touch others.

Not surprisingly, the power of touch to harm and to heal intimidates some people, but people are surrounded by touch. The difference in the health-care setting is that the poser of touch is harnessed with the goal of improving the well-being of others. This requires the learning and careful development of skills that others may not have. The ability to touch people purposively costs nothing, but it has the ability to profoundly impact on those who receive it.

For all its mystical virtues, however, touch is obviously not always good. The harsh reality is that if the intent of the person is to be cruel, to hurt or to abuse, touch can be a profoundly harmful experience for the recipient. It is no surprise that centuries-old forms of torture involve the use of extreme physical punishment. However, not all forms of abuse involve the use of violence against the body. People can also experience trauma by being denied loving or healing touch as much as through the use of excessive force. To complicate matters further, there are occasions in health care where it is necessary to cause a person pain

to bring about healing; for example, performing surgery, administering medications via injections or stretching limbs and scar tissue. Once again, in these situations it is the intent implied in the touch that defines whether the work is ethically justifiable.

Touch and professional practice

The ability to touch people, as a necessary part of health-care practice, is often taken for granted. For example, a primary care practitioner uses touch to take blood pressure and examine ailments, while a visit to a dental professional is obviously going to involve touching the face and mouth. But not all practitioners are allowed to touch people freely, and there are strict social codes around how, where and when the touch can take place (Lawler, 1991).

Society has traditionally allowed some practitioners to touch only when they have demonstrated competence, completed extended training and gained registration with a licensing authority. For their part, these practitioners have restricted their forms of touch to purposeful or intentional touch. This form of touch is different from the kinds of touch that happen in everyday personal and public life. Often it is touch that requires training, skill, purpose and the acceptance of the person receiving it. Surgeons, for instance, can touch the body in areas physically inaccessible to others (like the hip joint or the heart) while the person is anaesthetised. Nurses often perform very intimate procedures involving touch that would be unacceptable in any social location other than a hospital ward or clinic. Other practitioners use touch in the form of therapeutic manipulation (Oerton, 2004).

In recent years, the stranglehold that orthodox professionals had over the licensing of therapeutic touch has started to relax, and now a wider range of alternative and complementary practitioners use touch. The need for formal training and strict registration for practitioners has dissipated, and yet there remain some social conventions about where and when touch should take place. This increasing comfort with forms of therapeutic touch exists alongside an acute sensitivity to forms of **inappropriate touch**. Domestic violence and child abuse are widely acknowledged and condemned, although people young and old still experience physical and sexual violence, harassment and persecution. Physical violence need not involve another person: self-harm occurs when people inflict pain or injury upon themselves and may be considered a form of inappropriate touch.

Inappropriate touch Touch that is unwanted or of questionable intent.

Those who are given licence to touch in the course of their work have complex responsibilities. Not only are there shifting boundaries around who can and who cannot touch, but there are also considerations of the context, necessity and technical application of touch by the practitioner. Add to this the history and prior experiences of the giver and receiver, and the difficulties of navigating this complex social interaction are apparent. In the past, orthodox practitioners created rituals and cultural practices (like wearing white coats, working within hospitals and using special language that was reserved for those with special training) to sidestep many of these complex social tensions around touch. Latterly, however, society has shown an eagerness to dispense with these traditional practices, and has encouraged practitioners to look, talk and behave more like the people they serve, as well as leave their hospital wards and move out into the community.

With this change in the power dynamic between professionals and the lay public, a greater uncertainty has emerged about who can touch, when and where it can happen, and, indeed, when it is good or bad. Touch, like other aspects of the interactions between practitioners and patients or clients, requires consent and an appreciation of the appropriateness and potential interpretation of it.

Touch and human well-being

To be human and to be alive is to be in touch. We might well ask: 'Would we be able to survive without a sense of touch?' Clearly, people who have had neurological impairments—like spinal cord injuries and strokes—lack some ability to sense touch, but they survive regardless and often prosper. Equally, there are many that shy away from touch because it is hurtful or destructive, but they still come into contact with surfaces (chairs, beds, floors etc.) at every moment of their lives, and so have no choice but to move through a world of touch. All humans exist in a world of touch and navigate their way through it. In many ways, touch is the most dynamic sense, in that it brings people—literally and figuratively—into contact with the world and one another. It is vital that people engaging with the public in the provision of health care and disability support services grasp the complexity and importance of touch for others.

There are many issues to consider in relation to touch, including culture, touch through the lifespan, communication and professional practice. An understanding, curiosity and respect for the complexity of touch and its remarkable power to hurt and to heal is essential to good communication.

CASE STUDY 16.1

Touch in practice

Think of a situation in your own practice where you would need to touch another person physically. Now, follow this exercise as a way to show just how much the success of that experience depends on the context you find yourself in.

1 Keep the 'encounter' as it is, but imagine it takes place in a village in sub-Saharan Africa. You no longer have the white clinic room, or the technical equipment, but a dirt floor and a mud hut.

2 Now, remove the protection you carry as a health practitioner (your uniform, training and discipline). You are now just a neighbour.

3 Now ask yourself how your touch would be different.

Try to list at least five changes you would have to make given the new situation you find yourself in.

The purpose of such a task (and it is one you can simulate for any number of aspects of your practice) is to make you think the elements of touch that you might otherwise dismiss.

Touch is—on the one hand—so obvious and everyday it is easy to ignore its complexity and power. Practitioners need to be mindful of the value of it.

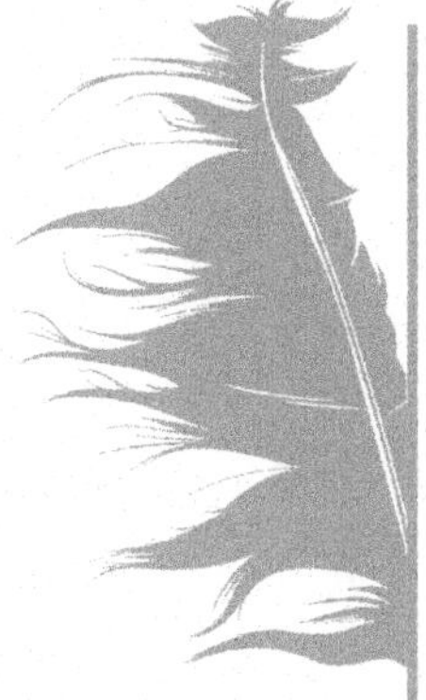

{ SUMMARY }

This chapter has considered the cultural significance of touch, the role of touch in technology and touch throughout the lifespan, and its role in defining professional practice. Touch is an essential component in practice and also plays a key role in communication. It is critical to have a broad appreciation of the power of touch—regardless of whether it is used as a primary mode of healing, or incidentally in the routine act of their everyday practice. Touch has profound significance for people, culture and society, and is able to profoundly impact on health and well-being. It is imperative that people working in the health care and disability support sector have a sound appreciation of the power and importance of touch, and equally that they are able to reflect on their practice and interactions in terms of appropriateness.

REFLECTION POINTS

16.1 Intention (motivation, message, meaning, emotion)

How does purposeful touch differ from other forms of casual touch?

16.2 Reception (received message, response, feedback)

How would you gain feedback in regard to whether touch is perceived as welcome or unwelcome?

16.3 Perception (style, manner, impression, analysls)

How does our use of touch help to define us as professionals?

QUESTIONS FOR REVIEW

1 How has touch influenced our culture as humans?
2 What role does touch play in modern technology?
3 How do children, adults and the elderly experience touch differently?
4 How can the language of touch help us express our feelings?

REFERENCES

Calvert, R. N. (2002). *The history of massage: An illustrated survey from around the world*. Rochester, NY: Inner Traditions/Bear & Company.

Lawler, J. (1991). *Behind the screens: Nursing, somology, and the problem of the body*. London, UK: Churchill Livingstone.

Nouwen, H. J. M. (1990). The *road to daybreak: A spiritual journey*. New York, NY: Doubleday.

Oerton, S. (2004). Bodywork boundaries: Power, politics and professionalism in therapeutic massage. *Gender, Work and Organization, 11*(5), 544–65.

WEBSITES

DePauw University Touch and Emotion Lab: www.depauw.edu/learn/lab
General Council for Massage Therapies (UK): www.gcmt.org.uk
Massage New Zealand: www.massagenewzealand.org
University of Miami Touch Research Institute: www6.miami.edu/touch-research

Environmental Worldviews

W. LINDSEY WHITE

CHAPTER OVERVIEW

This chapter covers the following topics:

- Environmental worldviews
- How does the world work?
- Ecosystem economics
- Ecosystem services
- Ecological footprint

KEY TERMS

Anthropocentric
Biocentric
Degraded
Ecocentric
Ecological overshoot
Ecologist
Ecosystem
Ecosystem services
Environment
Environmental health
Instrumental values
Intrinsic values
Maximum sustainable yield
Principles
Resource
Sustainability
System
Values

Environment can be defined in many ways. People talk about a family environment or the political environment of the country; that is, all the elements that surround you and of which you are a part. In the last few decades the word environment has taken on quite a specific meaning. It has come to mean 'nature'. So when we hear about environmental issues, we usually understand these to be issues related to the natural world. Global environmental issues include global warming, pollution, extinction of animals and deforestation. This chapter introduces some of these issues, particularly the ones that have an impact on human health.

Personal health and **environmental health** are linked in many ways. This is because our earth is a **system** with many interconnected components; if one component is changed it may have an impact on others. To visualise how this might work for humans, imagine a small island that has a limited amount of land to grow crops and feed the human population. The components of the system might be population, nutrition and the ability of the land to provide food. If the population increases too much, the land will have great demands put on it and may become **degraded**. Eventually it may become unable to produce enough food for the growing population, and the nutrition of the humans will decrease. On the other hand, if the environment changes (through increasing levels of rainfall, fire or drought), the ability to produce food may be either reduced or enhanced, again having an impact on human nutrition and the ability of the population to grow. So these factors are linked; if you change one, you change the others. The earth is a very complex system with millions of interacting parts. This means that changes made to one part may have very unpredictable outcomes on multiple other parts of the system. As the system becomes more complex, it becomes more difficult to predict the effect of changes.

Human actions can have a dramatic impact on the environment, and the environment can have dramatic impacts on people. There are some basic requirements that humans cannot live without, such as air, food and water. All of these come to us via the world around us, and the quality of these things can vary markedly depending on the state of the environment, which can in turn have an impact on our health and quality of life.

Before examining our environmental worldviews and some of the current important global environmental issues, it would be useful to have an understanding of what humans get out of the environment. **Ecologists** like to talk about **ecosystem services**, which are things that the environment provides to humans (and other organisms on earth). They are called services, because they would actually cost us money to obtain or carry out if the natural environment did not do it for us. Ecosystem services include (modified from Daily et al., 1997):

- cycling and movement of nutrients
- control of the vast majority of potential agricultural pests
- maintenance of biodiversity

- protection of coastal shores from erosion by waves
- stabilisation of climate
- moderation of weather extremes and their impacts
- provision of aesthetic beauty and intellectual stimulation that lift the human spirit
- production of **ecosystem** goods
- purification of air and water
- mitigation of droughts and floods
- generation and preservation of soils
- detoxification and decomposition of wastes
- pollination of crops and natural vegetation
- dispersal of seeds.

These services that are provided to humans (and the rest of the earth's organisms) are vital to our health and wellbeing. Therefore it is important to understand how our activities are having an impact on the provision of these services, and how changes in the ability of ecosystems to provide these services will have an impact on our health.

ENVIRONMENTAL WORLDVIEWS

Environmental worldviews have three main components:

- how people think the environment works
- the role of human beings in the environment
- what people believe is right or wrong environmental behaviour.

Fundamentally, it is important to examine thoughts and beliefs about the world but also try to figure out why people think that way. Do beliefs just mirror those of parents, wider family or peers? Have you really considered why you hold the beliefs that you do; taken them out, teased them apart and perhaps even considered other points of view? Tertiary education provides the opportunity to examine beliefs, opinions and actions, to interrogate, evaluate and form a response to them.

In this particular case, it is important that we learn about our environmental worldviews because:

- these views influence the way people interact with their environment; for example: do they eat meat? wear fur? litter? All of these behaviours stem from environmental worldviews
- as well as understanding choices, other people's environmental worldviews are the basis for how they understand the world and so can be a good predictor of their judgments and behaviour about the environment

- these views dictate the questions we ask and the answers we give about the environment. For example, do we ever ask the question about whether it is right or wrong to eat whale meat or mine for gold on conservation land; and if so, how do we answer these questions?

VALUES

Instrumental and **intrinsic values** underpin our views about the environment. If we assign instrumental value to something, it means we value it for what it can give to us; that is, it is an instrument of some sort. For example, think about the value of a car or a steak. They both have instrumental value to a human, the former as a transport mechanism; and the latter as a source of nutrition. Conversely, if we assign intrinsic value to something in the environment, we are saying it has value without any consideration to humans; it has value in and of itself. An easy example of something that might have intrinsic value is human life itself. Most people would agree that a human life has value over and above its usefulness to other humans; it has inherent or intrinsic value.

While the examples above might be easily understood, when you examine why you think certain things should be conserved or protected in the environment, it is useful to unpack their meaning, and ask whether we do this for their intrinsic or instrumental value. For example, you may feel that it is wrong to force whales into extinction. But why do you value whales? Do they have some intrinsic value, a right to life that humans should not affect? Is it because you want to preserve them so future generations can also experience a world with lots of biodiversity? You may have noticed that the latter of these two reasons, while sounding very nice, is actually assigning instrumental value to the whales. They have value because they might make future generations happy. Likewise, maintaining landscape in its pristine form so one can enjoy the beauty is giving it instrumental, not intrinsic value. As we go through this course and you examine your views and values of environmental issues, try to examine them through the lens of your **values**.

WHAT IS YOUR ROLE IN THE ENVIRONMENT?

Are people a part of the earth's environment? Do they sit outside of 'nature' as humans, exercising more of a management role than a participatory role? The way people answer these questions can be classified as anthropocentric, biocentric or ecocentric.

An **anthropocentric** environmental worldview puts humans in the centre of any decisions they might make about what is right or wrong environmental behaviour. In contrast to anthropocentric views, **biocentric** worldviews suggest that all life has instrinsic value, and humans are merely one part of that. They have no more rights than any other life form, and thus people should ensure their actions do not have an impact in a negative way on other forms of life. Another form of this is the **ecocentric** worldview, which values the environment without reference to human wants or needs. It recognises not just the importance of maintaining life, but the entire ecosystems needed to support life on earth.

HOW DOES THE ENVIRONMENT WORK?

People's understandings of how the world works reflect their fundamental beliefs about how things happen in the environment. Think about your understanding of global warming, species extinction, pollution and disease, for example. Do you understand the underlying processes that have an impact on these things? Do you believe that these things are driven by underlying scientific **principles** that can be understood with enough research, or that they are so complex that human science will never really understand what is going on—or do you believe that they are instead conditions set up by a higher power?

People may take an anthropocentric view, no matter how they think the world works. For example, if you believe in evolution, you might think it is all about survival of the fittest. Obviously humans are the fittest as we are the ones getting to make the decisions; therefore it is only right that we make decisions that are centred on our needs. On the other hand, if you believe in a more theologically based explanation for the way the world works, you can also place humans at the centre and think that the world has been created for us to use as we see fit. In either of these cases it is what humans need that sits at the centre. Don't think that the anthropocentric view always means environmental degradation and species extinction, though. Those who take this view may indeed be thinking ahead to the future survival of humanity, and thus ideas of long-term **sustainability** may come into play here. The key is that this long-term sustainability has value to humans first and foremost.

CASE STUDY 3.1

HOW THE WORLD WORKS: EVOLUTION

In many university biology textbooks, it is common to put in a famous quote from a Russian evolutionary biologist, Theodosius Dobzhansky: 'Nothing in biology makes sense except in the light of evolution' (Dobzhansky, 1964, p. 125).

Many biologists believe that evolutionary processes are central to the biological world. So what is this thing called evolution? How does it work? How can species change the way they look or act over time, and how can new species arise from existing ones? This case study provides a thought experiment that will allow you to visualise how evolution might take place.

Imagine a small population of mice living on a tiny island. The island can only support 100 mice at any one time, as there are limited resources. So each generation, even though mice produce litters of six babies, on average only two of each litter can survive, or the population would keep growing, which we have already said it doesn't. This is an example of 'survival of the fittest'. Of the six babies, only the strongest, smartest or luckiest two will survive. But more than this; if one family produced six offspring that were, on the whole, more fit than their competitors from other families, perhaps all six would survive to breed themselves, and this is the root of evolution. One more thing you need to know about our mice, and this is that they are mainly a tawny brown colour, but as with many traits, there is variation in the population, with some slightly darker and some slightly lighter. Every once in a while one mouse will be born with a mutation in the gene for fur colour and will be pure white, or pure black, but as the mutations are rare, and it is somewhat random as to which two of the six from each litter survives, these mutants are generally eliminated; that is, they don't leave offspring for the next generation.

So imagine a predator arrives on our little island. It is an owl that mainly feeds at night and loves the taste of little mice. Our mice are mainly a tawny brown colour, but as in any population, there is natural variation, so some are slightly lighter and some slightly darker. Unfortunately for the lighter ones, the owl finds them easier to see at night, so they start being eaten more often than their darker relatives. At the same time the darker mice seem able to escape the attentions of the predator. Consequently, after one generation, there are more dark mice than light ones, and the population has changed a little. But wait, I hear you say, this is not evolution; the dark ones already existed in the population; this process is merely weeding out some lighter variation.

But now imagine that one mouse appears with the mutation for black fur. When it breeds, all six of its offspring have this mutation and are also black. Because they are hard for the owl to see, four out of the six survive through to the next season to breed themselves, and again four out of six of their offspring survive. In just five generations, all 100 mice on our island would be black. Even if our predator dies or leaves the island, the natural variation would have been lost and the population would have changed from tawny to black. The predation exerted selective pressure, which caused a mutation for black fur colour to become 'fixed' in the population.

So this shows how, over successive generations, populations can change through mutation and selective pressure. You can use this thought experiment and tell a similar story of change about many 'traits' of an organism that could confer some advantage over their competing relatives. What if some new, highly nutritious food arrived on the island (think coconuts), but only animals with stronger jaws than their relatives could access the food? In this case, the selective pressure would be for jaw strength and any mutation for stronger jaws might become fixed in the population.

This kind of change in a population is called anagenesis, but it doesn't fully explain evolution, because they are still mice and if they happen to get together with the tawny mainland mice, they can interbreed. But imagine if the island mice not only changed their colour while on their island, but other things about their physiology changed, such that they were not able to interbreed with mainland mice. In this case they would have become a new species. This splitting of species based on geographical boundaries and subsequent mutation is called allopatric speciation.

ECOSYSTEM ECONOMICS

The idea of viewing an ecosystem in terms of its economics allows us to utilise parts of an ecosystem, while ensuring ongoing sustainability. We are all perhaps used to the idea of protecting the principal of an investment and living off the interest. For example, if you had 1 million dollars and were able to get a bank to pay you 10 per cent interest, you would get $100 000 per year, forever. The principal (the original 1 million dollars) would last forever, and thus the 'sustainable yield' would be $100 000. However, if you spent $200 000 per year, all of your principal would be gone after just seven years.

This concept of the **maximum sustainable yield** (MSY) is used in managing environmental resources as well. Consider grass from the lawn as a resource. How much grass could be sustainably harvested? Lawns are mown week after week for years, so obviously this is a sustainable **resource.** The idea underpinning this it that most species produce more offspring or growth than what is needed to sustain a constant level of population (think of the example of the mice in Case study 3.1).

In Aotearoa New Zealand we have a very good and world-leading example of managing a resource sustainably: our management of our fisheries. We use the MSY method to set the amount of all species of fish that can be harvested in each area around New Zealand in each year. To do this, information on the parent population, growth rates, age at sexual maturity and other aspects of the population must be known. Then a complicated set of calculations can determine how many fish can be taken from the population that will leave enough remaining to breed so the same amount can be taken the next year and forever; in other words, the maximum sustainable yield.

Of course it is important that the base information, such as how large the population is and the age demographics, is correct. The orange roughy fishery is an example of this, where the total allowable catch (TAC) set by the Ministry of Fisheries was based on incorrect information, which assumed that the fish were fast growing and had a short lifespan. It turned out that the fish being harvested lived long lives (up to 100 years old), were slow to grow and slow to mature. Once this became known, the TAC was reduced drastically to ensure a sustainable harvest (although there is still controversy over the harvest of this species; see Lack et al., 2003).

CASE STUDY 3.2

POPULATION, FAMINE AND POLITICS

The world's population has been increasing exponentially for the last 200 years (Cohen, 2003). The main reasons for this growth rate over this short period of time are:

- increased life expectancy through advances in sanitation and health
- the use of fossil fuels to meet our increasing energy requirements.

For tens of thousands of years, humans have been migrating into new ecosystems and habitats until they occupied a large proportion of the planet. Around 10 000 years ago we developed agriculture, enabling more people to be supported by less land.

In terms of environmental issues, many researchers think that human population is the most important. It is estimated that the world's population will not continue to grow at its current rate. The United Nations projections suggest (Food and Agriculture Organization, 2002) that the population will grow at an average of 1.1 per cent per year until 2030, compared to 1.7 per cent over the past three decades. As countries become more developed, the birth rate tends to decrease. The most populous country in the world, China, has had population growth control methods in place since the 1970s, and has slowed its annual growth to just 0.629 per cent. They have done this through restricting couples to having only one child, a practice that has been controversial for a number of reasons. One effect of this 'one child' policy, linked with a Chinese preference for boy children, has been a large gender imbalance in China, with 117 boys born in China for every 100 girls. This is much higher than the international norm of 106 boys for every 100 girls.

It is common to hear in the media that famines in Africa demonstrate what happens when a population exceeds the limits of its resource base. In other words, as large populations grow and increase their demands on resources, they damage the environment and reduce the capacity to support those populations. At some point there will not be enough food to support the humans present. This is a basic ecological principle called the carrying capacity.

It would be simple to look at the famines in Africa in terms of carrying capacity. There is a large population and not enough food to feed them; therefore the population must have exceeded the ability of the land to support its growing numbers. However, this is too simplistic a view, and ignores the political roots of famine. For example, in 1985 the worldwide series of Live Aid concerts raised millions to support African famine victims. But in the same year the 29 poorest countries of Sub-Saharan Africa paid back to the World Bank, the International Monetary Fund and Western commercial banks a total of US$6.7 billion, more than twice as much as they received in emergency aid. But where did this money come from? If these countries were producing goods and crops that could raise this much money, why couldn't they use it to purchase food for their citizens? The reason they could not do this was that they had to grow cash crops that could be exported for cash to service their debt. So it was not about carrying capacity of the land, but rather the way the land was being used.

Another example of politics playing a role in famine was in Ethiopia in 1984–85, during some of the worst famines in recent African history. While poor rains were partially responsible for the lack of crops produced in these years, the political conflicts in Ethiopia at the time were the ultimate cause, with various insurgencies taking place throughout the country. But while these facts contributed to the lack of crops produced in Ethiopia, international politics were in a large part responsible for the huge death toll of over one million lives. In early 1983 the United Nations Food and Agricultural Organization's Early Warning System clearly pointed out the impending food shortages in Ethiopia, but Western governments continued to withhold aid. Why did they do this?

ECOLOGICAL FOOTPRINT

It is not just the number of people on earth that creates environmental problems. The key is how much they consume. In the early 1990s William Rees, a Canadian researcher, and his doctoral student Mathis Wackernagel came up with the concept of an ecological footprint. This is a way to measure human demand on the earth's ecosystems, and is closely related to the concept of ecosystems services. The ecological footprint can be used to calculate how much biologically productive land and ocean is needed to regenerate the resources used and clean up the wastes produced.

There are many websites that provide tools for people to calculate their own ecological footprint. They take into account what kinds of foods are eaten, the type of housing and types and usage of transportation. People living in developed nations have large footprints; there is not enough biologically productive land on earth to allow everybody on earth to live that way. It would take more than five of our planets to support the current world's population in the average New Zealand lifestyle.

When the ecological footprint of every person on earth is calculated, we would need the equivalent of 1.4 planets to support our current lifestyles. So the earth's resources are being used faster than nature can replace them. This is called **ecological overshoot**. Humans first went into overshoot in 1986. Every year the Global Footprint Network (2010) calculates how far into the year we go before we are into overshoot and name this day Earth Overshoot Day, or Earth Debt Day. Unfortunately this day comes earlier and earlier each year. In 1996 it was in November, while in 2008 it fell on September 23, as humans used the entire capacity of the biosphere in just 267 days.

GLOBALISATION

The term **globalisation** is usually used to describe economic globalisation, which is the integration of local or national economies into an international economy. Economic globalisation has the ability to have a great impact on the environment, in either a positive or negative way, and it is important to introduce each possibility. Most environmental issues do not actually respect national boundaries, and so by their very nature are globalised.

The relationship between global trade and environmental degradation is complicated. Economists argue that global trade helps the environment, as wealthy countries can better afford to protect natural areas. On the other hand, environmentalists suggest that when a country pursues national wealth it increases global environmental degradation, and that free trade accelerates the process. Both of these points of view have some validity. As Aotearoa New Zealand has become more affluent, more land and seas have been put into reserve status. However, if we stop cutting our own forests down (except for sustainable ones), but we are wealthy enough to import timber goods (such as furniture) made from non-sustainable forestry of hardwoods in another country, do we not just export the degradation of our forests to another country, globalising our environmental impact?

International trade is a big part of globalisation, which creates greenhouse gas through transporting goods around the world. At least some of it seems quite pointless. For example, in 1998 Britain imported 240 000 tonnes of pork and 125 000 tonnes of lamb, and at the same time exported 195 000 tonnes of pork and 102 000 tonnes of lamb (Barker, 2002). Wool is grown in New Zealand and exported to Asia where it is made into cloth, which is then imported back to New Zealand to be sewn into garments.

Environmentalists also cite the idea of a 'race to the bottom', where liberalising trade and investment will cause governments to weaken or eliminate environmental protection laws, so as to increase their competitiveness. The idea is that companies that produce pollution or environmental degradation will move to countries with weaker environmental regulations. This has a twofold impact. First, as with the wood furniture example above, it exports the environmental degradation. But more importantly, it could set up a situation where national governments literally 'race to the bottom' to have the most relaxed environmental laws, dramatically increasing the rate of environmental problems.

In contrast to this view, some researchers suggest that globalisation and the environment are inextricably linked and must be understood together. This argument reasons that economic growth is underpinned by the use of natural resources, and a sound environment is needed to fulfil the promises of economic prosperity through globalisation. Therefore, better global governance with sustainable development at its core is the key to recognising the potential for humans in a global community.

SUMMARY

This chapter has introduced differences in environmental worldviews and explained why it is important to understand your own approach to the environment. In addition, we examined some of the global environmental issues that have an impact on our daily lives. Humans receive many 'services' from our environment, and if we degrade the ability of the earth to provide us these services, it will cost us.

The human population has undergone exponential growth, fuelled by industrialisation and the use of fossil fuels. The downsides of this are that we will of course run out of fossil fuels, and their use almost certainly contributes to global warming. We are not yet sure of the impacts of global warming, but many believe that the impacts will mostly be negative.

Globalisation will continue to have an impact on the environment, and vice versa. Finding ways to increase global governance is of primary importance to managing our way forward in the global economic and environmental community.

CRITICAL QUESTIONS

Cultural lens

- **Discuss** how culture can have an impact on environmental views.

Social lens

- **What** is your role in the environment?
- **What** is right or wrong environmental behaviour?

Gender lens

- **Describe** gendered perceptions of environmental issues.

Political lens

- **What** are your views on population growth?

Moral lens

- **Is** globablisation a good thing or not?

Media lens

- **How** does or should the media present environmental issues?

FURTHER READING

Common, M. & Stagl, S. (2005). *Ecological Economics: An Introduction.* New York: Cambridge University Press.

Daly, H. & Townsend, K. (eds) (1993). *Valuing the Earth: Economics, Ecology, Ethics.* Cambridge, MA; London: MIT Press.

Lenzen, M. & Murray, S. A. (2003). The ecological footprint: issues and trends. ISA Research Paper 01–03.

Wackernagel, M., Schulz, N.B., Deumling, D., Linares, A.C., Jenkins, M., Kapos, V., Monfreda, C., Loh, J. et al. (2002). Tracking the ecological overshoot of the human economy. *Proceedings of the National Academy of Sciences, 99*(14), 9266–9271. doi:10.1073/pnas.142033699. PMC 123129. PMID 12089326

REFERENCES

Barker, D. (2002). Globalization and industrial agriculture. In A. Kimbrell (ed.), *The Fatal Harvest Reader: The Tragedy of Industrial Agriculture* (pp. 249–263). Washington, DC: Island Press.

Cohen, J.E. (2003). Human population: the next half century. *Science*, *302*(5648), 1172–1175.

Daily, G.C., Alexander, S., Ehrlich, P.R., Goulder, L., Lubchenco, J., Matson, P.A., Mooney, H.A., Postel, S., Schneider, S.H., Tilman, D. & Woodwell, G.M. (1997). Ecosystem services: benefits supplied to human societies by natural ecosystems. *Issues in Ecology*, *1*(2), 1–18.

Dobzhansky, T. (1964). Biology: molecular and organismic. *American Zoologist*, *4*(4), 443–452.

Food and Agriculture Organization (2002). *World Agriculture: Towards 2015/2030 Summary Report*. Rome: Food and Agriculture Organization, United Nations.

Global Footprint Network (2010). *Climate Change Is Not the Problem: 2010 Annual Report*. Oakland, CA: Global Footprint Network.

Lack, M., Short, K. & Willock, A. (2003). *Managing Risk and Uncertainty in Deep-Sea Fisheries: Lessons from Orange Roughy*. TRAFFIC Oceania and WWF Endangered Seas Program <http://www.traffic.org/species-reports/traffic_species_fish10.pdf>.

WEBSITES

<http://www.fish.govt.nz>

New Zealand Ministry of Fisheries.

<http://www.footprintnetwork.org>

Global Footprint Network.

<http://www.med.govt.nz>

Views on globalisation.

<http://www.mfe.govt.nz/environmental-reporting>

The New Zealand Ministry of Economic Development, for facts on New Zealand energy sources and consumption.

<http://www.ren21.net/>

The Renewable Energy Policy Network for the 21st Century.

Urban Issues

SUSAN McNAUGHTON

CHAPTER OVERVIEW

This chapter covers the following topics:

- Urban design and public health
- Urban design and the role of central government
- Urban design effects on health
- Transport and public health
- Transport and employment
- Transport and economic growth
- Transport and air pollution
- Suggested alternatives to car transport
- Auckland Council and transport

KEY TERMS

Air pollution
Commuting
Indigenous
Mortality
Public health
Transport
Urban
Urban design

In 2007, the Auckland Regional Growth Forum published a sustainability framework that outlined the future direction for the growth of Auckland city. It included the following:

> The Auckland region must address disparities in opportunities and incomes, particularly for the most disadvantaged people living in the most disadvantaged communities. Decreasing access to affordable housing, poor health status and educational failure has resulted in endemic problems in some communities, particularly Māori, Pacific peoples and some recent migrant groups. At the same time disadvantage has a geographic dimension, resulting in concentrations of relatively poor people in what are becoming quite deprived neighbourhoods. Such concentrations can result in long term social polarisation, and anti-social or criminal behaviour. This could undermine sustainability efforts and potentially threaten the region's economic prosperity and social cohesion. The ongoing challenge is how to lift incomes across the board, reduce social/economic extremes and prevent the region from having geographic areas of deprivation.
>
> (Auckland Regional Growth Forum, 2007, p. 13).

If the Auckland Regional Growth Forum's comments are a reality for a significant number of **urban** dwellers, and if there are distinct issues and problems related to urban health, what is at the root of these problems? Who will offer workable solutions to them, and how? These questions are significant for all New Zealand's urban populations. This chapter explores what it means to be a city (urban) resident in Aoteraroa New Zealand at this point in history and the impact it has on health and illness experience. It also explores some of the factors that link urban living and health, asks some pertinent questions about these links, and examines what is being done to address the health needs of city dwellers in Aotearoa New Zealand.

Urban health issues result from the interaction of a number of factors. Aside from the wider socioeconomic and political influences, there are important local factors, some of which are presented in Figure 5.1 on the following page. There is intersection and interaction between these factors, and at any given moment in the history of a city some factors will be more significant drivers of urban health experiences than others. There are strong links between urban structure and design and **public health**. **Transport** and other uniquely urban issues also have a significant impact on the health of people living in cities. Interwoven throughout are mainly Auckland-based examples of current efforts to address some of these issues and some important human factors that may influence the success of these efforts.

URBAN DESIGN AND PUBLIC HEALTH

People have lived in towns and cities for thousands of years and, significantly, public health and town planning or housing have been closely associated in the past. Unfortunately, during the middle part of the twentieth century, when urban renewal was common in many older Western cities, the relationship between public health and town planning

Figure 5.1: Urban factors contributing to health issues

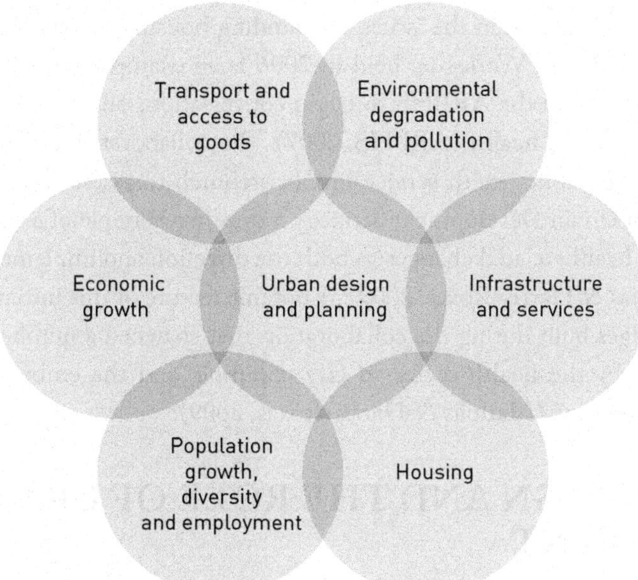

authorities was weakened (Sharp, 2009). Sometimes the consequences have been disastrous for minority communities, especially when the demolition of unfit housing has taken place before sufficient replacement housing has become available (Sharp, 2009). Urban renewal is a more recent phenomenon in New Zealand, but inner city renewal has been noticeable here since the early 1990s. Murphy (2008) notes that a relaxed regional authority attitude to the building of apartments in inner city Auckland before 2007 resulted in a number of poorly designed, cramped apartment blocks. This happened at a time when large-scale developments were seen as key to economic prosperity, and growing numbers of students were seeking cheap accommodation in the central city (Murphy, 2008). Paradoxically, this pursuit of economic prosperity has at the same time produced what has been called 'gentrified' redevelopment in Auckland (Murphy, 2008, p. 2521), such as the upmarket residential spaces of the Viaduct Harbour.

New Zealand's history records the involvement of health professionals in public health and **urban design** as a noticeable feature of city development. Dr Maui Pomare became Māori Medical Officer in 1901, and was instrumental in taking the government campaign of the day to address poor quality water supplies, sanitation and housing to Māori communities (Ministry for Culture and Heritage, 2009). His success in this endeavour led to twenty years of tireless campaigning to improve hygiene practices, particularly in maternity facilities, and much legislation aimed at improving sanitation infrastructure. In recent years, the scope of involvement of regional public health services with local councils has been growing. Auckland Regional Public Health Service (ARPHS) now provides advice on specific urban issues such as water quality, spray drift and **air pollution**, and has become intensively involved in the issues surrounding housing quality. The Public Health and Urban Development Workshop held in 2006 is an example of a collaborative effort between the council and the ARPHS to begin conversations and planning around urban design issues that affect health (ARPHS, 2007). The collaborative project between local authorities and the public health service in Christchurch to assess the health impacts of the Christchurch Urban Development Strategy is another example of a successful effort to produce specific health-related changes to both the direction and implementation of urban planning (Mathias & Harris-Roxas, 2009). A notable feature of this initiative has been the cross-sector bridges built during the collaboration that spawned a number of new forums for contribution by the health sector to city planning, and the embedded consultative involvement of local iwi (Mathias & Harris-Roxas, 2009).

URBAN DESIGN AND THE ROLE OF CENTRAL GOVERNMENT

City planning is a complex task. Communities are diverse, widely separated geographically and culturally, and with a range of needs that stretches the budget and imaginations of those involved in governance. A critical review of New Zealand's urban planning and design initiatives notes several salient points. First, while there is interaction between Māori and traditional Western value systems in planning and design there is still 'a disjuncture between Western individualised ownership on the one hand, and the **Indigenous** Māori communal valorisation of connectivity with the land, on the other' (Higgins, 2010, p. 4). Second, there has been a failure to include either urban design or planning in the *Resource Management Act* 1991 (RMA) (New Zealand Government, 2011), and therefore in many District Plans, leading to a failure in the implementation or adequate consideration of pressing urban design issues (Higgins, 2010). The Urban Design Protocol 2005 (Ministry for the Environment, 2010) sought to redress some of this oversight, and to tackle the urban gaps in the RMA by promoting the seven 'Cs' of urban design: context, character, choice, connections, creativity, custodianship and collaboration. While four main city councils and five others have signed up to this protocol, it does not have the legal or political weight of the RMA. Monitoring of the protocol in action by central government in 2007 showed encouraging signs of raised awareness and some improved design projects, but fewer than half the respondents felt urban design considerations were affecting policy development (Higgins, 2010). As of 2009, the development of a national policy statement on urban design has become part of a resource management reform package that may address some of these problems (Ministry for the Environment, 2009).

URBAN DESIGN EFFECTS ON HEALTH

The connections between urban planning and design and health are multiple. Work done by Badland and Schofield (2006) suggests that the size of the urban area significantly affects the type of physical exercise done and the perceived barriers to this; environmental barriers such as a lack of footpaths and lighting restrict small town residents, while social barriers such as motivation and time constraints are more significant in large cities. For older adults, the neighbourhood is a central context, and urban design has an impact on already existing issues related to the reduced income, mobility limitations and health needs of older adults (Michael et al. 2006). The safety of footpaths, accessibility of facilities such as shops and transport, and the general attractiveness of the neighbourhood have all been identified as significant indicators of both general satisfaction with the urban environment, and of the likelihood of older adults getting out and about independently. A similar study conducted in Christchurch (Giles-Corti & Donovan, 2002) showed that older adults were twice as likely to remain physically active in high rather than low socioeconomic status neighbourhoods, and this was directly linked to feeling that the neighbourhood was safe and attractive with low levels of crime or antisocial behaviour. The safety and attractiveness of local precincts where pedestrian traffic is encouraged is a noticeable feature of the vision presented in the Auckland Regional Land Transport Strategy 2010–2040 (Auckland Regional Council, 2010).

Urban design also affects health indirectly. In a large scale study of healthy food availability and cost across a wide variety of New Zealand food retail outlets, Wang and colleagues (2009) found that, while most healthy food choices were more readily available in urban rather than rural areas, the average cost of the same healthy basket of food was 14.3 per cent higher in urban areas compared with rural areas. The researchers concluded that difficulties adopting healthy eating for those on lower incomes might result therefore not only from economic considerations, but also from issues with the food environment (Wang et al., 2009). Considerations of the food environment in urban areas would include where and how healthy food options are offered. Availability and convenience are not the same, and for families on low incomes with limited time to shop because of work commitments or limited access to suitable transport for shopping, convenience may restrict the choice and affordability of healthy food even further. Urban design that discourages the inclusion of food shopping and preparation as collaborative, health-affirming activities also plays a significant role in reinforcing a disconnection from food that is characteristic of urban dwellers (Manzini & Jegou, 2003). A move towards education and shared experiences around food purchase and preparation could help to counteract the current consumerist attitudes towards food as a commodity that is produced and transported to a convenient location in an unknown way, prepared with as little effort as possible and assumed to have appropriate nutritional value (Manzini & Jegou, 2003; Miles & Miles, 2004).

CASE STUDY 5.1

URBAN DESIGN

In 2008, Auckland City Council published a framework for high quality urban design for Auckland that included ideas for growing a sustainable, vibrant city centre, similar to cities such as Melbourne and Brisbane. The six goals for Auckland city were: distinctive, compact, connected, sustainable, beautiful and human (Auckland City Council, 2008, p. 3).

Think carefully about each of these goals and decide:

- To what extent is Auckland achieving the goal? What role has urban design had? What should be the future role of urban design?
- If this goal is being achieved, what has been done, and has this been through citywide or local efforts?
- If this goal has not been achieved, what are the primary social, cultural and physical barriers to its achievement? Can these barriers be overcome?
- From a health perspective, what six urban framework goals would you set for Auckland?

TRANSPORT AND PUBLIC HEALTH

Transport plays a significant role in urban wellbeing. The networks of road, rail, bus, cycle and pedestrian routes that traverse a city connect its people with each other, employment, goods and services and leisure activities. Urban transport is constantly changing in response to the social and physical influences and needs of a city's inhabitants, but also the environmental and economic constraints that dictate how and when movement around the city can happen. In sixty years, rail transport has gone from the primary mode of moving people and freight throughout the nation to almost complete redundancy. This decline was a result of the availability of cheaper options for freight movement and improved roads in the period before 2000. A resurgent interest in rail is now apparent in response to environmental and health concerns for people and the planet as well as the search for clean, low-emission energy alternatives as the price of fossil fuels continues to rise. Transport plays an important role in health, both as a provider or limiter of access to health and disability services, and as a producer of damaging secondary health effects.

Figure 5.2 provides a simple illustration of some of the interactions between transport and health. The diagram shows four inner circles linked to transport—air pollution, economic growth, lack of exercise and the commuter culture. These are aspects of urban life that are of current concern and have direct links to urban transport. The outer circles represent some of the direct and indirect health effects of these four aspects, most of which are identified in the next section. The relationships between transport and employment, economic growth and air quality are explored in this section as examples of

Figure 5.2: Transport factors and associated health issues

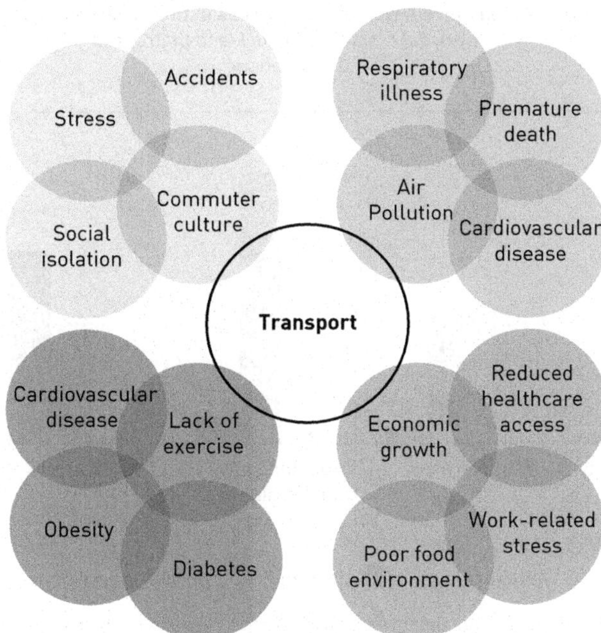

these interactions. Some current initiatives to address the health concerns in each area, and some of the urban social factors linked to these are presented. A brief consideration of some alternative transport options is also included.

TRANSPORT AND EMPLOYMENT

Workplace location is probably the single greatest contributor to the transport complexities of most city residents' lives. The 2006 census data from Statistics New Zealand on **commuting** patterns in Auckland showed large variations in terms of where people lived and worked among what were then separate cities within the Auckland region. While each city employed people who lived in that city, Auckland city was the destination workplace for more people from each of the other cities (see Figure 5.3.). Around 80 per cent of Auckland city residents also worked in Auckland city, compared with 40 per cent of Waitakere city (West Auckland) residents who worked in their home city. An almost equivalent number of Waitakere residents worked in Auckland city. Commuting patterns indicate clear 'corridors of transit' in each city. In the Auckland region, high-density employment regions are particularly noticeable in the Auckland city centre and in suburbs close to the motorway, such as Mount Wellington and Albany (Statistics New Zealand, 2011a).

Figure 5.3: Commuting patterns in Auckland, 2006

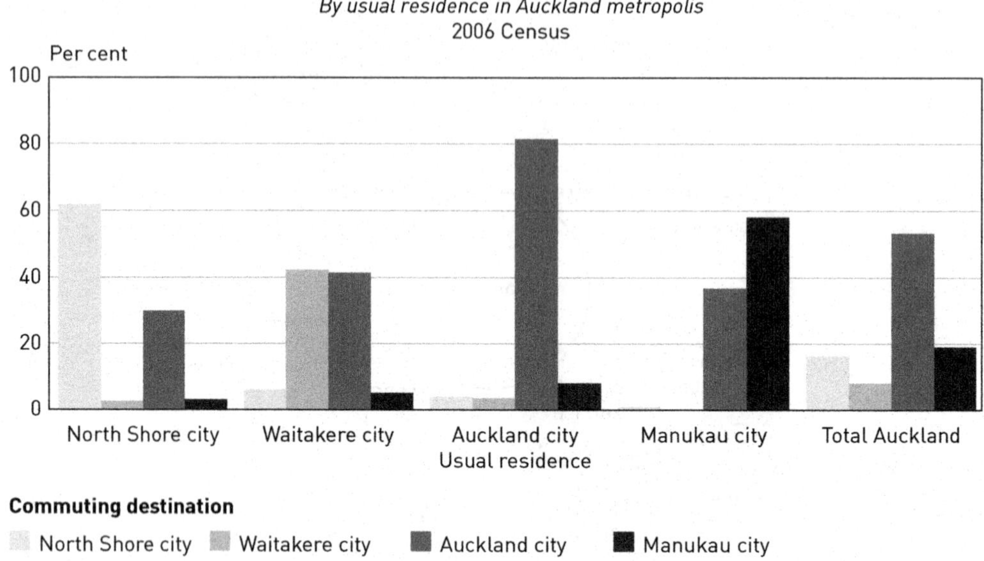

Source: Statistics New Zealand (2011a) and licensed by Statistics New Zealand for re-use under the Creative Commons Attribution 3.0 New Zealand licence.

TRANSPORT AND ECONOMIC GROWTH

Since 2008, economic conditions in New Zealand have deteriorated and unemployment has risen (Statistics New Zealand, 2011b), reducing the likelihood of people being able to consider only job positions that are close to home. Young people aged eighteen to twenty-four have been particularly affected by the loss of employment opportunities (Statistics New Zealand, 2011b), and this may have an effect on future transport problems as this age group becomes accustomed to commuting long distances to whatever work is available. Transport has become an integral part of the lives of urban dwellers, and it is possible that the long-distance travel patterns of the working day may also be present in travel associated with social activities. A survey of public life in Auckland (Auckland Council, 2010) noted that the central city has become dominated by the need to provide for traffic capacity and quick movement for up to 200 000 cars daily. This has resulted in the prioritisation of space to improve traffic flows to the point that the pedestrian network has become disconnected and associated with safety issues that create barriers. These issues make social activity in the city centre revolve around access by car, further reinforcing the transport patterns of city residents.

The cost of transport is also important to consider. Statistics New Zealand (2011b) reported that the price of transport rose by 11 per cent between June 2010 and June 2011, mostly as a result of a 20 per cent rise in the cost of petrol, which also pushed domestic air travel costs up. For the below-average wage earner, this huge rise in the cost of transport will have had equally large indirect effects on health. The overall cost of living increase was similar to the increase in transport costs for the 2010–2011 year (Statistics New Zealand, 2011c), reflecting the direct links between transport and the price of goods and services. Rises in the price of transport, food and accommodation lead to reduced money in the weekly budget for other items; for some this will include important health and wellbeing needs, such as visits to practitioners or medications for chronic illnesses, such as asthma and arthritis. In a study of the social and economic barriers to access to health care, Jatrana and Crampton (2009) found that significant financial barriers existed for low-income earners, especially females, who were foregoing visits to the doctor or dentist or paying for prescription medicines. The unsubsidised portion of a general practitioner visit of 25 dollars or more represented unaffordable care for many, and oral care was seen as even further beyond their financial means (Jatrana & Crampton, 2009). The Auckland Regional Growth Forum (2007) noted that those on low incomes are frequently living in disadvantaged areas, meaning that access to transport to these healthcare services is also likely to be an issue, especially for those with chronic conditions or disabilities.

TRANSPORT AND AIR POLLUTION

The connection between urban air pollution and health, particularly respiratory health, in New Zealand has been well documented (Pearce & Kingham, 2008; Richardson et al., 2011), and the Ministry for the Environment has implemented guidelines around acceptable levels of airborne particulate matter (PM) to address some of these effects. Large particulate matter, a concern with home heating emissions, is not the primary concern. Vehicle emissions that contain very fine particulate matter (PM2.5) and substances toxic to humans, including hydrocarbons, carbon monoxide, sulphides and nitrates (Levy et al., 2010), are the greatest concern. The contribution of each of these components to vehicle emissions has been shown to be highly variable, but a small number of well-conducted studies have provided strong evidence linking exposure to vehicle emissions with premature **mortality** (Levy et al., 2010), cardiovascular disease and the exacerbation of asthma (Health Effects Institute, 2010). Levy and colleagues (2010) concluded that the premature mortality effects related to PM2.5 emission concentrations were not only considerable in terms of deaths, but also in overall cost—around 18 billion dollars for 2010 in the United States. These findings suggest that the financial costs for the health effects of traffic congestion have remained significant despite improvements in vehicle emissions. The New Zealand experience is likely to be similar, given that central government still funds the bulk of healthcare and transport-related spending.

In a recent large review of the available evidence, the Health Effects Institute in the United States (2010) suggested that while the toxicity of emissions has improved through emission reduction efforts and regulations (such as those implemented in New Zealand), the real issue that remains is the pattern of exposure to emissions, and the concentration of the effect due to congestion and proximity to traffic and roadways. Exposure to emissions is a direct function of how many people live, work or travel on or near major arterial routes, and how many vehicles are on the road and for how long. In any urban situation, the question of where and why congestion occurs is critical. There is some conflicting evidence as to whether lower socioeconomic groups are at greater risk of higher exposure than higher socioeconomic groups (Health Effects Institute, 2010; Richardson et al., 2011), but for all those exposed to vehicle emissions on a regular basis, the effects of time and activity patterns combined with the presence of other sources of air pollution are not disputed.

SUGGESTED ALTERNATIVES TO CAR TRANSPORT

Based on findings from New Zealand surveys of light passenger vehicle urban travel, Lindsay and colleagues (2010) have suggested that most trips made by householders are of less than 7 kilometres, and that converting these to cycle trips would amount to significant health and cost benefits that heavily outweigh the risk of injury. Lindsay and colleagues (2010) suggested that a 5 per cent annual shift of short trips to cycling would save around two hundred million health dollars and 120 lives annually, and added to this, would reduce fuel expenditure and carbon dioxide emissions. It is interesting to note, however, that the researchers commented that the cost of life did not take age into consideration; since young people are more likely to die from a cycle accident than the health effects of lack of physical exercise, statistical measures of life cost may not be sufficiently convincing, particularly for parents.

New Zealanders, and especially Auckland residents, have been represented as over-reliant on cars and motorways (Bean et al., 2008) and prone to commuting long distances, often with only one occupant in the vehicle. While there are some sobering statistics behind some of these views, surveys and studies of the attitudes of city dwellers to transport have shown that the issue is not simple, and that using alternative methods of transport is not always an obvious or acceptable choice. Murray and colleagues (2010) investigated environmental attitudes and public prejudice towards public transport among drivers in Wellington, Christchurch and Auckland, as indicators of the social norms associated with public transport use in each region. Environmental concern was significantly related to positive attitudes towards public transport, as one might expect, but prejudice against it was more strongly related to beliefs and social norms around the use of public transport than to actual contact with or use of the bus or rail networks. Auckland drivers had higher levels of prejudice than those in Wellington and Christchurch, but the researchers suggested that this was primarily because of the actual and perceived quality of service, while the smaller differences between Christchurch and Wellington were related to the social norms around public transport (Murray et al., 2010). These findings suggested that there are a number of reasons why people choose to use public transport, but that prevailing attitudes towards it are of significance if the 'car culture' is to be changed.

The social narratives of dependence on cars, of walking, and the contradictions between them for Auckland residents have also been studied in an effort to expand the understanding of the place of walking in the lives of Auckland people. Bean and colleagues (2008) used a series of focus groups to investigate the social meanings of driving and walking for Auckland residents. While for some participants life without a car was unthinkable, a number expressed having conflicting relationships with the car as a necessity, while finding it environmentally and socially disagreeable. For parents, narratives of guilt and pressure to walk with children conflicted with narratives of time pressures, long commutes and child safety (Bean et al., 2008). Related to this, the car was frequently represented as an integral part of social responsibility and caring for others (Bean et al., 2008), confirming the researchers' prior understandings that cars both facilitate the expansion of social networks and also create the expectations of increased responsibility to maintain them. The researchers were somewhat surprised to find that attitudes towards walking were very positive across all age groups, especially for areas designated or designed for pedestrian activity, such as regional parks and malls. Walking had significant social values attached to it, and awareness of the need for walking to improve or maintain health was high, although many respondents cited poor public transport networks, road safety and car-dominated environments as reasons why walking as transport was a less attractive or feasible option (Bean et al., 2008).

The attitudes of parents with school-age children are of particular interest in the alternative transport debate. In contrast to the guilt parents felt from chauffeuring children across town by car, walking to primary school was seen as a desirable activity (Bean et al., 2008). Data collected between 2002 and 2006 on the Walking School Bus (WSB) movement, which provides adult-supervised walking groups to and from local primary schools along set routes at timetabled hours, has been recently reviewed by Collins and Kearns (2010). While the number of schools, routes and children participating in WSBs grew, WSBs were found to be more common in high- than in low-decile schools, and were used more often in the morning than the afternoon. The WSB movement was found to be both well established and sustainable, and appeared to be recreating a norm of independent walking to school for children beyond primary school, which in turn was felt to be a part of re-establishing social imperatives to value walking space in cities (Collins & Kearns, 2010). Some issues raised by this study were that typically WSBs were supervised by women, and that the availability of supervisors was a critical component of the success of the WSBs. Previous work had suggested that low-income neighbourhoods, where the need for the health and safety benefits of the WSB were greater, were underrepresented in participation in the WSB scheme (Collins & Kearns, 2005), and this trend did not appear to have changed (Collins & Kearns, 2010). Less flexible working arrangements for women in lower-income areas are a possible reason for the lack of WSB uptake in lower decile schools.

AUCKLAND COUNCIL AND TRANSPORT

The Auckland Regional Land Transport Strategy 2010–2040 states that 'transport is the number one issue of concern for more than 90 per cent of businesses' and 'Freight volume trips are projected to double by 2020' (Auckland Regional Council, 2010, p. 7). This highlights the major role played by transport in the economic growth of the Auckland area and, since Auckland contributes about one-third of New Zealand's Gross Domestic Product (GDP), of the whole country. There is an unstated but evident tension between this very real economic need and the equally pressing health needs of Auckland people, who are calling on the Auckland Council to respond to 'a strong need for significantly greater investment in public transport (both infrastructure and services), walking, cycling, and behaviour change measures to counter long term underinvestment in these modes' (Auckland Regional Council, 2010, p. 8). The vision and plan of the transport strategy is to see this imbalance redressed through ongoing targeted investment in cycleways, pedestrian access and improved networking of the public transport system. There are significant statements of intent and plans outlined to achieve these ends. What is not clear in all of this is how the major shifts in attitudes towards transport that the strategy frequently mentions will be achieved. Currently, economic constraint is already severely testing the resources and resilience of many low-income communities. Similarly, there is no mention of how the council plans to encourage businesses in economically conservative times to make changes to currently successful and cost-effective modes of transport. Without real traction on these fundamental social and economic issues, it is unlikely that the Auckland Council will be able to effect major changes to the way transport is perceived and used.

CASE STUDY 5.2

PUBLIC ADVOCACY FOR ACTIVE TRANSPORT

Transport issues are not ignored by the general public in New Zealand. Quietly persistent health advocacy, the active lobbying by individuals and groups for policy changes to improve health, does occur but seldom attracts media attention. In the period 2007–2010, city councils around New Zealand received around 2700 written submissions on active forms of transport from city residents wanting improvements in design and infrastructure to support walking and cycling (Richards et al., 2011). These residents cited health concerns over safety and the risk of injury, but also concerns around problems associated with physical inactivity (Richards et al., 2011), suggesting that the positive health benefits of active transport are known. Local advocacy groups for active transport, such as Cycling Advocates Network and Living Streets Aotearoa, can be found in most New Zealand towns and cities, but do not have a high profile. Interviews with advocates conducted throughout New Zealand revealed some common experiences—that advocacy is hard voluntary work but often motivated by concerns for health (Richards et al., 2010). Advocates also felt hampered by acute awareness of the physical dangers of active transport in a country without the infrastructural support for safe cycling and walking (Richards et al., 2010). On the whole, the relationships between these advocacy groups and local councils are positive; both parties are aware of the need to work towards political commitment and community mobilisation to see advocacy properly supported and active transport inititatives moved forward (Richards et al., 2010). There is room, however, for the health sector to use its professional leverage to a much greater extent in support of this advocacy, and to develop strategic alliances with local councils to increase the political power behind it (Richards et al., 2010, 2011).

SUMMARY

Urban design, planning and transport have significant, intertwined and longitudinal effects on both the nature of city living and the way in which health is both experienced and perceived. Both are linked to each of the other factors that shape the urban health experience: population growth, diversity, employment, housing, infrastructure, services, economic growth and environmental degradation and pollution. Unless quite radical changes are made, city dwellers in Aotearoa New Zealand can expect the predominance of particular ways of providing for the needs of their cities to continue to create tension between what is good for the economy and what is good for health. It is to be hoped that city authorities will look beyond short-term economic gain to long-term improvements in the experiences of those identified in the opening quote as disadvantaged. Cities must show themselves to be reducing social polarisation rather than contributing to its increase.

Urban design and planning are central to many issues, and the relationship between public health authorities and urban planners is critical to future health improvements for urban dwellers. Transport is linked directly and indirectly to health access, air pollution and to the dominant commuter culture that exists in larger cities. Strategies to address the problems created by urban planning and transport issues require significant social change, but are also likely to remain inextricably tied to the prevailing economic climate, which is currently unpredictable and volatile.

CRITICAL QUESTIONS

Cultural lens

- **Discuss** how culture can be nurtured in urban environments.

Social lens

- **What** elements in society converge to have an impact on health and wellbeing—how and why?

Gender lens

- **Is** there a need for gendered perspectives in urban design?

Political lens

- **What** is the purpose of national policy and strategy, and what influences its impact and effectiveness?

Moral lens

- **What** are the challenges and inherent considerations in identifying statistics in relation to cultural groups?

Media lens

- **What** roles do the media play in urban design and development?

FURTHER READING

Manzini, E. & Jegou, F. (2003). *Sustainable Everyday: Scenarios of Urban Life.* Milan: Edizione Ambiente.

Miles, S. & Miles, M. (2004). *Consuming Cities.* London: Palgrave Macmillan.

REFERENCES

Auckland City Council (2008). *Designing a Great City Centre for Our People* <http://www.aucklandcity.govt.nz/council/documents/urbandesigncbd/docs/cbdframework.pdf>.

Auckland Council (2010). *Auckland Public Life Survey* <http://www.aucklandcouncil.govt.nz/SiteCollectionDocuments/Auckland_Public_Life_Survey_July_2010_Pages_25-53.pdf>.

Auckland Regional Council (2010). *Auckland Regional Land Transport Strategy 2010–2040* <http://www.arc.govt.nz/albany/fms/main/Documents/Transport/RLTS/RLTS%202009/Regional%20Land%20Transport%20Strategy%20(RLTS)%202010-2040.pdf>.

Auckland Regional Growth Forum (2007). *Auckland Sustainability Framework: An Agenda for the Future* <http://www.arc.govt.nz/albany/fms/main/Documents/Auckland/Sustainability/Auckland%20Sustainability%20Framework.pdf>.

Auckland Regional Public Health Service (2007). *Public Health and Urban Development Workshop* <http://www.arphs.govt.nz/Publications_reports/reports/sophar06/Sophar_WorkshopDec06 asp>.

Badland, H. & Schofield, G. (2006). Understanding the relationship between town size and physical activity levels: a population study. *Health and Place, 12,* 538–546. doi:10.1016/j.healthplace.2005.08.007.

Bean, C.E., Kearns, R. & Collins, D. (2008). Exploring social mobilities: narratives of walking and driving in Auckland, New Zealand. *Urban Studies, 45,* 2829–2848. doi:10.1177/0042098008098208.

Collins, D. & Kearns, R. (2005). Geographies of inequality: child pedestrian injury and walking school buses in Auckland, New Zealand. *Social Science and Medicine, 60,* 61–69. doi:10.1016/j.socscimed.2004.04.015.

Collins, D. & Kearns, R. (2010). Walking school buses in the Auckland region: a longitudinal assessment. *Transport Policy, 17,* 1–8. doi:10.1016/j.tranpol.2009.06.003.

Giles-Corti, B. & Donovan, R. (2002). Socioeconomic status differences in recreational physical activity levels and real and perceived access to a supportive physical environment. *Preventive Medicine, 35,* 601–611.

Health Effects Institute Panel on the Health Effects of Traffic-Related Air Pollution (2010). *Traffic-Related Air Pollution: A Critical Review of the Literature on Emissions, Exposure, and Health Effects.* (HEI Special Report No. 17). Boston, MA: Health Effects Institute.

Higgins, M. (2010). Urban design and the planning system in Aotearoa New Zealand: disjuncture or convergence? *Urban Design International, 15,* 1–21.

Jatrana, S. & Crampton, P. (2009). Primary health care in New Zealand: who has access? *Health Policy,* 93, 1–10. doi:10.1016/j.healthpol.2009.05.006.

Levy, J.I., Buonocore, J.J. & von Stackelberg, K. (2010). Evaluation of the public health impacts of traffic congestion: a health risk assessment. *Environmental Health, 9,* 65 <http://www.ehjournal.net/content/9/1/65>.

Lindsay, G., Macmillan, A. & Woodward, A. (2010). Moving urban trips from cars to bicycles: impact on health and emissions. *Australian and New Zealand Journal of Public Health, 35,* 54–60. doi: 10.1111/j.1753-6405.2010.00621.x.

Manzini, E. & Jegou, F. (2003). *Sustainable Everyday: Scenarios of Urban Life.* Milan: Edizione Ambiente.

Mathias, K. & Harris-Roxas, B. (2009). Process and impact evaluation of the Greater Christchurch Urban Development Strategy Health Impact Assessment. *Biomed Central Public Health, 9,* 97. doi:10.1186/1471-2458-9-97.

Michael, Y., Green, M. & Farquhar, S. (2006). Neighborhood design and active aging. *Health and Place, 12,* 734–740. doi:10.1016/j.healthplace.2005.08.002.

Miles, S. & Miles, M. (2004). Consuming Cities. London: Palgrave Macmillan.

Ministry for Culture and Heritage (2009). *Maui Wiremu Piti Naera Pomare* <http://www.nzhistory.net.nz/people/maui-wiremu-piti-naera-pomare>.

Ministry for the Environment (2009). *Resource Management Act* <http://www.mfe.govt.nz/rma/central/nps/urban-design/index.html>.

Ministry for the Environment (2010). *New Zealand Urban Design Protocol* <http://www.mfe.govt.nz/issues/urban/design-protocol/>.

Murphy, L. (2008). Third-wave gentrification in New Zealand: the case of Auckland. *Urban Studies, 45,* 2521–2540. doi: 10.1177/0042098008097106.

Murray, S.J., Walton, D. & Thomas, J.A. (2010). Attitudes towards public transport in New Zealand. *Transportation, 37,* 915–929. doi: 10.1007/s11116-010-9303-z.

New Zealand Government (2011). *Resource Management Act* 1991 <http://www.legislation.govt.nz/act/public/1991/0069/latest/DLM230265.html>.

Pearce, J. & Kingham, S. (2008). Environmental inequalities in New Zealand: a national study of air pollution and environmental justice. *Geoforum*, *39*, 980–993.

Richards, R., Murdoch, L., Reeder, A.I. & Amun, Q. (2011). Political activity for physical activity: health advocacy for active transport. *International Journal of Behavioral Nutrition and Physical Activity*, *8*, 52. doi: 10.1186/1479-5868-8-52.

Richards, R., Murdoch, L., Reeder, A.I. & Rosenby, M. (2010). Advocacy for active transport: advocate and city council perspectives. *International Journal of Behavioral Nutrition and Physical Activity*, 7(5). doi: 10.1186/1479-5868-7-5.

Richardson, E., Pearce, J. & Kingham, S. (2011). Is particulate air pollution associated with health and health inequalities in New Zealand? *Health and Place*. Advance online publication. doi:10.1016/j.healthplace.2011.05.007.

Sharp, D. (2009). Public health and advocacy: lessons from and for urban regeneration. *Journal of Urban Health: Bulletin of the New York Academy of Medicine*, *87*, 5–7. doi:10.1007/s11524-009-9412-1.

Statistics New Zealand (2011a). *Commuting Patterns in Auckland* <http://www.stats.govt.nz/browse_for_stats/people_and_communities/geographic-areas/commuting-patterns-in-nz-1996-2006/commuting-patterns-in-auckland.aspx>.

Statistics New Zealand (2011b). *Linked Employer–Employee Data: March 2010 Quarter* <http://www.stats.govt.nz/browse_for_stats/income-and-work/employment_and_unemployment/LEED_HOTPMar10qtr.aspx>.

Statistics New Zealand (2011c). *Consumers Price Index: June 2011 Quarter* <http://www.stats.govt.nz/browse_for_stats/economic_indicators/CPI_inflation.aspx>.

Wang, J., Williams, M., Rush, E., Crook, N., Forouhi, N.G. & Simmons, D. (2009). Mapping the availability and accessibility of healthy food in rural and urban New Zealand: Te Wai o Rona: Diabetes Prevention Strategy. *Public Health Nutrition*, *13*, 1049–1055. doi:10.1017/S1368980009991595.

WEBSITES

<http://can.org.nz>

Cycling Advocates Network.

<http://www.livingstreets.org.nz/>

Living Streets Aotearoa.

Water, Soil and Food

LORETTA WHITE AND W. LINDSEY WHITE

CHAPTER OVERVIEW

This chapter covers the following topics:

- Freshwater
- Oceans
- Soil
- Soil degradation and land productivity
- Soil quality and food security
- Global food production

KEY TERMS

Agriculture
Aquifer
Arable land
Conservation
Contaminated
Cropland
Decomposed
Degradation
Detritus
Erosion
Eutrophic
Eutrophication
Food security
Food webs
Freshwater
Genetic engineering
Genetically modified
Nutrients
Organic farming
Pasture
Pollution
Saltwater intrusion
Soil
Soil organic carbon
Soil quality
Sustainable
Topsoil

Global environmental issues have direct impacts on human health and wellbeing. These include water resources, soil degradation and loss of **arable land**. These also have an impact on global food supplies. **Conservation** of these valuable resources is thus vital to human health in general.

FRESHWATER

Freshwater is needed for a variety of human uses: drinking and hygiene, **agriculture**, industry, recreation and transportation. Access to safe drinking water is vital to humans, but approximately 20 per cent of all people do not have this access, while 50 per cent lack adequate sanitation (United Nations, 2006). Even here in New Zealand, 2007 figures show that more than 13 per cent of people receive drinking water that is not compliant with bacterial levels (such as *E. coli*) required by our national drinking water standards (Ministry for the Environment, 2007a).

Worldwide freshwater consumption increased sixfold between 1900 and 2000, while the population growth rate was only half of this rate (United Nations, 2000). Freshwater makes up a very small proportion of the water on earth. The World Wildlife Fund (2006) notes that:

- the vast majority (97.5 per cent) of the world's water is saltwater, and two-thirds of the freshwater is frozen in the polar ice caps or in glaciers
- of the remaining portion of freshwater, the majority is groundwater, with only 0.3 per cent on the surface in lakes, streams and rivers. In essence, only 0.003 per cent of the water on earth can theoretically be used for drinking, agriculture, hygiene and industry
- agriculture uses 70 per cent of all freshwater withdrawals around the globe.

While humans need 2–4 litres of drinking water per day, it takes 2000–5000 litres of water to produce the daily food intake for one person (Food and Agriculture Organization of the United Nations, 2002).

Groundwater is water located underground in the pores, gaps and fractures in rocks. An **aquifer** is a layer of underground rock, with lots of pores and gaps, that holds water that can be extracted by drilling a waterwell. Groundwater is recharged from the surface, by rain, rivers and lakes, and can remain underground for lengths of time from days to millennia. The recharging process is very slow, and it is very easy to pump it out faster than having it replaced. This poses a major threat of water overuse, and is obviously non-**sustainable**. Unfortunately, the overuse of groundwater is taking place throughout the globe. Since much of the freshwater used globally comes from groundwater, it is very important to understand the threats to this resource, including overuse, **saltwater intrusion** and contamination.

SAN JOAQUIN VALLEY, CALIFORNIA

CASE STUDY 6.1

The San Joaquin Valley in California is a vast flat desert that was once an inland sea. The soil is good for growing crops, but as it is desert, there is little rain or surface water. Because of the geology of the area, there are vast sources of groundwater. To fuel the massive increase in agriculture (this valley produces up to 15 per cent of the total United States agricultural production), massive amounts of groundwater have been taken.

Groundwater use began in earnest in the 1920s, and by the 1950s the problem of land subsidence became obvious. In 1956 the US Geological Survey found that the water table had dropped over 100 metres in places. At that time, at least 35 per cent of the valley floor showed signs of subsidence, at rates of up to 45 centimetres per year in some places. By 1972, over half of the valley was found to be subsiding, by up to 9 metres.

Another impact of the overuse of groundwater is saltwater intrusion. Most of the world's population relies on groundwater for agriculture, household use and industry. Saltwater intrusion happens when the groundwater aquifer is in contact with the sea (this is quite common) and the rate of water being taken from the aquifer is greater than the recharge rate. In this case, as the aquifer is depleted, saltwater is drawn into the aquifer along a concentration gradient. The saltwater can move a significant distance inshore. In Madras, India, saltwater has moved 10 kilometres inland in the aquifer, making wells in the entire area useless. Saltwater intrusion is a particular problem in small islands, where the aquifer is in close contact with the surrounding oceanic water. The only way to control this is to balance withdrawal from the aquifer with the recharge rate, but very few aquifers worldwide are being managed in this sustainable fashion.

Groundwater contamination can take place when human-made products such as gasoline, oil and chemicals get into the groundwater and make it unsafe and unfit for human use. Some of the main sources of these contaminants are septic systems, landfills, hazardous waste dumps, pesticides, fertilisers and other chemicals. The risk of groundwater contamination in New Zealand is growing, along with increases in agricultural development and expansion in extra-urban growth. Micro-organisms and chemicals can be transported from surface water into the groundwater as a result of farming. Recently research was undertaken on the transmission of pathogens from animals into groundwater in the Waikakahi catchment in South Canterbury, which has many dairy farms. The study found that *E. coli* and Campylobacter from stock could make their way into groundwater that is used for drinking water at local farms (Close et al., 2008). Chemicals from industrial processes can also make their way into groundwater aquifers.

Many industries discharge wastewater with a high nitrogen content into local rivers and streams. It is assumed that these wastes will make their way to the sea, but recent studies have shown that not only does groundwater feed streams and rivers, but that there are water and chemicals going from streams and rivers back into groundwater aquifers. Studies of three meat-processing plants on the Canterbury Plains tested the nitrate content of the water in wells surrounding the disposal sites. Nitrate concentrations well over the Ministry of Health's maximum acceptable level were found extending into the groundwater some kilometres from the disposal site, with this area affected extending year after year (Hayward & Hanson, 2004).

Surface water, such as streams, rivers and lakes, can also become **contaminated** through increased **nutrients** and/or toxins. It might seem strange to talk about nutrients as a bad thing, but too many nutrients in water can lead to depletion of oxygen and the subsequent death of any organism that relies on it. **Eutrophication** is the term used for water that is high in nutrients, usually nitrogen and/or phosphorous. You might think that in nutritious water there should be lots of algae or plants, and therefore lots of oxygen because of increased photosynthesis. In fact, the exact opposite is the case. For example: algae grow very fast. Initially this leads to more oxygen in the water, but as the algae grow and die they sink to the bottom of the water where they are **decomposed** by bacteria. As the bacteria rot the algae, they use more oxygen than is produced by the algae and the result is a loss of oxygen from the water, which leaves it black and smelly. There are many sources of nutrients in surface waters. Sewerage, industrial wastes, household cleaners and farm wastes are all high in nutrients. If they are allowed to run into streams, rivers and lakes, they can cause the waters to become **eutrophic**.

OCEANS

The oceans provide many ecosystem services that have an impact on our health, most notably providing food and oxygen and taking up carbon dioxide. The Joint Group of Experts on the Scientific Aspects of Marine Environmental Protection (GESAMP) outlines the significant role of oceans (GESAMP, 2001):

- the ocean provides around 100 million tonnes of food every year
- the marine, fishing and aquaculture industries employ some 140 million people
- around 20 per cent of the global population derives at least 20 per cent of its animal protein from fish, while some island states depend on fish almost exclusively for their protein requirements.

This group has also identified vulnerable areas and the sources of their problems (GESAMP, 2001):

- some 60 per cent of all people live in coastal areas
- **pollution** and marine contaminants are a rising problem in terms of human health

- the risk of disease from consuming contaminated shellfish is responsible for 11 per cent of outbreaks of disease in food in the United States, 20 per cent in Australia, and a huge 70 per cent in Japan
- the main sources of marine pollution are:
  - run-off and discharges from the land (44 per cent), including fertilisers, sediment, sewerage and refuse from streams and rivers
  - discharges from land through the atmosphere (33 per cent), including toxins from industrial smoke stacks and car emissions
  - maritime transport activities (12 per cent), such as oil spills and dumping bilgewater
  - direct dumping of garbage and wastes (10 per cent), including dredged material, garbage, construction waste and waste chemicals
  - offshore oil and gas productions (1 per cent).

As with our atmosphere, the world's oceans contain a lot of carbon dioxide (CO_2). As the concentration of CO_2 in the atmosphere increases, so does the concentration of CO_2 in the ocean. Studies suggest that the oceans have taken up 48 per cent of all carbon dioxide from fossil fuel burning between 1800 and 1994 (Sabine et al., 2004), which is another example of an ecosystem service provided by the world's oceans. But this service is coming at a cost. It appears that increasing the CO_2 content of the oceans is making the water more acidic. If seawater is too acidic, animals that make shells or other hard parts of their bodies from calcium carbonate can no longer make these protective coverings, so continued acidification could have an impact on many marine organisms. Corals, crustaceans, echinoderms and molluscs are all marine animals that rely on calcium for parts of their skeleton or exoskeleton. These animals are the most common in the oceans, and are critical in many **food webs**.

In Aotearoa New Zealand we administer the sixth largest marine environment in the world of over 4.4 million square kilometres. Over 90 per cent of New Zealanders live within 50 kilometres of the coast (Ministry for the Environment, 2007b), therefore our coastal resources are at risk from many factors. Over the last 60 years, there have been increasing amounts of pollutants, nutrients and sediments entering our coastal waters, in a large degree as a result of urban growth. In the past twenty years, the government has been trying to reverse this. Under the *Resource Management Act* 1991, a 'Resource Consent' is required to discharge anything into streams, rivers or the ocean. Other control measures include mandatory settlement or holding ponds for new developments, to control the amount of sediment that reaches the sea.

SOIL

Soil is not simply the earth or dirt that roses are planted in. It is a system, an environment that is home to a large proportion of the biodiversity on Earth (Barrios, 2007), and which acts as a medium to provide nutrients and water to agricultural plants for life support (Wilding & Lin, 2006; Bennett et al., 2010). Soil contains complex layers of chemical and biological constituents; it is a mixture of inorganic particles, such as minerals, and organic particles, such as decomposed and decomposing plants and animals. Soil starts as a thin layer of weathered material (mineral eroded from bedrock), which is stablilised by primitive plants and colonised by microorganisms. Animals then add nutrients as they excrete, and as they die and decompose. Over centuries, animals living above and within the soil deposit more organic material and also mix the soil by burrowing and digging. The growth of larger plants with deep roots increases the weathering of bedrock, so soil increases both from the top (material such as leaf litter and dead organisms) and from the bottom (weathering of bedrock) (White, 2006). Although the physical and chemical characteristics of soil have been studied intensively, to clearly define and classify soil is difficult. Soil types are dependent on geology, climate, vegetation, resident organisms and surface features; for example, in hotter and wetter climate, **detritus** decays at a higher rate and results in richer soil, and a variety of soil colours develop from different weathered bedrock materials.

Soil is essential to life and critical to terrestrial ecosystems. Most food chains start from plants that grow in soil; we breathe the oxygen produced by plants; and we eat the plants and plant-eating animals (herbivores), as well as other products (such as eggs and dairy products) that animals produce. Humans have been using soil for food production since 12 000 to 13 000 years before the present era (BP), when the primitive agriculture of late Neolithic peoples advanced the development of human civilisation. Soil surveys were carried out in China as early as 4000 years BP to show soil fertility, which was used as the base of levy taxes for landowners. Studying soil properties was not just a practical exercise for peasants and landowners in ancient times, but also is relevant and very important for us today. The productivity of world soil has a direct impact on our survival on Earth.

SOIL DEGRADATION AND LAND PRODUCTIVITY

One of the largest environmental issues related to the future global production of food is soil degradation. Much of the earth's **topsoil**, which contains the nutrients in which crops grow, is eroded and ends up in the ocean, carried by rivers, streams and the wind. This is becoming an alarming issue as more and more of the topsoil that we rely on is eroded. Soil **erosion** could occur through natural causes, such as water and wind; however, it is mainly the result of chemical and physical **degradation** of the environment by humans (White, 2006).

Agricultural activities, such as monoculture planting, ploughing, the use of strong chemicals for weed killing and pests and overgrazing of cattle, all contribute to soil erosion.

Fertilisers other than that of an organic nature gradually destructure the soil. Intensive deforestation is also related to soil degradation. Soils in **croplands** are usually around 25 centimetres deep, and weigh about 400 000 tonnes per square kilometre. So the total amount of cropland topsoil is 4000 gigatonnes (Gt). The erosion rate for cropland topsoil is approximately 88 Gt/year. The rate of topsoil formation on croplands is about 17 Gt/year, meaning that every year 71 gigatonnes is lost. At this rate, nearly one-third of the world's arable land has been lost by erosion in the past four decades. Soil degradation has become the worst threat to land productivity and **food security**.

Land productivity is defined as the capacity of agricultural lands to produce biomass on a sustainable long-term basis under the constraints of each agroecological zone (FAO, 2003). Developing countries with larger populations rely heavily on their crop production to survive and to profit from exportation. To meet the high demand of food quantity and quality, fertilisers, pesticides, soil conditioning such as lime amendments and intensive mechanical agitation (tillage) are some of the methods used to overcome soil limitations and increase the crop productivity (Barrios, 2007).

Maintenance and improvement of soil fertility and land productivity through sustainable processes is the key to agricultural sustainability and global food security. **Soil organic carbon** (SOC) pool (Lal, 2004; Lal et al., 2007), soil organisms (Barrios, 2007) and tillage operations (Bennett et al., 2010) are some of the factors considered critical to land productivity. These are based on the principles of (a) the increase of available water; (b) the improvement of nutrients supply; and (c) the improvement of soil structure and other physical properties (Lal, 2004; Barrios, 2007; Lal et al., 2007). Land productivity is not the only factor to ensure food security. Food price is also critical to food security. As food prices soar around the world, this is becoming a more pressing issue, and one directly related to the health and wellbeing of our growing population.

SOIL QUALITY AND FOOD SECURITY

The quality of food is directly linked to the quality of soil. The indicators of **soil quality** include nutrient availability, total and convertible organic carbon, texture, plant-available water capacity, soil structure and strength (bulk density or penetration resistance), maximum rooting depth and pH values. Overfarmed lean soil produces food that lacks essential micronutrients such as iron, iodine and copper (Reeves, 1997; Lal et al., 2007). Deficiency of micronutrients leads to potential health issues, which can be devastating to people. Soil pollution caused by industrial activities, chemical pesticides and fertilisers also has an impact on food quality and human health.

Organic farming has become increasingly popular as a sustainable alternative to conventional farming. While it is not realistic for developing countries with large populations to feed, it is widely promoted in developed countries. Farmers in Germany and France are even subsidised to convert from conventional farming to organic farming. In Switzerland and Austria, organic production makes up 10 per cent of the total food production. Organic food production is also increasing at a 20 per cent per year rate in the USA and Japan (FAO, 2010). Organic food production in New Zealand has increased dramatically since 1990.

CASE STUDY 6.2

THE REVOLUTION OF SMALLHOLDERS: ESCAPE TO RIVER COTTAGE

Hugh Fearnley-Whittingstall, a TV personality from the United Kingdom (UK), moved to a countryside cottage named River Cottage in Dorset in 1998, to start a whole new lifestyle as a smallholder. A smallholding is a piece of land and adjacent living quarters that is used for the production of cash crops and/or subsistence farming; in New Zealand the equivalent is called a lifestyle block. While he was somewhat unique, in that he had television cameras follow him around and produced a television series examining his progress, he is not alone in shifting to an organic farming lifestyle. It has become a growing trend in developed countries such as the UK to pursue the passion for home-grown food.

Urban people picking up on the desire to grow their own food and produce has, in the West, spawned numerous organisations to assist them. Landshare is an organisation spearheaded by Fearnley-Whittingstall in collaboration with the TV broadcaster Channel 4 in the UK. Landowners with land not being currently farmed and potential growers who don't have any land are put together via a website, which has led to a community of over 66 000 members with more than 100 000 people on the waiting lists to join the programme. Not only do people grow food in other people's gardens, they also utilise unused spaces in the city, such as deserted car parks, to grow vegetables.

Another successful story was created by an Australian named Rodney Dunn. He and his wife started a farm-based cooking school in Tasmania in July 2001 named Agrarian Kitchen, with sustainable farming practices at the core of their philosophy. They encourage local farms to grow and keep a range of crops and animals that complement each other. All the crops are grown based on organic principles without the use of chemicals or artificial fertilisers.

Such programmes and smallholders may have little impact on solving global food shortages; however, the popularisation of the organic concept will help slow soil degradation and global starvation in the long run. Organic farming can be affordable, when combined with programmes such as Landshare. Through the promotion of the concept on television, the members of the general population are becoming more aware of the benefit of having healthy and sustainable soil and food. That holds the possibility of a revolution in conventional farming. With better use of city land, farmers may feel a reduced pressure to farm using conventional methods, and could feel free to switch to organic farming.

GLOBAL FOOD PRODUCTION

Food security is when all people in a population have access to sufficient, safe and nutritious food that:

a. meets their dietary needs
b. satisfies their food preferences
c. allows them to lead an active and healthy life.

Physical and economic access to food is important for human health. For a nation to have food security it must make sure that there is enough food available, that the supplies are stable and people have access to it. To achieve this, a country must either grow enough food or have enough money to purchase it. In the same way, food security from an individual perspective means that people should have sufficient income to buy the food that they are unable to grow.

According to the Food and Agriculture Organization of the United Nations (FAO) (2010), the total land area on earth is around 130.69 million square kilometres, but only 13.81 million square kiometres is arable land, and only 1.46 million square kilometres is permanent cropland. Approximately half of the cropland produces grain, and 37 per cent of the world's grain production goes to feed livestock, poultry or fish. Cereal grains provide half of the world's protein and calories, and developing countries such as China and India are the two major cereal producers. Around 847.5 million (13 per cent) of the world's population were classed as undernourished between 2005 and 2007. In African countries such as Congo, the proportion of starving population is as high as 69 per cent.

New Zealand has a land area of 263 310 square kilometres, of which 4530 square kilometres is arable and only 690 square kilometres is permanent cropland. However, we have 108 520 square kilometres of **pasture** land (41 per cent of total land area), and we produced 637 000 tonnes of cattle meat and 15 million tonnes of milk in 2009 (FAO, 2010). New Zealand is not only one of the biggest exporters of cattle meat and dairy products, but one of the few countries that are net exporters of food. That is, we export more food than we import; produce more food than we consume.

Genetic engineering of food is another environmental issue that may have an impact on human health and wellbeing. Genetic engineering involves direct manipulation of the genes of the target species, usually inserting genes that add new properties, creating a **genetically modified** (GM) organism. The New Zealand government's policy is to proceed with caution with GM while ensuring that opportunities for increased production are preserved. Coexistence between GM and non-GM agriculture is envisaged with a rigorous regulatory regime on a case-by-case approach, taking into account the entire production chain. So far there are no commercially produced GM organisms in New Zealand and no GM fresh produce is on sale, although some processed food may contain GM ingredients that have been assessed as safe for consumption.

CASE STUDY 6.3

GOLDEN RICE: ANGEL OR DEVIL?

'Golden rice' is a GM strain of rice with a much higher than normal vitamin A content. It was designed as a fortified food for people living in areas with vitamin A deficiencies. Golden rice was made by taking two genes from daffodils and one from a soil bacterium and inserting them into rice.

There is much opposition to genetically modified crops and foods, and we can use the example of golden rice to explore some of the supporting and opposing views. A lot of the opposition to GM arises from the problem of intellectual property rights; that is, the large multinational companies own the rights to the GM organism, and so farmers have to buy the seed at whatever price the company sets. The creator of golden rice, Professor Ingo Potrykus, wanted to provide the rice free of charge to the people who needed it, and was able to create Humanitarian Use Licences, which enable farmers to grow the rice without paying licensing fees. This was a complex issue, as he had used over 70 intellectual property rights from 32 different companies to create golden rice.

Other opposition to GM is about the long-term effects of consuming them and environmental health. Certainly, there have been examples of GM products being unsafe and causing sickness and even death in humans. In terms of environmental health concerns, consider crops that are modified to resist herbicides. Farmers can apply amounts of weed killer that would normally kill the crops to eradicate weeds without harming the crop, which is resistant. Consider also crops that are modified to be toxic to insects. Both of these situations can have impacts on whole ecosystems by eradicating sections of food chains; for example, the food of birds that eat the seeds of weeds or birds that eat insects. While there are no immediate concerns in relation to either of these for golden rice, critics object to it on the grounds that having it will open the door to more, potentially unsafe, GM organisms in the future.

Another argument against using GM crops is that there is actually plenty of food on Earth, and that it is merely a distribution problem that is creating shortages in some places, and if this is the case, why create food that has any risk at all? In terms of golden rice, while it is addressing a real problem of vitamin A deficiency, some scientists have pointed out that the only reason there is such a deficiency is because the people are not eating a balanced diet, because in their region farmers are no longer growing a diverse range of crops. This view holds that by focusing on vitamin A deficiency, the larger point is being missed, because people in these areas no longer have access to a range of nutritionally adequate sources of food.

SUMMARY

Some of the global environmental issues that have an impact on daily life have been introduced. Humans receive many 'services' from the environment, and any degradation in the earth's ability to provide these services will be costly.

Access to healthy food and clean water are very basic human requirements. A major issue facing the world in terms of food production is the loss of topsoil. Without soil, there can be no crops. In developed nations, methods of farming that retain topsoil are being instituted and this has slowed the erosion in these areas. In the rest of the world, the erosion continues at an alarming rate. The world's oceans provide us with much of our food, and yet they continue to be depleted by overfishing, pollution and perhaps from a new threat from acidification linked to increased carbon dioxide emissions. Freshwater resources are being stretched, both by overuse and salination of groundwater, and by pollution from industrial and agricultural activities.

CRITICAL QUESTIONS

Cultural lens

- **Does** New Zealand's position as a net exporter mean all people in New Zealand have food security?

Social lens

- **What** choices you make at a grocery store or garden centre can have an impact on soil? Should you buy organic products? Will you use chemical fertilisers in your own garden?

Gender lens

- **What** environmental issues are gendered?

Political lens

- **Is** organic farming practical for developing countries, or is it just a luxury for developed countries?

Moral lens

- **What** are your views on genetically modified foods?

Media lens

- **Is** there a particular perspective that the media should take?

FURTHER READING

Ableman, M., Wisehart, C. & Bittman, S. (1993). *From the Good Earth: A Celebration of Growing Food Around the World.* Ithaca, NY: H. N. Abrams Books.

Byrne, P., Ward, S., Harrington, J. & Fuller, L. (2010). *Transgenic Crops: An Introduction and Resource Guide.* Retrieved 8 March 2010 from <http://Cls.casa.colostate.edu>.

Lamkin, N. & Padel, S. (1994). *The Economics of Organic Farming: An International Perspective.* Guildford: CAB International.

Montgomery, D.R. (2007). *Dirt: The Erosion of Civilizations.* Berkeley, CA: University of California Press.

Montgomery, D.R. (2007). Soil erosion and agricultural sustainability. *Proceedings of the National Academy of the Sciences, 104*(33), 13260–13272.

REFERENCES

Barrios, E. (2007). Soil biota, ecosystem services and land productivity. *Ecological Economics, 64*(2), 269–285.

Bennett, L.T., Mele, P.M., Annett, S. & Kasel, S. (2010). Examining links between soil management, soil health, and public benefits in agricultural landscapes: an Australian perspective. *Agriculture, Ecosystems & Environment, 139*(1–2), 1–12.

Close, M., Dann, R., Ball, A., Pirie, R., Savill, M. & Smith, Z. (2008). Microbial groundwater quality and its health implications for a border-strip irrigated dairy farm catchment, South Island, New Zealand. *Journal of Water Health, 6*(1), 83–98.

Food and Agriculture Organization (FAO) (2002). *World Agriculture: Towards 2015/2030 Summary Report.* Rome: Food and Agriculture Organization of the United Nations.

Food and Agriculture Organization (FAO) (2003). *AEZWIN: An Interactive Multiple-Criteria Analysis Tool for Land Resources Appraisal.* FAO Land and Water Digital Media Series, vol. 15.

Food and Agriculture Organization (FAO) (2010). *FAO Statistical Yearbook 2010.* Retrieved from <http://www.fao.org/economic/ess/ess-publications/ess-yearbook/ess-yearbook2010/yearbook2010-reources/en/>.

GESAMP (IMO/FAO/UNESCO-IOC/WMO/WHO/IAEA/UN/UNEP (2001) (Joint Group of Experts on the Scientific Aspects of Marine Environmental Protection and Advisory Committee on Protection of the Sea). A sea of troubles. *Reports and Studies,* GESAMP No. 70, 35 pp.

Hayward, S.A. & Hanson, C.R. (2004). *Nitrate Contamination of Groundwater in the Ashburton-Rakaia Plains.* Canterbury: Report No. R04/9, Environment Canterbury.

Lal, R. (2004). Soil carbon sequestration impacts on global climate change and food security. *Science, 304*(5677), 1623–1627.

Lal, R., Follett, R.F., Stewart, B.A. & Kimble, J.M. (2007). Soil carbon sequestration to mitigate climate change and advance food security. *Soil Science, 172*(12), 943–956.

Ministry for the Environment (2007a). *Proposed National Environmental Standard for Sources of Human Drinking-water Resource Management Act, Section 32: Analysis of the Costs and Benefits.* Report No. ME 798. Wellington: Ministry for the Environment.

Ministry for the Environment (2007b). *Environment New Zealand 2007.* Report No. ME 847. Wellington: Ministry for the Environment.

Reeves, D.W. (1997). The role of soil organic matter in maintaining soil quality in continuous cropping systems. *Soil and Tillage Research*, *43*(1–2), 131–167.

Sabine, C.L., Feely, R.A., Gruber, N., Key, R.M., Lee, K., Bullister, J.L., Wanninkhof, R., Wong, C.S., Wallace, D.W.R., Tilbrook, B., Millero, F.J., Peng, T.H., Kozyr, A., Ono, T. & Rios, A.F. (2004). The oceanic sink for anthropogenic CO. *Science*, *305*(5682), 367–371.

United Nations (2006). *Factsheet on Water and Sanitation* <http://www.un.org/waterforlife decade/factsheet.html>.

White, R.E. (2006). *Principles and Practice of Soil Science: The Soil as a Natural Resource* (4th edn). Malden, MA: Wiley & Sons.

Wilding, L.P. & Lin, H. (2006). Advancing the frontiers of soil science towards a geoscience. *Geoderma*, *131*(3–4), 257–274.

World Wildlife Fund (2006). *Living Planet Report 2006*. Gland, Switzerland: World Wildlife Fund.

WEBSITES

<www.iisd.org>

The International Institute for Sustainable Development.

<http://www.landshare.net/>

Landshare brings together people who have a passion for home-grown food, connecting those who have land to share with those who need land for cultivating food.

<http://www.mfe.govt.nz/>

New Zealand Ministry for the Environment, where you can find the latest *State of the Environment* report.

<http://soilandfood.org/>

The Soils, Food and Healthy Communities (SFHC) project in northern Malawi works with over 4000 farmers to improve soil fertility, food security and nutrition.

<http://www.theagrariankitchen.com>

The Agrarian Kitchen is committed to reconnecting the kitchen with the land. Its aim is to create a place where people can rediscover the pleasure of gathering and cooking with produce as close to its source as possible.

READING 24

Climate Change

W. LINDSEY WHITE AND ROGER WHITING

CHAPTER OVERVIEW

This chapter covers the following topics:

- The Greenhouse Effect
- What is the evidence?
- Intergovernmental Panel on Climate Change
- Doubts about the theory
- Global dimming
- The future

KEY TERMS

Carbon dioxide
Fossil fuels
Glacial periods
Global dimming
Global warming
Greenhouse Effect
Ice ages
Industrialisation
Interglacial ages
Nonrenewable
Particulate material
Peer review
Photosynthesis
Renewable
Scientific

The temperature of the earth's climate has undergone many changes in the last billion years. We have had **ice ages**, where lower surface temperatures resulted in the expansion of polar and continental ice sheets. In between these ice ages have been periods of warm surface temperatures where there are no ice sheets at all, even at the poles. Over the last 3 billion years there have been four major ice ages, and in fact we are currently in an ice age, as there are significant polar ice sheets. Within the ice ages there are periods when it gets even colder, resulting in increased continental ice sheets and alpine glaciers. These are called **glacial periods**, with the warmer periods being **interglacial ages**. The last glacial age started around 110 000 years ago and ended around 10 000 years ago. Since then the earth has been warming. The sea level changes dramatically between glacial and interglacial ages. During glacial ages water is taken from the oceans to form the polar and continental ice sheets, so the sea level drops up to 120 metres. For the last 10 000 years the earth has been warming up, glaciers have been retreating and the sea level has been rising.

The basic theory of **global warming** is that:

- a planet that is as far from the sun as our earth is should be at a temperature below zero degrees centigrade
- as the earth is not as cold as that, something must be keeping it warm
- factors that could be keeping the planet warm could include heat from the centre of the earth and/or something that is stopping the heat from the centre of the earth and the heat from the sun from escaping into space
- the something that prevents the heat from the earth escaping into space is the atmosphere, which acts like a blanket around the Earth.

Thus far the theory is not contentious. However, it does suggest that changes to the composition of the atmosphere will change the extent to which it holds in the heat of the earth. At this point questions arise regarding how much the atmosphere is changing, whether the changes are humanmade and whether anything can be done about it. There are clearly a number of competing influences on the atmosphere. Some of these will warm it and some will cool it. Unfortunately, unlike most **scientific** questions, humankind cannot carry out experiments on the planet to see what could happen. Therefore we must rely on evidence of past eons and measurements from the present, together with theoretical modelling.

While it is well known that the earth is indeed warming up, there are differences in opinion regarding whether the rate of warming has increased beyond what is 'natural'. According to the Intergovernmental Panel on Climate Change (IPCC), the earth has been warming since the mid 1800s and the global average temperature of the surface air has increased by about 0.6 degrees Celsius since the early 1900s (more information on the IPCC below).

While this might not seem like a very great change, the variation in temperature between ice ages and the earth's warmest periods is only around 10 degrees (IPCC, 2007). Some scientists point out that just because this increase in temperature is correlated with **industrialisation,** it does not mean industrialisation is the cause. They argue that scientists started accurately measuring global temperatures just as the earth started to warm up from probably the coldest period for a thousand years, so maybe what we are seeing is simply a normal heating up because of natural causes. So what are the human activities that could cause global warming? Most of it is attributed to the **Greenhouse Effect.**

THE GREENHOUSE EFFECT

The Greenhouse Effect centres on the concept that there are certain gases in the earth's atmosphere that trap solar energy inside the atmosphere. The main gases are **carbon dioxide** (CO_2), methane (CH_4), nitrous oxide (N_2O) and halocarbons (a group of gases containing fluorine, chlorine or bromine). So if more of these gases accumulate in the atmosphere and everything else stays the same (net amount of solar energy), the earth's temperature will increase.

Figure 7.1: Mean concentrations of CO_2 in the Earth's atmosphere (parts per million) derived from in situ air measurements at the Mauna Loa Observatory, Hawaii

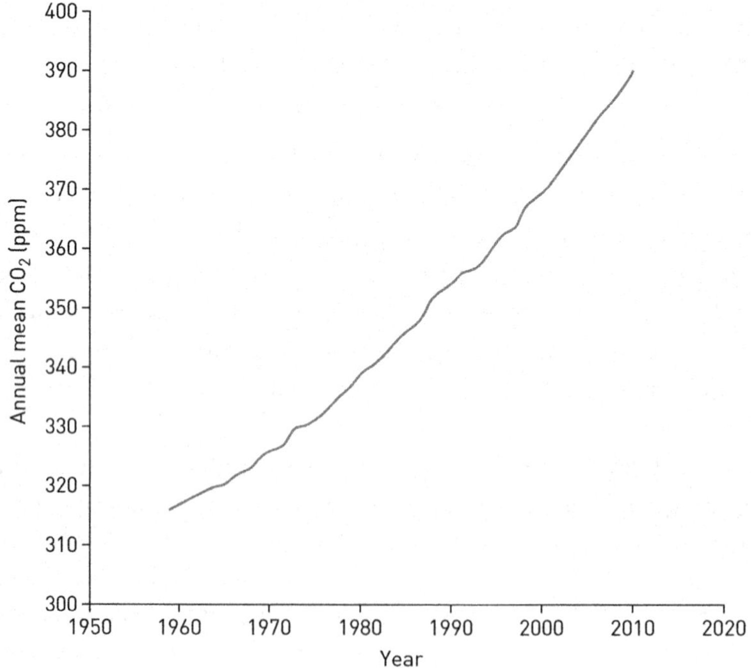

Source: <http://scrippsco2.ucsd.edu/data/atmospheric_co2.html>.

WHAT IS THE EVIDENCE?

Much research has been done looking at rocks laid down in the sea and in lakes and rivers. The composition of these rocks can indicate the temperature at which they solidified and the composition of the water from which they arose. From the composition of the water it is possible to calculate the amount of carbon dioxide (CO_2) in the air above the water. Thus a chart of atmospheric CO_2 levels and global temperatures can be constructed. These charts show that the earth has been through a number of cold and warm eras. Humans have arrived quite recently and have spread over the globe as it warmed up after a long cold period.

Of particular interest in this work is the way in which the warming and cooling of the planet have coincided with the increasing and decreasing CO_2 levels. This sort of historical mapping does not automatically indicate whether the warming caused the CO_2 or CO_2 caused the warming. However, it does indicate they are related. This type of connection is where a lot of scientific development starts.

The temperature of the planet has changed over the last thousand years. The CO_2 levels have increased to levels not seen for several million years. This has been put down to the burning of forest and grassland by early humans and finally gradually moving to the burning of coal and oil over the last 200 years. However, the global temperature has not increased greatly over this time. This has called into question the connection between the CO_2 levels and global temperatures, and has enabled possible connections between them to be ignored.

Another way to explore the issue of global temperatures is to measure a large number of possible parameters relating to the world's climate, then try to create a mathematical computer model of the world temperature. This involves obtaining data from a wide range of sources (see Figure 7.2).

Most countries have a meteorological service that measures and records temperatures, rainfall, wind speeds and air pressure. This is normally used to make weather forecasts. This data is often pooled with that for other countries, and provides a continually increasing source of weather data. Data are also available from historical records (such as church records, diaries and ships' logs). It also includes data from ice cores in Antarctica and Greenland, which can be used to obtain information on dust levels, temperatures in the past (for example, by measuring radioactive isotope ratios in the ice) and atmospheric composition (from bubbles trapped in the ice).

From this, a mathematical model of the earth's climate can be developed and its behaviour studied. The models work by dividing the planet's surface into cells, and then calculating how the flow of energy, air and water will take place between the cells. If a model gives a good description of the past climate, it will probably give a good prediction of the future climate. Currently the models developed are rather coarse (dividing the world into squares a thousand kilometres across). However, as computing power increases these are being refined, and more and more data is becoming available on what factors affect our climate.

Figure 7.2: Observed changes in (a) global average surface temperature; (b) global average sea level from tide gauge (blue) and satellite (red) data; and (c) Northern Hemisphere snow cover for March–April

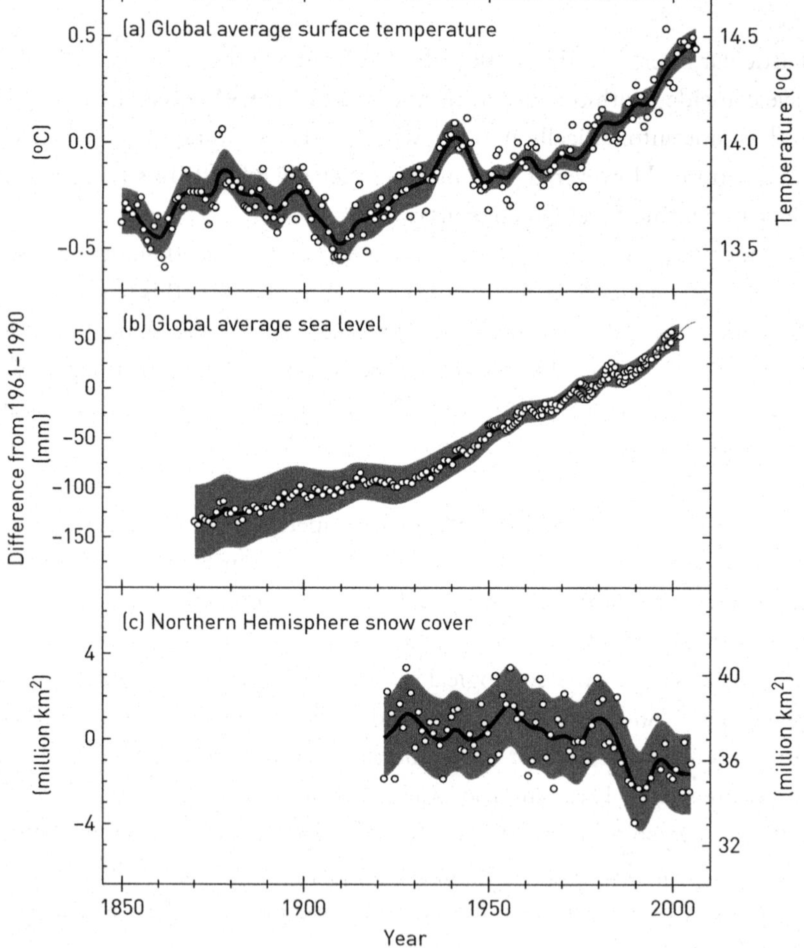

Source: IPCC, 2007, Figure 1.1, used with permission.

All differences are relative to corresponding averages for the period 1961–1990. Smoothed curves represent decadal averaged values while circles show yearly values. The shaded areas are the uncertainty intervals estimated from a comprehensive analysis of known uncertainties (a and b) and from the time series (c).

CASE STUDY 7.1

WHERE DOES ENERGY COME FROM?

Much of the talk around climate change and global warming has to do with our use of **fossil fuels** and other energy sources, so let's take a look at just where this energy comes from.

A large proportion of energy comes either directly or indirectly from the sun, and much from the burning of fossil fuels (Ministry of Economic Development, 2008). Every day, the sun delivers to the earth around 7000 times the amount of energy we use globally. Wind power is generated through heating and cooling of air masses associated with the sun and global weather patterns. Almost all hydroelectric power comes from harnessing the energy of water as it moves downhill, and it is energy from the sun that evaporates the water and takes it uphill in the first place. Fossil fuels also rely on the sun's energy. Coal, oil and natural gas are all formed from the breakdown of organic matter. Coal comes from the fossilised remains of forests that grew in the Carboniferous period, some 300 million years ago. Oil is formed by zooplankton and algae that settled to the bottom of seas or lakes. These deposits become covered by sediment, and through heat and pressure transformed into oil. Much of today's oil formed during the Jurassic period, around 150 million years ago. Natural gas is associated with coal and oil deposits and is also formed from the decay of organic material. So the fossil fuels we are burning today are the result of **photosynthesis** that was carried out millions of years ago, driven by the sun's energy.

We are able to collect very little solar power for our needs. So our energy requirements are being subsidised by solar energy that fell to earth millions of years ago. Our complete industrial history, the massive growth in human population and our ability to have an impact upon the environment has been enabled by the use of these fossil fuels.

Fossil fuels are **nonrenewable** resources, as once the supplies have been used they are not able to be replaced. While coal and oil are undoubtedly still being formed by the same processes that have occurred for millions of years, the process is very slow, and they are being consumed at a much faster rate. While there is much debate over just how long the oil will last, even the most optimistic estimates state that, at current rates of consumption, we will reach a peak of production within 25–45 years, after which the supply will decrease dramatically, being entirely exhausted by the end of this century (Wood et al., 2004). Natural gas, at our current rate of use, will last between 60 and 65 years, and there is about 200 years of coal left, but, of course, if it were used to replace oil and natural gas, this would drop to less than 100 years (British Petroleum, 2008).

New Zealand's energy use is quite different to that of global averages. We import around 35 per cent of the energy used in the form of oil or oil products. While the global average for fossil fuels is around 86 per cent, in New Zealand this is 70 per cent, as **renewable** energy plays a big part (30 per cent) in our energy requirements. This ranks us third in all OECD countries in terms of renewable energy use, behind only Iceland and Norway. Our renewable energy comes from geothermal

(42 per cent of NZ renewable energy use), hydroelectric (37 per cent), woody biomass (19 per cent), wind (1 per cent) and others making up the remaining 1 per cent, including solar, biogas and landfill gas (Ministry of Economic Development, 2008).

INTERGOVERNMENTAL PANEL ON CLIMATE CHANGE (IPCC)

This is an international scientific body that reviews and assesses the most relevant and up-to-date scientific information relating to global climate change. Thousands of scientists from all over the world contribute on a voluntary basis to this review and assessment. The IPCC was established in 1988 by the United Nations Environment Programme (UNEP) and the World Meteorological Organization (WMO).

The IPCC does not carry out the climate research or monitor climate or weather. Its main activity is publishing special reports on subjects that are seen to be relevant to the United Nations Framework Convention on Climate Change (UNFCCC), which is an international treaty acknowledging the potential of harmful climate change. The most recent report from the IPCC on global climate change was the *IPCC Fourth Assessment Report: Climate Change 2007* (IPCC, 2007).

The main findings from this report were:

- Warming of the climate system is unequivocal.
- Most of the observed increase in globally averaged temperatures since the mid-twentieth century is very likely (more than 90 per cent) due to the observed increase in anthropogenic (human) greenhouse gas concentrations.
- Anthropogenic warming and sea-level rise would continue for centuries due to the time scales associated with climate processes and feedbacks, even if greenhouse gas concentrations were to be stabilised, although the likely amount of temperature and sea level increase varies greatly, depending on the fossil intensity of human activity during the next century.
- The probability that this is caused by natural climatic processes alone is less than 5 per cent.
- World temperatures could rise by between 1.1 and 6.4 degrees Celsius during the twenty-first century, and that:
    - sea levels will probably rise by 18 to 59 centimetres
    - there is a confidence level of more than 90 per cent that there will be more frequent warm spells, heat waves and heavy rainfall
    - there is a confidence level of more than 66 per cent that there will be an increase in droughts, tropical cyclones and extreme high tides.

- Both past and future anthropogenic carbon dioxide emissions will continue to contribute to warming and sea-level rise for more than a millennium.
- Global atmospheric concentrations of carbon dioxide, methane and nitrous oxide have increased markedly as a result of human activities since 1750, and now far exceed pre-industrial values over the past 650 000 years.

DOUBTS ABOUT THE THEORY

Doubts about the theory behind the concept of global warming are generally centred around two main issues. The first is that the climate has changed a lot in the past, both colder and warmer, and this does not always correlate with carbon dioxide levels in the atmosphere. The second is that there has been a significant increase in carbon dioxide in the atmosphere over the last decades without any significant increase in temperature.

From these arguments it might seem rash to significantly hamper economic growth by campaigning to stop something that is not proved to be happening. It should also be noted that a significant number of individuals and organisations support the approach that we do not yet have any proof of climate change being a product of burning fossil fuels. Critical thinking is to be encouraged when considering information and the sources of it. Critical consideration of some of the messages arguing against the notion of global warming uncovers conflicts of interest, as organisations are set up or supported by the companies producing and marketing fossil fuels.

CASE STUDY 7.2

HOW DOES SCIENCE WORK? PEER-REVIEWED PUBLICATIONS

In the section on the IPCC, it was noted that they compiled, reviewed and assessed tens of thousands of peer-reviewed studies to come to their conclusions—but what is a peer-reviewed study? Why do scientists think this kind of publication is better than other types of publication, such as books or websites? To answer this, we can examine what a scientist goes through to publish in a peer-reviewed journal.

Our scientist, let's call her Jane Smith, is a marine biologist who studies the impacts of rising seawater levels on coral growth. She designs her study, applies for some funds to carry it out, completes the study, analyses her results and comes to her conclusions. She feels that she has found something that is of interest to the wider **scientific** community so wants to publish in a good international scientific journal, for example *Science* or *Nature*.

What makes a 'good' journal? One indicator is the citation index, generated by an electronic analysis of published reference lists of scientific papers, noting how many times the journal is found in each reference list. The journal that is listed in the most reference lists of all has the highest citation index (that journal has been cited the most). The idea is that, if articles from a given journal are cited most often, the journal must be publishing the most important articles in the world.

Now back to Dr Jane. She goes to the *Nature* journal website and looks up the instructions to authors, where she finds out what kind of articles will be accepted, the editorial process and the particular format she needs to follow in submitting her manuscript. She writes her manuscript and sends it off to the editor of *Nature*. The editor receives the paper and, based on the subject, selects two scientists who are in the same field as Dr Jane and sends them the manuscript to review. This is the '**peer review**' part; the two reviewers are usually given a few weeks to carry out the review, and then they send a report back to the editor. They can recommend that the paper should not be published, should be published with some alterations or should be published as is. If it is not a really terrible paper, they generally recommend the middle option and give a list of particular changes that should be made. The editor then removes the reviewers' names from the reports (so Dr Jane will not know who they were) and sends the reports to Dr Jane. She either makes the changes they suggest or does not, if she happens to disagree with the reviewers. She sends the revised manuscript back to the editor, along with a letter outlining how she has addressed the issues raised by the reviewers. The editor then decides if the reviewers' issues have been adequately addressed and if so, accepts the paper for publication. This whole process from first submission to the journal to publication can take several months, depending on the journal.

So now you know how peer-reviewed publications make it into journals, but there is one more point to make here. You may be surprised to find out that researchers generally do not receive any money for their publications (in fact, some journals ask them to pay a fee to get published). The reviewers receive no money either; usually they are scientists at universities and it is considered part of their role as a scientist to contribute to science by reviewing articles. In many cases the editor is also a voluntary role, with no salary attached. This is why peer-reviewed publications are seen as robust. They have been independently and anonymously reviewed by at least two experts in the same field.

GLOBAL DIMMING

It has been suggested that one of the phenomena that could be preventing the global temperature from rising could be an effect called **global dimming**: the effect by which **particulate material** in the upper atmosphere can reduce the amount of sunlight reaching the ground. Historical records show significant changes in weather in various parts of the globe at different times. For example, 1815, 'the year without a summer' in Europe, is now known to have been caused by the eruption of Tambora in what is now Indonesia. Also, Roman records report unusually red sunsets the year the Taupo volcano here in New Zealand erupted. More recently, the eruption of Mount Pinatubo was followed by a two-year drop in temperature of several degrees in the southern hemisphere.

The effect is not only caused by volcanoes. Human industrial activity has greatly expanded over the last hundred years. Most industrial activity tends to produce gases and/or dust. To prevent gases and dust being a nuisance to local populations, industry tends to pick the cheap option of getting it high in the air so that it disperses. This has become more common since the mid twentieth century, when Clean Air Acts started to be adopted. However, this effect merely spreads the dust over a wider area.

Stratospheric aircraft have also contributed to the material in the upper atmosphere. These aircraft burn a lot of fuel in the stratosphere and leave trails of water–ice particles to circulate the globe. The sunlight hitting the earth is reflected by these particles, so the energy arriving at the earth's surface is reduced. The magnitude of this effect was noted in 2001. Immediately after September 11, all civilian aircraft in the USA were grounded, and so the aircraft contrails gradually dispersed and an increase in surface temperature of several degrees was measured.

Overall, it would seem that over the last hundred years there has been a gradual increase in particulates in the upper atmosphere, which has probably decreased the amount of sunlight reaching the ground and thereby prevented surface temperatures from rising.

THE FUTURE

Clearly, if the world climate is going to change significantly in the next few decades the population of the world will be severely affected. However, if industries and governments are to commit large proportions of their resources to changing industrial practices, certainty is needed. An international consensus is also needed to ensure that all countries make a commitment to effect some change. This is not likely until the scientific evidence is much stronger. Arriving at that point requires much research and debate. This has been generated in the last few years, and the work is carrying on at an increasing pace. Improved computer capacity will enable climate models to be refined, and ongoing research on the climate processes will inform those models to deliver usable data.

To ignore the issue is to court disaster. The predicted effects of global warming vary, but if seawater temperatures rise and the polar ice caps melt, the level of the sea may rise several metres. This might be a minor problem for Aotearoa New Zealand, but it would be devastating for countries such as Bangladesh and the Netherlands.

SUMMARY

The issue of global warming is still a contentious topic, with conflicting evidence being cited. There are a number of competing influences on the climate, including the Greenhouse Effect and reflectance from aerosols and global dimming. Much more research needs to be done to find a consensus so that worldwide action can be taken to limit the risks associated with global warming, which have the potential to have a radical and negative impact on a substantial proportion of the world's population and much of its economic development.

CRITICAL QUESTIONS

Cultural lens

- **How** would rising sea levels have an impact on leisure activities and expectations of kiwis?

Social lens

- **How** does human activity (including aeroplane travel and the burning of carbon-based fuels) contribute to global dimming and warming?

Gender lens

- **Debate** the relative contribution of various groups within the community to global warming.

Political lens

- **How** should the international community come to some consensus on how to deal with global sea level rise?
- **Given** the massive amount of peer-reviewed literature on global warming, do you think all those scientists could be wrong?

Moral lens

- **Why** can no country in the world decide to solve the problems of global warming or global dimming?

Media lens

- **How** does the media present 'solutions' such as collecting and burying carbon dioxide emissions?

FURTHER READING

IPCC (2007). Summary for policymakers. In: S. Solomon, D. Qin, M. Manning, Z. Chen, M. Marquis, K.B. Averyt, M. Tignor and H.L. Miller (eds), *Climate Change 2007: The Physical Science Basis. Contribution of Working Group I to Fourth Assessment Report of the Intergovernmental Panel on Climate Change*. Cambridge and New York: Cambridge University Press.

REFERENCES

British Petroleum (2008). *BP Statistical Review of World Energy June 2008* <http://www.bp.com>.

Intergovernmental Panel on Climate Change (IPCC) (2007). Pachauri, R.K. & Reisinger, A. (eds and core writing team), *Climate Change 2007: Synthesis Report. Contribution of Working Groups I, II and III to the Fourth Assessment Report of the Intergovernmental Panel on Climate Change*. Geneva: Intergovernmental Panel on Climate Change.

Ministry of Economic Development (2008). *Energy Information and Modelling, Energy Data File June 2008*. Wellington: Ministry of Economic Development.

Wood, J.H., Long, G.R. & Morehouse, D.F. (2004). *Long-term World Oil Supply Scenarios: The Future Is Neither as Bleak or Rosy as Some Assert*. Washington, DC: Energy Information Administration: Official Energy Statistics from the US Government <http://www.eia.doe.gov/>.

WEBSITES

<www.climate-skeptic.com>

Read the other side to the global warming debate.

<www.footprintnetwork.org>

Work out your ecological footprint.

<http://www.globalissues.org/article/529/global-dimming>

Global dimming.

<www.iisd.org>

The International Institute for Sustainable Development.

<http://www.ipcc.ch/>

Intergovernmental Panel on Climate Change (IPCC).

<http://www.skepticalscience.com>

Global warming sceptics.

<http://www.youtube.com/watch?v=zORv8wwiadQ>

Action on Global Warming.

READING 25

Biodiversity

LEN GILLMAN

CHAPTER OVERVIEW

This chapter covers the following topics:

- Biodiversity
- Global patterns of biodiversity
- Evolutionary speed hypothesis
- Origins of New Zealand biodiversity
- Other contributions
- Low species richness in New Zealand
- Unique indigenous New Zealand flora
- Unique indigenous New Zealand fauna
- Biogeographic context

KEY TERMS

Biodiversity
Biota
Divaricating
Ecology
Elevational diversity gradient
Endemic
Evolutionary speed hypothesis
Exotic
Fauna
Flora
Generation time
Genetic evolution
Gondwana
Latitudinal diversity gradient
Plate tectonics
Speciation
Species richness
Taxonomic
West Wind Drift

The natural world is important to people because it contributes strongly to our sense of wellbeing. Humans derive enormous pleasure from the beauty of nature and its diversity. Furthermore, the unique component of **biodiversity** to a particular homeland can add to our sense of belonging and identity. Some say humans have a moral obligation to protect biodiversity on the basis that we don't have the right to destroy other species.

BIODIVERSITY

Biodiversity includes the diversity within species, between species and among ecosystems. Diversity among ecosystems includes the variety of forests, grasslands, lakes, rivers, wetlands and marine ecosystems. There are many different ways of characterising biodiversity, but the simplest measure is **species richness**, or the number of species in a given area:

Global patterns of biodiversity

Even the most unobservant person travelling from the cold Arctic region at high latitudes down to tropical rainforest near the equator could not help but notice the dramatic change in the variety of species. The enormous number of different species living together at the equator is almost overwhelming; just about every plant and animal encountered seems to be of a different species. Moving away from the equator towards the poles the number of species within a given area declines slowly at first and then plummets steeply with increasing latitude. This **latitudinal diversity gradient** is the most fundamental and spectacular pattern of nature on Earth.

Consider trees as an example. We might expect to find up to 265 tree species in every tenth of a hectare in an Amazon rainforest near the equator (for comparison, a rugby field is about seven-tenths of a hectare), but at mid latitudes in temperate forest near Auckland, New Zealand, tree species richness drops to about 10 to 12 species in the same area. Further south, in parts of the South Island, or in boreal forest at high latitudes in the Northern Hemisphere, it drops to 1 to 5 species in an entire region. Similar declines in species richness with latitude are found in freshwater and marine ecosystems, and the full range of life forms, including plants, reptiles, mammals, birds, fish, invertebrates, parasites and micro-organisms (Hillebrand, 2004). Perhaps most amazing of all, we know from the fossil record that this pattern has existed for more than 270 million years, and persisted through countless shifts in climate (Stehli et al., 1969).

A similar pattern is generally found with increasing elevation and is referred to as an **elevational diversity gradient**. For example, in New Zealand there is a decrease of 3 to 4 woody plant species with every 100-metre increase in elevation (Ogden, 1995). Hot dry climates (such as deserts) have fewer species than hot wet climates (such as tropical rainforests) and in the Amazon tropical rainforest, areas with greater rainfall have a greater number of species (Gentry, 1988). However, wet climates that are cold (such as Fiordland in New Zealand's South Island) tend to have low species richness. Therefore, rainfall is only important for species richness in climates that are warm enough for water to be a limiting factor for growth.

EVOLUTIONARY SPEED HYPOTHESIS

It was first suggested more than 200 years ago by von Humboldt (1808) that energy might be the primary cause of global biodiversity patterns. The **evolutionary speed hypothesis** is one of the many theories that attempts to explain how energy might lie at the root of the latitudinal diversity gradient. Animals living in warmer tropical climates have shorter **generation times** than those living at higher latitudes in cooler climates. In 1959, Rensch suggested that because natural selection accumulates change with each generation, shorter generation times found among animals living in the tropics might increase the pace of natural selection and thereby the pace at which evolution progresses.

Rohde (1992) proposed that thermal energy might also influence the rate at which mutations are produced within a population. More mutations over a given length of time will increase the number of mutations that provide a selective advantage, and therefore increase the pace at which **genetic evolution** can occur. Genetic evolution is necessary for **speciation**, and therefore a greater rate of genetic evolution is likely to result in a greater rate of increase in the number of species. It follows that, over a given period of evolutionary time, more species will accumulate through the process of genetic change in areas where the rate of evolution is faster.

CASE STUDY 8.1

TESTING THE EVOLUTIONARY SPEED HYPOTHESIS

In recent years, staff and students at AUT University and University of Auckland have been testing and developing the evolutionary speed hypothesis. The first of these studies (Wright et al., 2006) produced impressive results. This study measured the amount of genetic evolution in closely related plants that occur at different latitudes. The study found that genetic evolution has been on average more than twice as fast in plants that occur naturally in the warmer tropics as it has been in plants that occur in cooler environments at higher latitudes such as in Aotearoa New Zealand. The differences in rates of evolution between sister plant species in some cases exceeded an order of magnitude. For example, in the gene studied, more than 13 times more genetic evolution was found for *Agathis borneensis* from tropical Borneo on the equator than in *Agathis australis* (kauri) which occurs at latitudes between approximately 35° and 38° South in Aotearoa New Zealand. The study included 45 independent comparisons from a broad range of flowering and non-flowering plant groups.

A larger study, involving 260 mammal species from 10 orders and 29 families, by the same research group tested for both latitudinal and elevational effects

(Gillman et al., 2009). Again, rates of genetic evolution were found to be faster for mammals living in warmer climates at both lower latitudes and at lower elevations. These researchers have since found similar results for amphibians, marine fish and birds.

Moreover, consistent with the idea that rates of genetic evolution determine patterns of species richness, they found that rates of genetic evolution in plants that grow in arid Australia, where diversity is low, was slower than in closely related plants that grow in wet Australia, where diversity is extremely high. The fossil record also shows us that rates of diversification have been greater in warmer latitudes (e.g. Jablonski et al., 2006), and that rates of diversification are greater where species richness is higher (Krug et al., 2007). These studies suggest that the evolutionary speed hypothesis may have merit. However, there is a lot more work required in this area.

ORIGINS OF NEW ZEALAND BIODIVERSITY

In order to understand the origins of New Zealand species, and indeed to understand the **ecology** of the species themselves, it is first necessary to understand something of New Zealand's geological history. As humans we are inclined to think of the land and its physical features, such as lakes, rivers and mountains, as permanent. However, the land has little permanence, and even the most striking geological features in New Zealand have formed only recently on an evolutionary time scale (Stevens et al., 1988).

The Southern Alps, for example, only began to rise five million years ago (MYA), and have only existed as high mountains for about two million years. And although five million years is an unfathomably long time from a human perspective, it is relatively short compared to the 3800 million year history of life on earth. There are two main components to the shaping and reshaping of the land: first, rain and wind constantly work to erode the land flat and the action of ocean waves eats away at the coastline; and second, **plate tectonics** can cause the uplift of mountains, where the plates move towards each other, and they can generate volcanoes where a plate margin is forced down to a depth where it melts. The shaping and reshaping of land through plate tectonics has had important implications for the evolution of **biota** on land. The movement of continental plates across the surface of the globe has also played a critical role in shaping the present-day life on earth, because of the effect of land masses and their biota separating as plates drift apart, and because of the effect of other land masses crashing together to unite species that have evolved separately in different locations. Again these processes have been extremely slow on a human time scale. The Pacific Plate, for example, is moving at about 4 centimetres per year, which means it will take over 100 million years to move 4000 kilometres.

As in other parts of the world, plate tectonics has had a major influence on the biota of New Zealand since it first rose from beneath the sea approximately 144 MYA. New Zealand's terrestrial environment has had approximately 80 million years of largely isolated biological history, punctuated with periods of biotic dispersal, mainly from Australia, but also from other areas of the Pacific. Plate tectonics has been causal in the process of generating three of the four major components of New Zealand's present-day biota.

It is thought that plate tectonics led to Aotearoa New Zealand becoming completely separated from **Gondwana** approximately 80 MYA. Although small mammals existed before then, the separation of New Zealand predates the extensive radiation of mammal species that followed the mass extinction event around 65 MYA. New Zealand did not receive modern placental mammals, monotremes, marsupials or snakes until very recently, when many mammal species were introduced by humans. However, after New Zealand separated from Gondwana it did continue to receive species from it that could disperse over the ocean. For example, wrens, wattle birds and thrushes all appear to have colonised New Zealand after separation from Gondwana.

The movement of tectonic plates led to the land masses of Australia, Papua New Guinea, Indonesia and Asia colliding approximately 24 MYA. The collision caused tropical currents to be diverted down to New Zealand. This produced sea temperatures of 5–7°C greater than at present. Sea temperatures strongly influence land temperatures, and therefore New Zealand's climate became much more tropical than at present. The currents from the tropics enabled tropical species to disperse to New Zealand. In addition, at this time a string of islands extended to the north of New Zealand up into the tropics, and many species were able to colonise these sequentially until they eventually reached New Zealand (Stevens et al., 1988).

Tectonic movement separated the Australian continent from Antarctica, and this enabled a circumpolar current to establish. This intensified as the separation grew. By about 35 million years ago (MYA), this current in turn began a circumpolar wind pattern that resulted in a strong prevailing wind from Australia to New Zealand. By 20 MYA the **West Wind Drift** was strong enough to disperse new species of plants and birds to New Zealand from Australia (Stevens et al., 1988).

Indigenous and **exotic** species coexist in our environment. These exotic introductions, along with hunting by early Māori, have been responsible for the extinction of many animals. The total number of complete extinctions of terrestrial bird species caused directly or indirectly by humans in New Zealand is 43. This is 33 per cent of our pre-human terrestrial bird diversity. In addition, 37 of the remaining 88 species are threatened with extinction. So many plant pest species have been introduced that there are now more exotic species that have established wild populations capable of self-dispersing in New Zealand than native species.

CASE STUDY 8.2

CONTRIBUTIONS TO NEW ZEALAND'S BIOTA

From Gondwana	From the tropics	From Australia	Human immigration
Plants Ancestors of kauri (*Agathis*) and totara (*Podocarpus*) **Animals** Ratites that diversified into three kiwi and nine moa (all extinct) species Ancestors of iconic and primitive New Zealand animals tuatara, frogs, *Peripitus* (velvet worm), the giant earthworm and the giant insects and snails, including the carnivorous snails (*Paryphanta* and *Powelliphanta*) Wrens, wattlebirds, thrushes (after separation from Gondwana) Bats	**Plants** Coral Mangrove Nikau palm Cabbage trees Coconut palms (these disappeared again during the Ice Age within the last two million years)	**Plants** Mountain daisies Australian gum (*Eucalyptus*)* Australian wattle (*Acacia*)* * These disappeared again during the Ice Age within the last two million years **Birds** Takahe Kakapo Robin **Insects** Monarch butterfly	**Plants** More than 2000 species now established as wild populations More than 25 000 species for ornamental gardening **Animals** Vast array of exotic mammals including: Polynesian rat (kiore) and dog (kuru) Ship rat Hedgehog Cats Possums Many other species, including: 25 species of earthworms 26 species of slugs and snails

Human activities and introduced animals have led to the extinction of many species, including native species of pelican, snipe, goose, swan, duck, moa, raven, coot and the giant Haast's eagle (Taylor & Smith, 1997), piopio, huia, wren and laughing owl, with saddleback, kakapo and stitchbird now extinct on the mainland.

OTHER CONTRIBUTIONS TO BIOTA

Mountains did not exist in New Zealand before about two million years ago, when the Southern Alps were uplifted because of the pressure created by two plates pushing against each other. More recently, volcanic activity in the North Island has also created mountains (50 major volcanoes in the last 50 000 years). The relatively sudden appearance of mountains in New Zealand provided new alpine environments that have enabled the evolution of new species, such as the ground-hugging alpine totara, which diverged from the lowland tall tree species. Mountains also provided a new habitat that enabled the capture of alpine plants dispersing across the Tasman Sea from Australia.

In the last 2.4 million years, there have been 20 glaciations—this is the so-called Ice Age. The last glaciation (22 000–14 000 years ago) was the coldest. During this time, temperatures were approximately 5°C lower than at present. The sea level was also 120–135 metres lower than today. The North, South and Stewart Islands were connected in a single landmass covered mainly by grasses and small shrubs; forest probably did not exist south of Auckland. The severe climate during these glaciations, and possibly during the cooling period before glaciations, resulted in the extinction of many plants in New Zealand, including *Eucalyptus*, *Acacia* and coconut palms (Stevens et al., 1988).

LOW SPECIES RICHNESS IN NEW ZEALAND

New Zealand has a wide range of habitats because of its topographic diversity (mountains up to 3754 metres above sea level) and soil diversity, and its wide range of climates derived from its large latitudinal span (13°) and differing rainfall regimes. Given this high habitat diversity, it might be expected that New Zealand would have a high species richness of native plants and animals for its size. However, this is not the case; New Zealand's species diversity is relatively poor. There are five possible reasons for this:

1. The landmass of New Zealand was greatly reduced 30 MYA.
2. The topographic diversity is relatively recent, having developed in the last two million years.
3. The extreme changes in climate that have occurred in the last two million years have caused many extinctions. Plants and animals have not been able to survive by migrating north and south to track changing climates as they have been able to do on continents.
4. New Zealand is more isolated than any other landmass of equivalent area on Earth, thereby restricting dispersal to New Zealand from continental sources.
5. Evolutionary speed and inherent capacity for speciation may be relatively low in New Zealand because of the cool climate that it has experienced over the last 20 million years.

UNIQUE INDIGENOUS NEW ZEALAND FLORA

The **flora** of Aotearoa New Zealand includes many **endemic** species; all indigenous gymnosperms (non-flowering, woody species) and 85 per cent of indigenous angiosperms (flowering species) are endemic. The fact that most of New Zealand's plant genera are shared with other countries suggests speciation has either occurred relatively recently or that it has occurred slowly. It is also likely that many old Gondwanan lineages that might have diverged into different genera have been lost, either during the time when little of New Zealand remained above sea level, or during the last 2.4 million years of the Ice Age.

New Zealand has few annual plants: only 5 per cent of the indigenous flora, compared with a global average of 13 per cent. A large number of New Zealand plants rely on birds for dispersal, presumably because there were no native mammals other than bats that could potentially fulfil this role. Perhaps the feature that most distinguishes New Zealand's indigenous flora from those of northern hemisphere temperate regions is the lack of deciduous trees (trees that drop their leaves in winter); the New Zealand indigenous flora is predominantly evergreen.

New Zealand has some species that are interesting because they are the largest in the world relative to the others in their **taxonomic** group. For example, New Zealand has the largest

- liverwort (*Schistochila appendiculata*, up to 1 metre in length)
- lichen
- moss (*Dawsonia superba*), which grows to approximately 60 centimetres
- buttercup (*Ranunculus lyallii* or Mount Cook lily)
- fuchsia (*Fuchsia excorticata*, the New Zealand tree fuchsia).

Another very distinguishing feature of the indigenous flora is that it contains a greater proportion of **divaricating** plants (10 per cent of species) than anywhere else in the world. These plants usually have relatively few and small leaves, which are mostly located towards the centre of the plant's tangle of stems, and the stems are very tough and springy. This divaricating form is thought to have been a defence mechanism against moa browse. Some have argued that the high rate of divarication is a response to harsh climatic environments. However, many species only have a divaricating form when they are young; once they are large enough not to be in reach of moa they develop a normal form with large leaves (Atkinson & Greenwood, 1989).

Much of the indigenous New Zealand flora is vulnerable to mammalian browsers because it has not co-evolved with them. The main radiation of mammals occurred only after New Zealand was isolated from Gondwana 80 MYA. As such, New Zealand plants lack many of the common chemical defences, such as 1080, found in exotic species that have evolved alongside mammals. The poison 1080 occurs naturally in Australian *Eucalyptus* but not in New Zealand pohutukawa, even though these plants belong to the same family (Myrtaceae).

UNIQUE INDIGENOUS NEW ZEALAND FAUNA

The indigenous **fauna** of Aotearoa New Zealand is unique as much for what it doesn't include as for what it does include. It is one of the few relatively large landmasses on Earth that does not have any indigenous mammals (other than bats and marine mammals). Nor does it have snakes.

New Zealand does, however, have a number of very interesting reptiles and amphibians. We know from fossil evidence dated 14–18 MYA—a time when the New Zealand climate was much warmer than it is today—that New Zealand had a native freshwater crocodile. It is assumed to have become extinct when the climate cooled. New Zealand's most unique living reptile is the tuatara (*Sphenodon punctatus*).

New Zealand has a number of interesting endemic gecko and skinks. New Zealand gecko (37 species) are thought to have their origins in Gondwana, before New Zealand separated from that continent 80 MYA. Gecko have a broad head, a distinct neck, velvety skin and wide flat toes with rows of fine hair that enable them to climb on smooth surfaces. They have very good sight and hearing (they can hear a pin drop 5 metres away) that enables them to see and hear an approaching fly (inaudible to humans), and then catch it on the wing. Gecko mainly eat invertebrates, but they also eat berries, nectar, seeds and carrion. They communicate with chirps, squeaks, barks and warning calls that are largely inaudible to humans. New Zealand gecko live for 45 years or more, and are among the most primitive, and therefore unique, in the world. They have vertebrae that are concave at both ends instead of having ball-and-socket vertebrae typical of exotic gecko, and all New Zealand gecko give birth to live young, whereas all but one exotic species lay eggs. The world's largest gecko (55 centimetres long) was the New Zealand species *Hoplodactylus decourti* (now extinct). New Zealand also has the southernmost occurring species, the harlequin gecko of Stewart Island (Hudson, 1994).

Skinks have an indistinct neck, shiny skin, a snake-like tongue and toes with sharp claws. Skinks range substantially in size and colour from 'spectacular oranges/creams/tans of the chevron skink at around 320 mm in total length, to bold stripes of moko and striped skinks' (Hudson, 1994). They mainly eat invertebrates and carrion, but they also eat berries, nectar and seeds. New Zealand has the two southernmost species, the southern skink and small-eared skink of Stewart Island.

Before the arrival of humans New Zealand had 131 species of terrestrial birds (excluding sea birds) living either on the mainland or islands; 71 per cent of these were endemic and many were flightless. The loss of flight in New Zealand birds is understood to be linked to the low risk of predation from snakes and mammalian predators during their evolution. Predation in New Zealand was largely restricted to that from other birds, such as hawks, eagles, adzebills and owls. The smallest of the flightless birds were the tiny mouse-sized wrens (now extinct) that hopped about on the forest floor, and were perhaps ecologically similar to mice. Large flightless birds included kiwi and kakapo (1–4 kilograms), the extinct goose (10–15 kilograms) and giant flightless birds such as the extinct adzebill (20–30 kilograms) and moa (25–250 kilograms).

New Zealand had some of the largest and heaviest birds for their particular groups in the world. These giant birds were particularly vulnerable to becoming extinct through being hunted after Māori arrived. Smaller New Zealand birds, such as the tiny flightless wrens, were vulnerable to the introduction of the Pacific rat, and other species fell to the many mammals introduced by Europeans, such as rats, cats and possums.

CASE STUDY 8.3

TRULY UNUSUAL FAUNA

New Zealand has a fascinating array of invertebrates, including five species of velvet worm (*Peripatus*) and approximately 2500 spiders. Again, many of these invertebrates are primitive and globally unique, many of them are giants. Giant New Zealand invertebrates include:

- giant carnivorous snails (*Powelliphanta* and *Paryphanta*), the largest of which is as big as a man's fist
- giant earthworms (more than 1 metre in length, one of 173 indigenous species of earthworm)
- seven out of 70 endemic weta species, which are huge, up to 9 centimetres long and 71 grams in weight. They are among the world's heaviest insects—comparable to the size of a rat
- the puriri moth, with a wingspan up to 15 centimetres
- giant flightless giraffe weevils.

New Zealand has four endemic frog species, all occurring in the genus *Leiopelma*. In addition, there are three introduced species. New Zealand's endemic frogs are unique, again because they are primitive. Indeed, they are of international significance as they differ greatly to almost all other surviving frogs in the world. New Zealand frogs:

- have vertebrae that are concave at both ends, instead of having the common ball-and-socket design
- have ribs that are not joined to the backbone
- lack the disc-like ear of other frogs
- lack a voicebox, and hence make no croaking sound
- have pupils that are round, while Australian frogs, for example, have horizontal pupils
- have two tail-wagging muscles

- produce froglets that develop inside the egg sac and emerge as a tailed adult, lacking a tadpole stage (Hudson, 1994).

The tuatara is not a lizard but the sole surviving species, endemic to New Zealand, of a separate order of reptiles, Rhynchocephalia. Tuatara differ from lizards because they:

- do not have teeth set in sockets, but instead they have a serrated jaw
- have bird-like ribs
- have a skin-covered ear
- have a third eye on the top of the head, with a lens and retina, but with a skin covering.

Tuatara live for 90 years or more and attain 610 millimetres in length (although there is fossil evidence of 1.2 metre-long tuatara).

BIOGEOGRAPHIC CONTEXT

Because Aotearoa New Zealand is a group of islands that have long been isolated from continental land masses, much of the evolution that has occurred here has occurred in isolation from the 'mainstream' evolution elsewhere in the world, and in particular, in isolation from mammals. This enabled birds, and in some cases invertebrates, to use habitat and resources in a way that is used by mammals elsewhere. In the absence of mammalian predators and competitors, birds and other animals in New Zealand have evolved characteristics that differ from similar animals elsewhere in the world, such as having a larger size, longer life spans and slower rates of reproduction.

Importantly, New Zealand's plants and animals did not co-evolve with mammals, and so they have not evolved 'strategies' to cope with the ability of mammals to locate plant and animal prey by smell and at night. Many indigenous New Zealand animals rely on staying still to avoid predation, which is not a very useful tactic when the predator can see with its nose almost as well as by sight; nor is it a good tactic to prevent predation from humans. The result is an indigenous flora and fauna in New Zealand that was, and still is, highly vulnerable to exotic species. Many New Zealand bird species were easy prey for humans, and their slow reproductive rate made losses due to predation difficult to replace.

The process of human colonisation followed by the extinction of a considerable proportion of the large animal fauna has occurred repeatedly over tens of thousands of years as humans have expanded across the earth. Furthermore, the vulnerability of island species that have evolved without mammals to the introduction of exotic mammals and human predation is not unique to New Zealand. Of the total number of bird extinctions recorded in the last 400 years, 93 per cent have been island species.

SUMMARY

Biodiversity is greatest in warm, wet tropical climates, and declines with increasing latitude and elevation as temperatures decline. Diversity is also lower in dry climates. Warm, wet climates are species rich, whereas cool or dry climates are species poor. This pattern of diversity on earth may be related to evolutionary speed and consequential rates of speciation.

The indigenous fauna and flora of Aotearoa New Zealand are truly unique, having some of the world's most primitive and giant species. Much of this uniqueness is a result of their long isolation from mainstream evolution and the lack of co-evolution of New Zealand biota with mammalian predators and snakes. The biodiversity of this land was influenced by tectonics (through the breaking up of Gondwana) and human immigration and activity. Humans have contributed to the extinction of many species, both directly by hunting and indirectly through the introduction of many exotic plant and animal pests.

CRITICAL QUESTIONS

Cultural lens

- **How** do people from different cultures value biodiversity differently? Is New Zealand's biodiversity relevant to the culture of New Zealanders today?

Social lens

- **Is** the unique nature of biodiversity in New Zealand something that society should value and promote? **Why** do we plant exotic species in our streets instead of indigenous species?

Gender lens

- **Do** men and women place different values on biodiversity?

Political lens

- **Do** those who make political decisions understand what is unique and important about New Zealand's biodiversity?

Moral lens

- **How** do we reconcile expenditure on protecting biodiversity with poverty and the impact that poverty has on people's health?

Media lens

- **How** do the media present issues relating to biodiversity conservation? Does the approach depend on the species in question (such as, kakapo versus snails)?

FURTHER READING

Parsons, S. (ed.) (2006). *Biology Aotearoa: Unique Flora, Fauna and Fungi.* Auckland: Pearson Education New Zealand.

Stevens, G., McGlone, M.S. & McCulloch, B. (1988). *Prehistoric New Zealand.* Auckland: Heinemann Reed.

REFERENCES

Atkinson, I.A.E. & Greenwood, R.M. (1989). Relationships between moas and plants. *New Zealand Journal of Ecology, 12*, 67–96.

Gentry, A.H. (1988). Changes in plant community diversity and floristic composition on environmental and geographical gradients. *Annals of the Missouri Botanical Garden, 75*, 1–34.

Gillman, L.N., Ross, H.A., Keeling, J.D. & Wright, S.D. (2009). Latitude, elevation and the tempo of molecular evolution in mammals. *Proceedings of the Royal Society B, 276*, 3353–3359.

Hillebrand, H. (2004). On the generality of the latitudinal diversity gradient. *American Naturalist, 163*(2), 192–211.

Hudson, B. (1994). *Reptiles & Amphibians in New Zealand.* Auckland, New Zealand: Print Media Specialists.

Jablonski, D., Roy, K. & Valentine, J.W. (2006). Out of the tropics: evolutionary dynamics of the latitudinal diversity gradient. *Science, 314*, 102–106.

Krug, A.Z., Jablonski, D. & Valentine, J.W. (2007). Contrarian clade confirms the ubiquity of spatial origination patterns in the production of latitudinal diversity gradients. *Proceedings of the National Academy of Sciences of the USA, 104*, 18129–18134.

Ogden, J. (1995). The long-term conservation of forest diversity in New Zealand. *Pacific Conservation Biology, 2*, 77–90.

Rensch, B. (1959). *Evolution Above the Species Level.* London: Methuen.

Rohde, K. (1992). Latitudinal gradients in species diversity: the search for the primary cause. *Oikos, 65*, 514–527.

Stehli, F.G., Douglas, D.G. & Newell, N.D. (1969). Generation and maintenance of gradients in taxonomic diversity. *Science, 164*, 947–949.

Stevens, G., McGlone, M.S. & McCulloch, B. (1988). *Prehistoric New Zealand.* Auckland: Heinemann Reed.

Taylor, R. & Smith, I. (1997). *The State of New Zealand's Environment.* Wellington: Ministry for the Environment.

von Humboldt, A. (1808). *Ansichten der Natur mit wissenschaftlichen Erlauterungen.* Tubingen.

Wright, S., Keeling, J. & Gillman, L. (2006). The road from Santa Rosalia: a faster tempo of evolution in tropical climates. *Proceedings of the National Academy of Sciences of the USA, 103*, 7718–7722.

WEBSITES

<http://www.doc.govt.nz/>

New Zealand Department of Conservation.

<http://www.forestandbird.org.nz/>

New Zealand Forest and Bird.

<http://www.massey.ac.nz/massey/research/centres-research/nz-wildlife-health-centre/nz-wildlife-health-centre_home.cfm>

New Zealand Wildlife Health Centre.

<http://www.newzealand.com/travel/media/features/naturesustainable-tourism/nature_tuatara-living-dinosaur_feature.cfm>

Sustainable tourism in New Zealand.

<http://www.wildlife.org.nz/>

Wildlife New Zealand.

READING 26

Political Context of Aotearoa New Zealand

SUSAN SHAW

CHAPTER OVERVIEW

This chapter covers the following topics

- National identity
- Political structures
- The welfare state
- A modified political landscape
- Government agencies
- Professional governance
- Economic perspectives
- Corporate stakeholders
- Legislation and strategy

KEY TERMS

Access
Contracts
District Health Board (DHB)
Egalitarianism
State
Welfare

Health and disability services and the people they serve do not exist in isolation. Aotearoa New Zealand has a heritage of public provision of these services, and the existence of and **access** to them is part of our national identity. The associated government expenditure means there is always interest in the nature and performance of health and disability services, and this often extends to debates about specific services and ways of working. Questions about what to provide and how to evaluate it are complex, and bring many contested concepts into sharp relief, engendering much scrutiny. An appreciation of the various competing interests and structures can assist people who work within and access services provided by the health and disability sector to navigate them.

NATIONAL IDENTITY

The current political system in Aotearoa New Zealand is founded on notions of **egalitarianism** and emancipation. The system of parliament and government is based on the English (Westminster) model. There is one house of parliament that is made up of representatives elected by the public. The nation prides itself on being the first in the world to enable women to vote, and has a significant history of women's participation and influence in political leadership compared to other nations with similar political structures (Korpi & Palme, 2003; Curtin, 2008). Since 1867 the New Zealand parliament has included a number of 'Māori seats' in the structure of its parliament, although debates about issues which are of great significance to Māori (such as ownership of the foreshore and seabed and the status of Te Tiriti o Waitangi) continue and are hotly contested (Humpage, 2006).

The image that a nation and its inhabitants have of itself can be analysed in terms of how it presents and promotes itself to the world. Over the last century Aotearoa New Zealand has gone from presenting itself as a colonised and male-dominated society to, more recently, associating with a sophisticated, progressive and urban image, with a subculture of risk and adventure (Atiljevic & Doorne, 2002).

POLITICAL STRUCTURES OF AOTEAROA

One of the enduring challenges of political systems is tension between two key elements: the sovereignty of the **state** and that of the individual. Political structures can be defined according to how these two elements are perceived and the balance between contested views of them.

The concepts of 'left' and 'right' are often used to provide simplistic descriptions of political perspectives. Right-wing politics is associated with an emphasis on the individual. This perspective holds that people have the talent and resources (physical, intellectual and financial) and motivation to provide for themselves and to take care of their own needs.

Such a view values competition and implies that the fittest and most able members of society will excel and aspire to making a profit and therefore deserve to succeed. When people provide for themselves the state is relieved of responsibility for their wellbeing and the need to provide support and resources. This leads to a reduced need for expenditure on health and disability services and has the potential to increase choice, especially for those who are the most fortunate. Right-wing beliefs contend that anyone is able to achieve well if he or she works hard enough. However, such a success- and profit-driven value system arguably requires that there are winners and losers, and the reality for many is that, no matter how hard they work, they cannot compete financially with others or achieve their goals.

The left-wing perspective holds that resources can and should be managed in a way that ensures access for all. The state is constructed as having the interest of all citizens at its centre and the infrastructure for organising and delivering services and resources. This creates an environment where the state becomes involved in the lives of individuals by mandating the resources that are available, and therefore ultimately defining how people will behave. The left-wing perspective presents the state as well positioned to decide what people need and to ensure that these needs are provided for. An accompanying notion is that of fairness, which implies that all people within the society are treated the same, and experience the same access to services and support. This view promotes the rights of the state as a whole over those of the individual, and positions the state as a primary decision-maker in people's lives. Within a left-wing context there is little scope for individual expression or choice, and likely to be minimal opportunity for people to think or act aspirationally, stifling innovation and creativity. The state can take on a paternalistic role in which it removes the opportunity for people to provide adequately for themselves by providing support, which may in turn restrict their ability or motivation to become more independent.

Any philosophical approach to the planning and provision of resources and services has advantages and disadvantages. All political structures have their merits and challenges, and contextual issues will invariably have an impact on their success or failure. Human nature also plays a part in the success of any political approach to the management of resources. Systems based on left-wing or right-wing perspectives may be undermined by the greed of individuals or groups within society as they strive to compete with one another for wealth, status or profile. It is also true that not all people are motivated or able to make their own way in the world. Both right-wing and left-wing perspectives encompass their own strengths and limitations. In reality it is difficult to identify any 'pure' example of either of these political views. The political landscape of Aotearoa New Zealand references both left- and right-wing concepts, but functions as a relatively centrist state.

THE WELFARE STATE

Many nations established **welfare** systems designed to ensure a basic level of wellbeing. In Aotearoa New Zealand this was based on a principle that all people (not just the poor) are able to access services, such as education and health, provided by the state. Germany can trace this political heritage to the late nineteenth century. The United Kingdom and New Zealand both created welfare structures in relation to health care in the 1940s. Approximately three-quarters of health care provision in Aotearoa New Zealand is provided by the state, while the remaining 25 per cent is privately funded, by individuals or their insurance providers. This universal welfare support is often contrasted with that of the USA, which provides centrally funded health care for approximately one-quarter of the population, including the poor, disadvantaged and defence force veterans, but not generic support for the vast majority of the population. The major criticism of the welfare state is the cost to taxpayers, particularly for those who also pay in addition for private insurance. Other models are effectively in place, with Singapore providing a particularly strong example of balancing access and cost, where the resources are linked directly to the individual rather than the providers of services.

The development of the welfare state in Aotearoa New Zealand in the 1940s became part of a national identity, with strong links to left-wing concepts as it emphasised provision of housing, education and healthcare for all members of society. This provision fitted well with egalitarianism, which had been politically evident in the establishment of the welfare state. Current discussion about 'welfare dependence' is an example of the concern that providing resources and other support for people within society may reduce their ability to engage with wider society.

CASE STUDY 9.1

ART AS A PUBLIC GOOD

A common criticism of conservative (or right-wing) political agendas is that the poor will be further marginalised by limited access to decreasing state resources. It is suggested that benevolence and philanthropy on behalf of the wealthy will contribute to society as they return some of their excess wealth to society for the good of all. Purchasing and providing access to works of art has long been considered a philanthropic endeavour evident throughout history. Art contributes to the wellbeing of a society. While Aotearoa New Zealand is a relatively small nation, we have had a history of philanthropy in the arts, but the future of this is being questioned. Sir James Wallace, patron of the arts, believes that upcoming generations of wealthy New Zealanders show little interest in philanthropy (Herrick, 2011).

A MODIFIED POLITICAL LANDSCAPE

From the mid 1980s a new interpretation of political systems emerged. This was starkly illustrated in Aotearoa New Zealand, with the election in 1984 of the fourth Labour government, led by David Lange. The country had been governed by a National (centre-right) government for the preceding years, and had seen an emphasis on costly large infrastructure projects. There was a palpable interest in moving emphasis back onto social care. In electing a Labour government New Zealanders would have believed the country was going to be led with an emphasis on support services. However, this left-wing government embarked on a programme of economic and social reform that resonated with a right-wing political ideal. This political dynamic came to be known as new-right politics, which may have appeared to be left-wing and yet behaved in a right-wing way. This heralded a period of radical political and social reform for approximately ten years from the mid 1980s. While the incoming Labour government of 1984 encountered a substantial economic crisis, there is debate about whether it required such extensive reform or approaching it in such a determined, unconsulted, fast-paced and culturally inconsiderate manner (Aberbach & Christensen, 2001).

A further conflation of left- and right-wing politics occurred in the 1990s, when the notion of 'third way' politics emerged (Porter & Craig, 2004). New Zealand again was identified with this trend, with the then Prime Minister, Helen Clarke, and the British Prime Minister Tony Blair considered to be trailblazers for this new perspective. This trend attempted to blend social responsibility with acknowledgment of environmental issues, while bringing private sector business values of efficiency and success to public sector government.

CASE STUDY 9.2

MIXED OWNERSHIP

The interest in state and business interaction has led to a proliferation of 'public–private partnerships'. This concept emerged in the UK in 2000 (Spackman, 2002), and implies that services traditionally provided by the state (such as health and education) were fundamentally inefficient and could benefit from the expertise of private sector business. These public–private partnerships have become popular in the United Kingdom, as schools and hospitals have been built, commissioned and managed through them. While this has obviously led to examples of hospitals being built or remodelled to meet needs, there is criticism of the ongoing costs and merits of this perspective. Many institutions carry with them long-term **contracts** that effectively constrain the service and the expenditure of the organisation for many years to come. In some instances it appears that the mixed ownership model has a negative impact on the resources available in the future (Hellowell & Pollock, 2009).

The role of the state in the planning and delivery of healthcare and disability support services is not limited to the provision of buildings and salaries of staff. The state asserts a role as arbiter of information about wellbeing. This information has the potential to be clouded by political agendas as it promotes some opinions and marginalises other expertise. In Aotearoa New Zealand there is a wide range of expertise in the health and disability sector and a good deal of rhetoric about choice. However, medical perspectives and delivery models prevail in terms of funding and provision of health and disability services. Medical practitioners are often positioned and portrayed as the gate-keepers to services.

GOVERNMENT AGENCIES

There are a number of government agencies involved in the planning, delivery and evaluation of our healthcare and disability support sectors. This intense political interest and scrutiny results from the amount of resources expended in these sectors, and cannot be isolated from the concepts of national identity that are connected with the welfare state. Some of these agencies occupy a particularly contentious space, as they wrestle with how to meet the expectations and need for services within the constraints of limited budgets and resources.

Ministry of Health

Within Aotearoa New Zealand the Ministry (previously known as the Department) of Health provides guidance to the public about wellbeing. It may be assumed that the Ministry is politically neutral and provides information, direction and advice based on sound expertise rather than political trend or favour. However, evidence of political agendas pervading the work of government agencies exists; for example, the role of market values in the provision of state housing (Murphy, 2003). Health and disability exist within political and social contexts, as do the science and expertise that are associated with them. It is impossible to dissociate images and information from agendas and current contextual issues. The emphasis on targets to measure health service performance in the United Kingdom, which has established some currency in Aotearoa New Zealand, has been critiqued in relation to its apparent political agenda (Bevan & Hood, 2006).

Knowledge also develops over time, and along with pervading political ideas can lead to changes in advice and information. Official advice published by the New Zealand Department of Health in the middle of the twentieth century about abortion illustrates attitudinal responses to the rights of women, parents and unborn children, and confirms that such action is illegal. The political role of the state includes the development and enforcement of laws, and this flyer suggests that a religiously inspired message about the sanctity of life may have informed the construction of abortion as a crime. In the late 1970s debate raged in relation to legislation specifically addressing contraception, sterilisation and abortion. This is a good illustration of the power of political agendas and processes to have an impact on even the most personal and intimate behaviour and choice of individuals.

National Health Committee

This agency (also known as the National Advisory Committee on Health and Disability) was originally established in 1992 and reformed in 2001. It is charged with providing the Minister of Health with advice and ensuring the public receive good value from the resources invested in the health and disability sectors.

Pharmac

Pharmac is the national pharmaceutical management agency. It is responsible for managing defined resources (financial budgets) to obtain the best value treatment (predominantly medicines) for all New Zealanders. Medicines consume a significant part of the healthcare budget, and there are significant challenges associated with choosing which ones to fund and provide to the population. These decisions can see the real-life crises and challenges of individuals and those they love pitted against the perception that corporations that manufacture and market pharmaceuticals are driven by a business model that emphasises profit.

Accident Compensation Corporation (ACC)

What is now known as the Accident Compensation Corporation came into being in the early 1970s as a result of consultation and debate (Woodhouse, 1967; Bismark & Paterson, 2006). The history of the organisation and the perception of it within the political environment can be seen in how the name of the agency has changed over its history. Initially it was constructed as a benevolent social agency (the Accident Compensation Commission), providing support in the form of expertise and financial contributions for those who became injured. Since then the agency has been redefined as a corporate organisation in the form of an insurance company. The role of ACC includes preventing injury, assessing and managing claims, funding the provision of rehabilitation services and functioning as an insurance company that gathers premiums and pays compensation. The agency also has a mandate to advise the government.

The ACC model of providing support for people with disabilities has received acclaim. However, there is a growing challenge to the disparities in the levels of support available for people according to the cause of their disability. The scheme does not cover injury or disability caused by illness, and as a result two people living with the same degree and type of disability within Aotearoa New Zealand may receive radically different support. For example, a person who is either born without a limb or loses it as a result of disease is not entitled to ACC funding or resources, while a person who loses the corresponding limb in a motor vehicle accident (even if he or she were at fault) is entitled to receive rehabilitation and earnings-related compensation. There is a view that the corporate nature of the agency establishes a culture of mistrust in relation to those receiving services, placing an emphasis on reducing costs (Moon, 2003).

District Health Boards

There have been a number of different structures charged with managing the centrally funded resources that address the needs of local communities. The current framework distributes central funds to **District Health Boards** (DHBs), which are responsible for ensuring the provision of health and disability services within their geographical area. Making decisions at local levels about what services are needed and how they should be provided is an attempt to acknowledge regional variations in needs and access. DHBs are expected to protect, improve and promote health within their populations in ways that effectively meet their needs. There is also an emphasis on integration between services.

Primary Health Organisations

DHBs in turn provide funding to Primary Health Organisations (PHOs). The emphasis on primary care is a particular feature of recent health and disability service development and delivery in Aotearoa New Zealand. Until fairly recently the provision of services emphasised the work of institutions. It was common for people to need to visit a purpose-built place such as a hospital to seek advice or expert care. This approach is a challenge from a cultural perspective, as such institutions are infused with their own cultural dynamics, including rules about how to interact and hierarchical conventions about the status of professionals. In addition, the need for health and disability services is increasing, and institutions are not physically able to meet the demand. The emphasis on primary care values the provision of support in the community, where people are supported to stay in their own environments and engage with health and disability services within the community rather than in institutions. Such an approach values wellness over illness and enables the development of culturally appropriate services. The primary healthcare model purports to bring professionals from a range of disciplines together and to encourage choice and access. In reality, this model centres on a medical view of health and wellbeing, with services mediated by general medical practitioners (GPs), and incorporating pharmacy, nursing, physiotherapy and other professions that are closely aligned with a medical perspective. There is scope for the community and primary care model of health and disability support to incorporate a broader view of health and wellness and to enable choice beyond the traditional medically based perspective.

Health Workforce New Zealand (HWNZ)

One of the biggest challenges for health and disability services across the world is the development of an appropriate workforce. The World Health Organization (WHO) has suggested there is a shortfall in the order of millions of health practitioners across the globe. Health Workforce New Zealand has been established to address the emerging workforce issues across the nation. This involves challenging conventions about scopes of practice and ways of working.

CASE STUDY 9.3

EMERGING ROLES

Health and disability services across the world are faced with dramatic demographic changes that require a radical review of workforce development. There are not (and cannot be) a sufficient number of practitioners to provide the type of care and support that we currently experience in the future. This has led to an emphasis on developing interprofessional education and collaborative practice, where practitioners are taught and expected to interact with one another for the benefit of the service users (see chapters 2 and 18). Workforce issues have also seen the emergence of new groups of practitioners. In the USA the 'physician assistant' (PA) role has existed for many years, and the existence of such a profession has redefined and redistributed some of the work of medical and surgical practitioners.

Health Workforce New Zealand (HWNZ) has funded a trial of physician assistants in Aotearoa New Zealand, and is now funding a project exploring the role of practice assistants in primary care settings. The project itself is the result of a partnership between two tertiary education providers (Unitec Institute of Technology and AUT University) and a PHO (Waitemata Health). The primary care practice assistant (PCPA) role is being developed to define and consolidate a range of various tasks currently carried out by people with a number of roles in general medical practices. These tasks include communicating with patients, taking observations and setting up clinical spaces. It is anticipated that having PCPAs working under the supervision of doctors and practice nurses will enable them in turn to work at the higher end of their scope of practice, and therefore contribute to the efficiency of general practice and primary care.

As with all changes in practice or role developments there are challenges in terms of how existing groups describe themselves and potential tensions about how new roles may encroach on scopes of practice, professional identities and aspirations. There is also a risk that an emphasis on efficiency may lead to a culture in which priority is placed primarily on the speed and cost of the services provided rather than the quality of them and meeting the needs of individual service users in ways that are appropriate and meaningful for them.

PROFESSIONAL GOVERNANCE

There are a number of potential risks associated with the delivery of health and disability services, as those seeking support are often vulnerable and many interventions require specialised skill and expertise. It is common for groups of practitioners to be defined according to their knowledge and skill, and it is in their interests to protect that expertise and the status that is attached to it. As many services are provided directly by the state or by agencies that are in part centrally funded, there is a political interest in maintaining oversight of the quality and potential risks of practice in the health and disability sector. Many professional groups have a long history of organising themselves for the purposes of maintaining a united voice, asserting their point of difference from others and establishing a critical mass that is able to communicate with power brokers and funding agencies (Shaw, 2011). Historically, professions with the highest profiles in the context of Aotearoa New Zealand had specialised legislation that defined their roles and set them apart from other groups of practitioners.

It became clear that other professional groups lacked this recognition, yet warranted the profile and oversight that such legislative acknowledgment afforded. In 2003 the *Health Practitioners Competence Assurance Act* came into being. This legislation repealed a number of Acts for specific groups and identified a substantial list of professionals who were to be registered and governed centrally. This has seen the establishment of responsible authorities (often called registration boards or councils) for a number of groups. These authorities are responsible for defining the scope of practice of the professions and providing oversight in terms of quality. They are also charged with the management of risk, and it is assumed that this ensures the safety of the public as they receive health or disability services provided by registered practitioners. The governance of these groups is mandated by central government, and is an example of how government agencies are involved in the design and delivery of service. HWNZ has indicated its interest in consolidating the administrative functions of regulatory authorities in order to make efficiency gains (HWNZ, June 2011).

The concept of governance is also used in relation to the management of clinical services. Health and disability services in Aotearoa New Zealand have experienced various models of leadership and management, and these have attempted to balance the tensions between the expertise of business management and clinical expertise and decision-making. The concept of clinical governance is now widely used, and conveys the belief that all stakeholders (including patients and practitioners) should be involved in the planning, management and evaluation of health and disability services.

ECONOMIC PERSPECTIVES

At the heart of many political principles and actions is the need to balance limited resources with the provision of services. This requires making judgments about what will be delivered and how, inevitably leading to situations where people in need miss out on support. Within the context of the health and disability sector, there is an unlimited need for expenditure, so structures are put in place to consider the use and delivery of resources.

CASE STUDY 9.4

BUSINESS, PUBLIC HEALTH AND THE PASSAGE OF TIME

One of the most striking examples of knowledge changing over time illustrates how political, health, professional and corporate messages have changed in relation to smoking. In the middle of the twentieth century cigarette smoking was popularised. Messages about smoking helping people to relax and socialise prevailed (Street, 2004). Health professionals were depicted in advertisements promoting smoking, and public health advice in Aotearoa New Zealand stated that it was not harmful to health. Knowledge and advice about smoking has since changed dramatically, and ironically, health professionals still feature in the messages but as experts stating that smoking is dangerous and they should be consulted to help people avoid or quit smoking in the interests of their health.

Recent debates in relation to smoking and public health focus on how information about smoking is conveyed. Advertising is a focus for discussions about how acceptable and accessible cigarettes are to the public and how people may be encouraged to smoke or accept smoking. Limitations have been placed on how products that are considered harmful are represented in the media and this has led to limitations on when and how advertisements are presented and, in particular, restrictions on how alcohol and cigarettes are promoted. In the past, there has been an emphasis on allowing advertising to inform the public about these substances while limiting specific influencing concepts such as connections between glamour, popularity and success, and the use of them. A current debate centres on the interest in requiring that cigarettes are sold in plain packaging. This is an extension of removing them from display and therefore reducing the opportunity for them to be promoted because it is believed this may reduce smoking. However, it is argued that promotional devices such as brand names, labels, and advertising images and messages are the intellectual property of businesses promoting legal products and that limiting the publication and presentation of these devices is breaching the rights of companies to promote their products. The history of how cigarettes and smoking have been portrayed, promoted, debated and controlled provides an interesting commentary on relationships and tensions between governments, business, health and individual choice. Health professionals have gone from promoting smoking to passing judgment on it, and holding the expertise on why and how to limit smoking and its effects.

Figure 9.1: Don't smoke too young

ISSUED BY THE DEPT. OF HEALTH
If you want to excel—
DON'T SMOKE TOO YOUNG!
Once acquired, the smoking habit is hard to break—don't acquire it too young if you want to excel in sport and learning.
Here is the case for tobacco smoking: for and against:—
FOR: It helps you to relax; it takes the strain off tired nerves and induces a feeling of relief from fatigue and irritability: it is an aid to sociability.
AGAINST: Excessive smoking can irritate the throat and lungs, shorten the breath; upset the action of the heart; set up and perpetuate catarrhal conditions and is a cause of morning cough. (There is no proof that it can cause permanent damage to lungs or heart, or induce cancer).
FACTS: Tobacco smoking is habit forming. The "fragrant weed" harbours poisons—nicotine and carbon monoxide. The nicotine content of dry tobacco smoke averages 0.6 per cent. Not very much, but a heavy smoker gets a little nicotine lots of times each day. And the effect is cumulative. Inhaling smoke into the lungs allows about 85 per cent. of the nicotine to be absorbed.
ADVICE: (1) Moderation in the use of tobacco by adults.
(2) Abstinence in adolescence—no tobacco until 21 years of age should be the rule. It does retard mental and physical achievement.
(3) Minimum inhalation.
HELP YOURSELF TO KEEP FIT!
KEEP THIS ANNOUNCEMENT FOR FUTURE REFERENCE.
FOR A HEALTHIER NATION

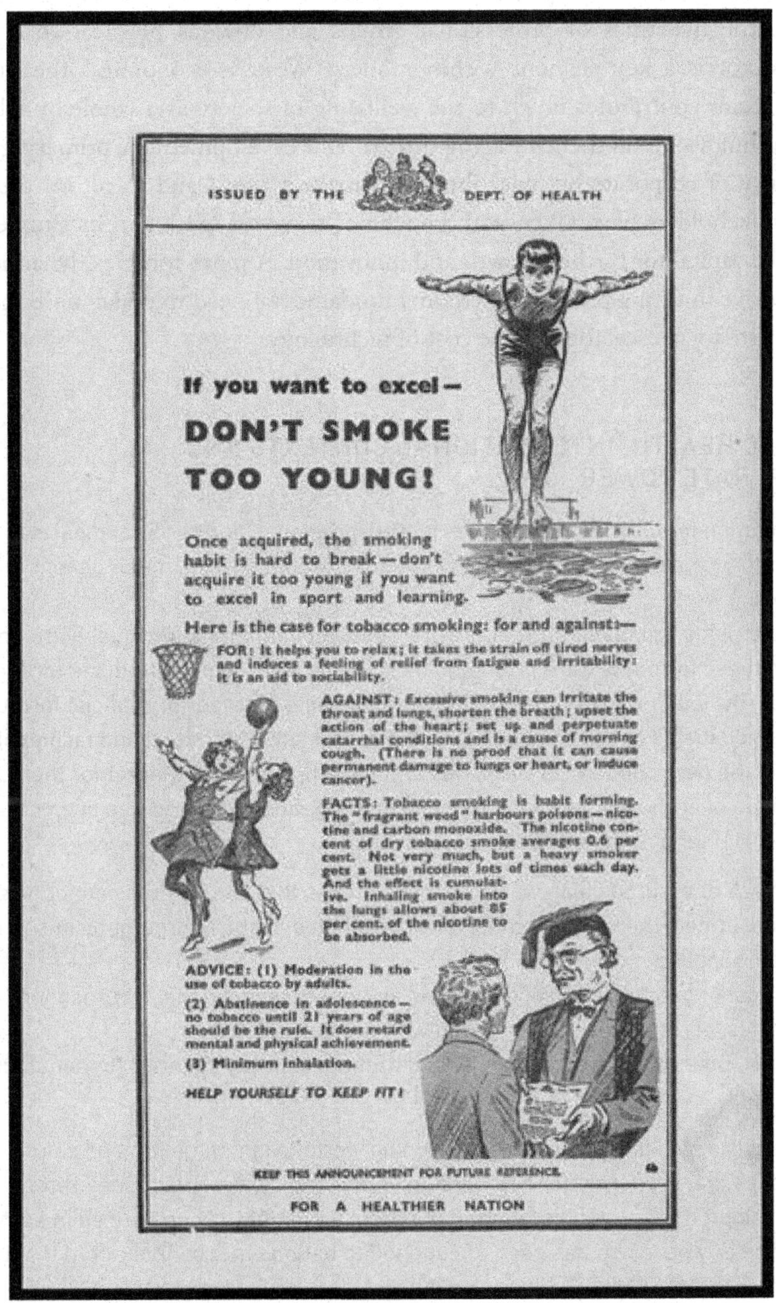

Source: *Don't Smoke Too Young*. New Zealand Department of Health, 1945 (Eph-B-HEALTH-NZ-DH-1945-01). Reproduced with permission from the Alexander Turnbull Library.

CORPORATE INFLUENCES

The ability of agencies and agendas to influence resources and decision-making is not limited to the dynamics of professional groups and obvious political structures. The business sector is a key element within modern Western economies. The business or corporate sector contributes much to the wellbeing of society as a whole by taking risks, supporting innovation and encouraging growth and development. A primary goal of the vast majority of corporate organisations is to make a profit and to return the financial risk that stakeholders have taken with benefits. This profit motive in its simplest format provides the capital for further growth and innovation. A more complex dynamic emerges when the drive to turn a profit is based on a fundamental need to make more money. This can contribute to an escalation in the cost of technology.

CASE STUDY 9.5

PUBLIC HEALTH, INTERNATIONAL CONTEXTS AND CORPORATE POWER

It is common for people and agencies in well-developed and resourced parts of the world to assume their decisions or products would have as much benefit in the developing world.

One striking example of this is the promotion of infant milk formula. For a period of time these formulas were promoted as scientifically superior products for feeding babies. This led to women abandoning breastfeeding in favour of artificial formula. When the benefits of breast milk became more widely understood and fashionable again in the developed world there was a need to find another market for them. The promotion of artificial infant milk formula in the developing world has been criticised (Boyd, 2011) for a number of reasons, including:

- the lack of assured clean water supplies means that the formula cannot be safely reconstituted, therefore the milk is contaminated by the microorganisims in local water supplies
- the cost of purchasing milk formula is an unnecessary financial burden for families, especially when compared with breastfeeding
- human breast milk is nutritionally and immunologically superior to manufactured formula.

There is also a tendency in the developing world to ignore health and safety messages that may emerge in relation to or accompany products. One example of this is the promotion and distribution of products that have been banned in some countries or whose use has been questioned to nations that cannot afford the 'better' alternative or lack the legislative or quality control infrastructure to evaluate or restrict such activities. The sale of poisons that have been banned in the developed world to developing nations is an example of this (Klenovsek & Mesko, 2011).

LEGISLATION AND STRATEGY

The most obvious forum for political messages about health and disability can be found in legislation that is passed by parliament and the strategy documents produced by relevant departments and government agencies. There is very specific legislation in Aotearoa New Zealand that relates to the work of practitioners and the quality of practice.

Table 9.1: Examples of legislation relating to health and disability sector practitioners in Aotearoa New Zealand

Legislation	Purpose
Health and Disability Commissioners Act 1994	Outlines rights of service users and responsibilities of practitioners
Privacy Act 1993	Outlines rules relating to the collection and use of personal information
Health Practitioners Competence Assurance Act 2003	Establishes the mechanism for formal governance of specific groups of practitioners (registration boards and councils)

Sources include Health Information Privacy Code (1994, 2008)

The Ministry of Health makes information available about the goals for the health and disability sector. This information often takes the form of strategy documents that are developed following consultation, and outline the current issues and responses to them within the context of Aotearoa New Zealand.

Table 9.2: Examples of strategy documents relating to the health and disability sector

Strategy	Web link for more information
New Zealand Health Strategy (2000)	<http://www.moh.govt.nz/moh.nsf/indexmh/new-zealand-health-strategy-2000>
Primary Healthcare Strategy (2001)	<http://www.moh.govt.nz/moh.nsf/indexmh/primary-health-care-strategy-2001>
New Zealand Disability Strategy (2001)	<http://www.odi.govt.nz/nzds/>
He Korowai Oranga: Māori Health Strategy (2002)	<http://www.moh.govt.nz/moh.nsf/pagesmh/2292>
The Pacific Health and Disability Action Plan (2002)	<http://www.moh.govt.nz/publications/pacificactionplan>
Good Oral Health for All, for Life: The Strategic Vision for Oral Health in New Zealand (2006)	<http://www.moh.govt.nz/moh.nsf/by+unid/229C4904287A71EDCC2571D3007BE4BE?Open>

SUMMARY

Within the health and disability sector tensions readily emerge in relation to how resources are developed and delivered. Challenges relate to fundamental differences between stakeholders as to the importance of health and wellbeing, access to services and funding. The welfare state, so much a part of the psyche of Aotearoa New Zealand, is grounded on the concept of egalitarianism, leading to a widely held belief that all people are entitled to the same services and that they will be of the highest quality. There is a conundrum when the majority of the society contributes to the services that are available to all and therefore everyone believes they have access. Such wide access to services may be criticised for overly advantaging those who are able to afford to pay for services, as they have more choice than others and perhaps their needs should not be a priority for publicly funded services.

Asking critical questions about the motives underlying programmes and initiatives may help to uncover the agenda of those developing or resourcing them. Any analysis of issues should involve critical questions about who the stakeholders are (including corporations, government, the public, professional groups and service providers) and which groups stand to benefit most from the outcome.

CRITICAL QUESTIONS

Cultural lens

- **Why** are determinants of health experienced differently by Māori?
- **Why** is culture on its own a simplistic explanation for health inequalities?

Social lens

- **What** elements in society converge to impact on health and wellbeing—how and why?

Gender lens

- **Why** are men and women differently represented in statistics about obesity and overweight?

Political lens

- **What** is the purpose of national policy and strategy, and what influences its impact and effectiveness?

Moral lens

- **What** are the challenges and inherent considerations in identifying statistics in relation to cultural groups?

Media lens

- **How** is the health of Indigenous people presented in the international media, and what purpose does this serve?
- **How** are people with disabilities presented in the international media?

FURTHER READING

Gauld, R. (2009). *Revolving Doors: New Zealand's Health Reforms: The Continuing Saga* (2nd edn). Wellington: Institute of Policy Studies Health Services Research Centre, Victoria University of Wellington.

REFERENCES

Aberbach, J.D. & Christensen, T. (2001). Radical reform in New Zealand: crisis, windows of opportunity, rational actors. *Public Administration*, *79*(2), 403–422.

Atiljevic, I. & Doorne, S. (2002). Representing New Zealand tourism, imagery and ideology. *Annals of Tourism Research*, *29*(5), 648–667.

Bevan, G. & Hood, C. (2006). What's measured is what matters; targets and gaming in the English public health system. *Public Administration*, *84*(3), 517–538.

Bismark, M. & Paterson, R. (2006). No fault compensation in New Zealand: harmonizing injury compensation, provider accountability and patient safety. *Health Affairs*, *25*(1), 278–283.

Boyd, C. (2011). The Nestle infant formula controversy and a strange web of subsequent business scandals. *Journal of Business Ethics* (in press).

Curtin, J. (2008). Women, political leadership and substantive representation: the case of New Zealand. *Parliamentary Affairs*, *61*(3), 490–504.

Health Workforce New Zealand (HWNZ) (2011). *Stakeholder Bulletin*, June, p. 2 <http://healthworkforce.govt.nz/sites/all/files/HWNZ%20stakeholder%20bulletin%20 July%202011.pdf>.

Hellowell, M. & Pollock, A.M. (2009). The private financing of NHS hospitals: politics, policy and practice. *Economic Affairs*, *29*(1) 13–19.

Herrick, L. (2011, 6 June). Knight worries about art funding. *New Zealand Herald* <http:// www.nzherald.co.nz/nz/news/article.cfm?c_id=1&objectid=10730486>.

Humpage, L. (2006). An 'inclusive society': a 'leap forward' for Maori in New Zealand? *Critical Social Policy*, *26*, 220–242.

Klenovsek, A. & Mesko, G. (2011). International waste trafficking: preliminary explorations. In NATO, *Understanding and Managing Threats to the Environment in South Eastern Europe Understanding and Managing Threats to the Environment in South Eastern Europe NATO Science for Peace and Security Series C: Environmental Security, 2011, 2*, 79–99.

Korpi, W. & Palme, J. (2003). New politics and class politics in the context of austerity and globalization: welfare state regress in 18 countries, 1975–1995. *American Political Science Review*, *97*(3), 425–446.

Ministry of Health (2000). *The New Zealand Health Strategy*. Wellington: Ministry of Health.

Ministry of Health (2001). *Primary Healthcare Strategy*. Wellington, New Zealand: Ministry of Health.

Ministry of Health (2006). *Good Oral Health for All, for Life: The Strategic Vision for Oral Health in New Zealand.* Wellington: Ministry of Health.

Moon, M. (2003). *Pain Poppies: The Human Ecology of Chronic Pain.* Lyttleton: InPress.

Murphy, L. (2003). To market and back: housing policy and state housing in New Zealand. *Geojournal*, *59*, 119–126.

Porter, D. & Craig, D. (2004). The Third Way and the Third World: poverty reduction and social inclusion in the rise of 'inclusive' liberalism. *Review of International Political Economy*, *11*(2), 387–423.

Shaw, S.M. (2011). Whence, why, how, and whither 'responsible authorities': professional registration boards and councils. In K. Tudor (ed.), *The Turning Tide: Pluralism and Partnership in Psychotherapy in Aotearoa New Zealand* (pp. 96–105). Auckland: LC Publications.

Spackman, M. (2002). Public-private partnerships: lessons from the British approach. *Economic Systems*, *26*, 283–301.

Street, A. (2004). Ask your doctor: the construction of smoking in advertising posters produced in 1946 and 2004. *Nursing Inquiry*, *11* (4), 226–237.

Woodhouse, O. (1967). *Royal Commission on Compensation for Personal Injury in New Zealand.* Wellington: Government of New Zealand.

WEBSITES

<http://www.hdc.org.nz>

The website for the Health and Disability Commissioner.

<http://www.healthsponsorship.co.nz>

The website for Health Sponsorship Council.

<http://www.moh.govt.nz>

The website for all the Ministry of Health documents.

<http://www.moh.govt.nz/moh.nsf/indexmh/Publications-Strategies>

Ministry of Health Strategy documents.

<http://www.nhc.health.govt.nz/>

National Health Committee.

<http://www.nzhis.govt.nz>

The website for the New Zealand Health Information Service.

<http://www.pharmac.govt.nz>

The website for Pharmaceutical Management Agency Ltd (PHARMAC).

Social Context

SUSAN SHAW

CHAPTER OVERVIEW

This chapter covers the following topics

- How people group themselves
- Defining difference
- Social constructs
- Culture and wellbeing
- Justice and fairness
- The power of relationship

KEY TERMS

Class
Community
Deviant
Diversity
Dominance
Equality
Equity
Eugenics
Health Reforms
Othering
Social capital
Society
Therapeutic relationship
Whānau Ora

Humans are social beings: they seek out and find themselves interacting with others in the course of their lives as they work, socialise and meet various needs. On any given day people associate with those around them in relation to their work, family, interests and cultural heritage. An appreciation of difference, **dominance** and **diversity** is essential to understanding why people respond and engage in any particular situation.

HOW PEOPLE GROUP THEMSELVES

Sociology is the study of how people interact with one another. In any **society** groups are defined and afforded status in relation to how their role or contribution is perceived or valued. Societies define norms, and individuals or groups who function outside of these can be marginalised, which invariably leads to them being less valued than their counterparts who conform. One of the fundamental elements within a society is that of **community**. Interaction between people within their communities creates **social capital** (Onyx & Bullen, 2000).

There are a number of ways in which people are stratified within society. These may relate to income, influence or other indicators of status, such as title and position. In many societies the place of individuals in the social hierarchy is defined before they are born, according to tradition and religious or **class** boundaries. Aotearoa New Zealand, a relatively young society, is known for its class mobility, as children often find themselves participating in more esteemed roles than their ancestors. This egalitarianism is evident throughout the recent history of the nation and is considered to be part of the national psyche. Concepts of class or caste may be used to define distinct differences between groups and their place in society. It has long been believed that Aotearoa New Zealand is a classless society. In reality there are clear and growing differences between those who are well resourced in this nation and those who are not.

CASE STUDY 10.1

DEFINING NEW ZEALANDERS

There are a number of characteristics that are used to define New Zealanders. The prevailing concepts are linked to a pioneering spirit and a lack of distinctions between groups of people based on their status or income. Some of these elements are promulgated in messages such as 'number 8 wire' and 'she'll be right'.

A lighthearted but insightful look at the characteristics of New Zealanders can be found in a book and website that identified New Zealand 'tribes':

- The North Shore Tribe: Achieving
- The Grey Lynn Tribe: Intellectual
- The Balclutha Tribe: Staunch
- The Remuera Tribe: Entitled
- The Otara Tribe: Community

- The Raglan Tribe: Freespirited
- The Cuba Street Tribe: Avant-Garde
- The Papatoetoe Tribe: Unpretentious.

(Caldwell & Brown, 2007)

There are a number of constructs that can be used to define difference within society. Four elements are often used to denote wellbeing in Aotearoa New Zealand: housing, health, employment and education. In the 1970s the Elley Irving scale was used in Aotearoa New Zealand to explain the structure of society. This scale was devised by analysing 500 occupations (Congalton, 1954; Elley & Irving, 1985) and identifying five groups. Class mobility was evident when children grew up to occupy a 'higher' position than their parents had held. More recently, the New Zealand Deprivation Index (Crampton et al., 2004) has been employed to analyse position in society from census data. The elements used within this index, which give insight into the development and predominant values in society, include: communication, income, employment, transport, support, qualifications, home ownership and the degree of crowding in living spaces. Socioecomonic status (SES) has a direct impact on the level of choice and access to services and expertise that people may have (Shaw et al., 2005). It is also true that social support systems and connectedness contribute to the overall wellbeing of society (Panelli & Tipa, 2007).

CASE STUDY 10.2

OFFICIAL INFORMATION: THE CENSUS

Every five years a census is undertaken to gather information about New Zealanders. This is an official process in which people are required to provide responses to very specific questions at a particular point in time. The New Zealand Deprivation Index is currently used in the design and analysis of census questions.

The formal nature of the census implies that it will take place regardless of other contextual factors, but in the last century the New Zealand government has postponed two planned census events. This first happened in 1941 during World War II, and more recently in 2011 following the major earthquake in Christchurch on 22 February. In both of these instances the personal experiences of New Zealanders and the impact of them on wider society was considered to be so significant that it would be inappropriate to impose the structure and requirements of a census on the public.

DEFINING DIFFERENCE

It is common and convenient to think of Aotearoa New Zealand as an egalitarian society with minimal differences between groups in society. However, the reality is that there are some significant differences within this society, and as a result people experience radically different levels of, and access to, care and wellbeing. The most obvious distinctions are apparent in relation to cultural heritage, disability and immigrant status.

Māori are the Indigenous first people of Aotearoa. The heritage of Māori prior to European colonisation was not of one defined group but of many separate nations interacting with one another in terms of trade and social and political development. Despite the presence of a number of imperial powers, Māori chose to sign a treaty with the British Crown in 1840 with the intention of maintaining sovereignty and governance over Māori while enabling British rule and leadership to govern the settlers. The expectation was that Māori would receive the benefits of British subjects, therefore it is reasonable to expect that they would enjoy the same health status as the settlers. As the health and disability sectors developed the emphasis on Western science, English language and culture and purpose-built institutions alienated Māori in many ways. While it could be argued that services are available to all, the predominant culture within these institutions alienates Māori worldviews and, along with deteriorating socioeconomic status, has contributed to substantially poorer health outcomes for Māori.

CASE STUDY 10.3

INDIGENOUS EXPERIENCES AFTER THE TREATY

Comments from Māori leaders about governance give insights into Indigenous experiences of living in Aotearoa New Zealand following the signing of Te Tiriti o Waitangi in 1840.

Hone Heke was the first of more than forty northern chiefs to sign the Treaty of Waitangi. By September, more than 500 chiefs in different parts of the country had signed. The treaty guaranteed Māori 'all the rights and privileges of British subjects'.

A visible message from Māori about their experience following the signing of Te Tiriti was created when Hone Heke cut down the flagpole in Kororareka in the Bay of Islands. Some maintain that the act was a public challenge to the British Crown. On 19 July 1844, Hone Heke wrote to the Governor explaining that he had made the flagpole for the native flag and that the Europeans had not paid for it (*The New Zealander*, 1845), which explains why he felt he had the right to protest in this way (see <http://freepages.genealogy.rootsweb.ancestry.com/~nzbound/nz1845.htm> for extracts from the weekly newspaper *The New Zealander*).

Other comments from Pakeha leaders provide insights into attitudes towards Indigenous Māori that illustrated a less than an equitable partnership. Two particular examples can be found in records of a parliamentary debate in 1867 about native schools (10 September):

- Hugh Carleton (school inspector) asserted that 'things had now come to pass that it was necessary either to exterminate the Natives or to civilise them' (New Zealand Parliamentary Debates, 1867 1, part 2, p. 862).
- Major Heaphy (VC) stated that 'Any expenditure in this direction would be true economy, as the more the Natives were educated the less would be the future expenditure in police and gaols' (New Zealand Parliamentary Debates, 1867 1, part 2, p. 863).

While it has been suggested that New Zealanders are particularly accommodating (Ward & Masgoret, 2008), there is evidence that non-European immigrants can experience health and disability support services in ways that are confusing and alienating. These experiences have an impact on practitioners and would-be service users. Immigrant practitioners may have knowledge and skills but lack the local understanding of working within the context of Aotearoa New Zealand. For example, there are tensions within nursing about what constitutes good quality nursing and among medical laboratory scientists about the scope of their role. Nursing practice in Aotearoa New Zealand is associated with technical knowledge and skill and a strong ethic of care, which encompasses the provision of intimate and personal care as part of comprehensive and professional practice. Nurses from other nations may not value the provision of basic care in the same way, as they are familiar with families providing such support and consider it a demeaning and unnecessary role for professional nurses. Medical laboratory scientists are educated in Aotearoa New Zealand to work primarily in laboratories without patient interaction. However, some immigrant medical laboratory scientists have studied and practised in environments where the role is considered from a more holistic perspective, where practitioners may take blood samples and then be responsible for preparing and interpreting the tests that result from them.

There are differences in health status in relation to geographical location. People living in poorer communities are likely to experience poorer health and life expectancy than those who are well resourced. These analyses invariably include ethnic and socioeconomic differences, and critique the ways funding is calculated and dispersed throughout society. It has been suggested (see Chapter 9) that New Zealand has at least partially abandoned the principles of universal welfare in favour of a market-driven approach to health (Pearce & Dorling, 2006).

Disabled people experience marginalisation in this society, as they are fundamentally singled out for their difference. People living with disabilities are not necessarily unwell, and yet services and support provided for them are predominantly funded and provided within the context of the healthcare sector. This defines them as in need of care rather than support, and implies that medical and scientific expertise may benefit them by way of a cure or treatment. For a large proportion of the disabled community, the emphasis is on engaging equitably within society rather than conforming to a sick role. There is great power in labelling people as **deviant**, as it creates a space for individuals and groups to be defined as less valued than others. Valued social roles are attributed to those who are seen as contributing to society, and this tends to be related to financial contribution; for example, employees and employers are considered to make a positive contribution as they pay tax. People who are considered to make a reduced contribution include beneficiaries, as they are constructed as costing rather than contributing to society. Having a less valued social role, such as that of a beneficiary, positions people as being less entitled to respect or support than those with 'positive' social roles, who are seen as contributing to society.

CASE STUDY 10.4

IDENTIFYING PEOPLE AS DEVIANT

Wolfensberger (1972) identified a number of historical misconceptions of people with disabilities. Any labels that may be attributed to people can be considered a marker of deviance, therefore setting them apart as 'others' within society.

The labels associated with these misconceptions include viewing people as:

- menace
- sick
- an object of pity, charity, ridicule or dread
- subhuman
- holy innocent
- eternal child.

There is a tendency to categorise people according to self and other (or 'them' and 'us'). This **othering** is particularly problematic within the health and disability sector, as it provides opportunities to marginalise individuals and groups within society. Identifying people as deviant within is particularly powerful, as it can establish people as less worthy than others. People may be considered deviant when they do not comply with the norms or stereotypes that prevail in society.

SOCIAL CONSTRUCTS

There are a number of concepts that have been used to describe Aotearoa New Zealand as a society. These concepts are primarily technical descriptions, but that they exist and are used means that to an extent they serve to define elements of our society.

The concept of **eugenics** was popular between the mid 1800s and 1900s. Promoted as a scientifically based view, it held that races could and should be kept pure by avoiding cross-cultural marriage and reproduction. Scientific papers were developed about this. Aotearoa New Zealand had its own high-profile proponent of these views. Sir Truby King is heralded as the founder of the New Zealand Plunket Society. The increased survival and wellbeing of women and children, at a time when giving birth and being born was a risky endeavour, has been at least in part linked to the emergence of Plunket. However, there is evidence that the work of Plunket only made positive differences for the settler families and did not have the same impact on Māori communities. Sir Truby's eugenic beliefs (Richardson, 2004) were closely linked to his personal view that the settlers should outbreed the natives. The view that some races are purer than others and have more right to wealth and success is no longer tolerated in the majority of societies today.

Messages about differences and similarities between people help define society. They encompass concepts of **equity** and **equality**, which are often conflated or used interchangeably. Equity is about fairness and impartiality, while equality relates to being equal, of the same size and value, having the same rights and status.

CASE STUDY 10.5

VALUING SUPPORT ROLES

Two examples of the resources available to support disabled members of our society have recently gained a public profile and raise questions about how equitable things really are.

The provision of resources and support for people who have been injured in accidents is overseen by the Accident Compensation Commission (ACC). There have been a number of changes to this scheme over the years, and there are examples of people receiving different levels of service from ACC when compared to others according to the rules that were in place at the time they were injured. However, more dramatically, the support that is available for people who become disabled as a result of injury (by ACC) is radically different to that provided (by the Ministry of Health) for those who are disabled as a result of illness.

The provision of community-based residential support often requires that staff are present in the homes of the disabled people they work with overnight. Following an extended debate about the role of caregivers who stay overnight in residential services it has been decided that they are entitled to be paid for the hours that they spend overnight at work. While much of the immediate debate has centred on the cost of paying for this work (and addressing the historical loss of income), there is a much more significant issue involved: the value that is placed on the provision for support of disabled members of New Zealand society.

CULTURE AND WELLBEING

Health and wellbeing encompass all the aspects of human existence, including physical, mental, emotional, spiritual and cultural. The importance of these elements is evident in studies that link wellbeing to a sense of attachment to social space (Witten et al., 2001; Wiles et al., 2009) and the importance of social engagement (Kaariaainen & Lehtonen, 2006). Modern and scientific views of people and their health often deconstruct human existence into disparate components. There is an increasing appreciation that the provision of good quality services requires that support is meaningful for those receiving it. There is also a growing sense that health and disability services should focus on the strengths and abilities of individuals, and value diversity rather than a negative or deficit-based perspective that emphasises problems and then asserts the ability to cure them.

CASE STUDY 10.6

A SPIRITUAL PERSPECTIVE ON PHYSICAL PAIN

An elderly man was admitted to a neurological ward for care near the end of his life. Members of his community (ashram) provided companionship, food and physical care for him while he was in hospital. His prevailing symptom was severe pain and the nursing staff responded to this by offering him medication, which he generally declined.

One evening a student nurse was particularly concerned about his wellbeing and asked him why he would not accept the offers of analgaesia. His response was to warmly and quietly suggest that the staff had failed to notice that while he was in pain this was of little significance to him and he was primarily focused on his spiritual wellbeing.

One of the enduring arguments about access to services and the wellbeing of Māori, as the Indigenous people of Aotearoa New Zealand, is that the same services are available across the community, therefore if people or groups do not appear to benefit from them it is a matter of choice, and perhaps demonstrates a lack of responsibility. Such perspectives disregard the importance of culture in the lives of people, and experiences of discrimination (Harris et al., 2006). They also demonstrate a tendency for people to not recognise the power dynamics within society, and in particular for those in dominant groups to overlook difference and diversity. The history of marginalising Māori perspectives, which has been evident in the loss of te reo and traditions such as tohunga, illustrates a lack of regard for cultural identity and wellbeing, and ultimately contributes to reduced participation in health and disability support services. The development of **Whānau Ora** is significant, as it seeks to connect separate support services and agencies with people within a culturally based philosophy of care and support.

CASE STUDY 10.7

WHĀNAU ORA

Whānau Ora is an inclusive approach to providing services and opportunities to whānau across New Zealand. It empowers whānau as a whole, rather than focusing separately on individual whānau members and their problems.

Whānau Ora will work in a range of ways, influenced by the approach the whānau chooses to take. Whānau Ora is not a one-size-fits-all approach. It is deliberately designed to be flexible to meet family needs.

'Stop the scenario of five Toyota Corollas in the driveway one each for the Plunket nurse, the truancy officer, the social worker, the probation officer and the district nurse' (*New Zealand Listener*, 2010, p. 5).

JUSTICE AND FAIRNESS

The perception of how people are treated can be used to judge a society. This extends to how the least advantaged members of the community are valued and supported, and how those who breach the trust or safety of the community are treated. It is important not to assume that the presence of a legal system automatically correlates with a fair and just society.

CASE STUDY 10.8

RESTORATIVE JUSTICE

In appreciation of the cultural contexts that people experience, new approaches to responding to crime were initiated in Aotearoa New Zealand. This enabled facilitated interactions between the victims and perpetrators of crime and the ability for whānau to be involved in the process.

A study comparing restorative justice programmes to traditional non-restorative approaches, in relation to offender satisfaction, restitution, compliance, and recidivism, found restorative programmes to be more effective.

(Latmer et al., 2005)

THE POWER OF RELATIONSHIP

The importance of social structures and relationships between people extends beyond the interactions that take place between patients and practitioners to the relationship between agencies and the public. Managing large-scale development and delivery of services can create an environment in which people are categorised into generic groups, encouraging generalisations about what they need. This compromises those who associate with marginalised groups and devalues diversity within society. While change can be imposed on people, consultation and engagement with communities can lead to more enduring change (Greenaway & Witten, 2005).

Power dynamics among professionals exist within and between groups of practitioners, and generally serve to maintain their identity and position within society. In some ways these dynamics create subcultures within society as they are defined by language and rules which are often only fully understood by those who are initiated into the groups. The more obvious distinctions are apparent in the use of titles, with the use of the title Dr being of particular interest in Aotearoa New Zealand, as it is conferred on medical practitioners who do not hold doctoral qualifications.

CASE STUDY 10.9

PROFESSIONAL INTERACTIONS

The United Kingdom has a health system providing a wide range of care to all members of society that has some similarities with the New Zealand model. In the middle of the last decade a documentary was screened in the UK in which a business leader (Sir Gerry Robinson) spent some time in a large National Health Service (NHS) hospital in Rotherham. The basic concept was that his business expertise could assist with increasing the efficency of the hospital. A year later a follow-up documentary was screened, revisiting parts of the first documentary. There are a number of perspectives from which to analyse these documentaries. One interesting perspective comes from considering statements made by practitioners about managers.

Consultant surgeon:

> I am the surgeon and I'm the one who is going to implement it. I know the details and ins and outs of everything. I don't claim I'm better than the general manager or other people but I know better than anyone else.

Junior doctor:

> Most of the managers here, and I can't think of a single one, has an MBA. Without being derogatory they probably have 3 O-levels and are managing people with 5 or 6 degrees each.

(*Can Gerry Robinson Fix the NHS?*, BBC, 2006)

Despite the need within health professional groups to define and distinguish themselves from others there is increasing interest in finding ways for practitioners to interact meaningfully. Service users do not make fine distinctions between the roles of particular practitioners. Patients and service users are likely to be able to identify which staff answer their questions adequately and interact with them in helpful ways; they are unlikely to appreciate the finer details of the role differences, territories and boundaries that exist and are maintained between named groups of practitioners (Sullivan, 2000; Willis, 2006).

The social nature of humans is an important factor in care and support. While technology and expertise play a role in the quality of service provision, the quality of interaction between practitioners and service users cannot be underestimated. When people feel respected and understood they are more likely to access services. Once people access services, social concepts such as the **therapeutic relationship** play a role in quality delivery at a very human level.

SUMMARY

Humans are by nature social beings; they constantly interact with others and social wellbeing has an impact on the general wellbeing of individuals, groups and the wider communities and society of which they are a part. However, interest in the values of business and profit-driven motives has clouded the notion of Aotearoa New Zealand as a fair, equal and classless society. There is evidence that culture, ethnic background, socioeconomic status and disability all have an impact on the wellbeing of individuals, as these elements all have an impact on the access to and meaningfulness of services. Good quality social engagement contributes to effective leadership and management, communication between practitioners and therapeutic interaction with service users.

CRITICAL QUESTIONS

Cultural lens

- **What** responsibility should there be for the impact of imported diseases on Indigenous populations?

Social lens

- **How** does the welfare state benefit society?

Gender lens

- **What** professional roles do women dominate, and why?

Political lens

- **What** is the purpose, impact and legacy of the 1990s **health reforms**?

Moral lens

- **How** do we balance human and resource considerations?

Media lens

- **What** role does the media play in representing egalitarianism?

FURTHER READING

Coxon, E., Jenkins, K., Marshall, J. & Massey, L. (1994). *The Politics of Learning and Teaching in Aotearoa New Zealand*. Palmerston North: Dunmore Press.

McLauchlan, G. (2012). *The Passionless People Revisited*. Auckland: David Bateman.

Moon, P. (2001). *Hone Heke Nga Puhi Warrior*. Auckland: David Ling Publishing.

REFERENCES

Caldwell, J. & Brown, C. (2007). *8 Tribes: The Hidden Classes of New Zealand.* Auckland: Wicked Little Books.

Can Gerry Robinson fix the NHS? (2006). Lord, D. (producer). London: BBC.

Congalton, A.A. (1954). Social grading of occupations in New Zealand. *British Journal of Sociology, 4*(1), 45–59.

Crampton, P., Salmond, C. & Kirkpatrick, R. (2004). *Degrees of Deprivation in New Zealand: An Atlas of Socioeconomic Difference: 2001 Edition.* Auckland: David Bateman.

Elley W.B. & Irving, I.C. (1985). The Elley-Irving socio-economic index: 1981 census revision. *New Zealand Journal of Educational Studies, 20,* 115–128.

Greenaway, A. & Witten, K. (2005). Meta-analysing community action projects in Aotearoa New Zealand. *Community Development Journal, 4*(2), 143–159.

Harris, R., Tobias, M., Jeffreys, M., Waldergrave, K., Karlsen, S. & Nazroo, J. (2006). Effects of self-reported racial discrimination and deprivation on Maori health and inequalities in New Zealand: a cross-sectional study. *Lancet, 368*(9529), 44–52.

Kaariaainen, J. & Lehtonen, H. (2006). The variety of social capital in welfare state regimes: a comparative study of 21 countries. *European Societies, 8*(1), 27–57.

Latmer, J., Dowden, C. & Muise, D. (2005). The effectiveness of restorative justice practices: a meta-analysis. *Prison Journal, 85*(2), 127–144.

New Zealander (1845). Narrative of events at the Bay of Islands. *New Zealander, 1*(1) <http://freepages.genealogy.rootsweb.ancestry.com/~nzbound/nz1845.htm>.

New Zealand Listener (2010). It's about families. 27 February, p. 5.

New Zealand Parliamentary Debates (1867).

Onyx, J. & Bullen, P. (2000). Measuring social capital in five communities. *Journal of Applied Behavioural Science, 36,* 23–42.

Panelli, R. & Tipa, G. (2007). Placing well-being: a Maori case study of cultural and environmental specificity. *Ecohealth, 4*(4), 445–460.

Pearce, J. & Dorling, D. (2006). Increasing geographical inequalities in health in New Zealand, 1980–2001. *International Journal of Epidemiology, 35,* 597–603.

Richardson, S. (2004). Aotearoa/New Zealand nursing: from eugenics to cultural safety. *Nursing Inquiry, 11*(1), 35–42.

Shaw, C., Blakely, T., Atkinson, J. & Crampton, P. (2005). Do social and economic reforms change socioeconomic inequalities in child mortality? A case study: New Zealand 1981–1999. *Journal of Epidemiology and Community Health, 59,* 638–644.

Sullivan, W.M. (2000). Medicine under threat: professionalism and professional identity. *Canadian Medical Journal, 162*(5), 673–675.

Waitangi Tribunal (1999). *The Wananga Capital Establishment Report (WAI 718).* Wellington: GP Publications.

Ward, C. & Masgoret, A.M. (2008). Attitudes toward immigrants, immigration, and multiculturalism in New Zealand: a social psychological analysis. *International Migration Review, 42*(1), 227–248.

Wiles, J.L., Allen, R.E.S., Palmer, A.J., Hayman, K.J., Keeling, S. & Kerse, N. (2009). Older people and their social spaces: a study of wellbeing and attachment to place in Aotearoa New Zealand. *Social Science and Medicine, 68,* 664–671.

Willis, E. (2006). Introduction: taking stock of medical dominance. *Health Sociology Review*, *15*, 421–431.

Witten, K., McCreanor, T., Kearns, R. & Ramasubramanian, L. (2001). The impacts of a school closure on neighbourhood social cohesion: narratives from Invercargill, New Zealand. *Health and Place*, *7*, 307–317.

Wolfensberger, W. (1972) *The Principle of Normalisation in Human Services*. Toronto: National Institute on Mental Retardation.

WEBSITES

<http://www.8tribes.co.nz/>

8 Tribes: The Hidden Classes of New Zealand. Auckland: Wicked Little Books.

<http://www.tpk.govt.nz/_documents/whanau-ora-factsheet.pdf>

Whānau Ora.

<http://www.waitangi-tribunal.govt.nz/reports/downloadpdf.asp?reportid=39e13093-2f4d-4971-aca0-28e811572755 (chapter 2)>

Waitangi Tribunal Te Ropu Whakamana i Te Tiriti o Waitangi: The Wananga Capital Establishment Report.

READING 28

The Treaty of Waitangi and Health Outcomes within Aotearoa

RENEI NGAWATI AND BEATRICE LEATHAM

CHAPTER OVERVIEW

This chapter covers the following topics:

- What is a treaty?
- Historical impacts of colonisation
- Pre and post treaty: setting the context
- Post treaty legislation
- Treaty in legislation and healthcare
- Māori health policy: inclusion and practice

KEY TERMS

Determinants of health
Disparities
Ethnicity
Health policy
Health Promotion
Kāwanatanga
Kuia
Pākehā
Participation
Partnership
Protection
Public policy
Rangatiratanga
Sovereignty

(cont.)

Taha hinengaro	Taonga
Taha tinana	Te Whare Tapa Whā
Taha wairua	Tertiary healthcare
Taha whānau	Treaty of Waitangi

The **Treaty of Waitangi** is broadly accepted as the founding document of Aotearoa, and therefore plays a significant role within **public policy**. Only in the last two decades has Aotearoa seen the inclusion of the Treaty within the health sector in an attempt to address the health inequalities between Māori and non-Māori. To understand the significance of the Treaty and its application to healthcare, we must appreciate the journey the Treaty has taken in our society and how impacts of our history have contributed to these existing inequalities. With that, we can move forward to using the Treaty as a platform for better health, social and economic outcomes for Indigenous peoples of Aotearoa, and therefore better outcomes for all members of our society. Within this chapter, examples will be provided of how the Treaty is applied in public policy and in practice.

WHAT IS A TREATY?

A treaty is an agreement between two parties that either promotes and/or promises the exercise of peace and cooperative living (cohabitation) (Arato, 2010). The rationale for entering treaty agreements can vary, including postwar devastation, prevention of pending war or to enable a colonising population to cohabitat with an Indigenous population. Treaty agreements can also be entered into in order to create opportuniities for sustainable trade and economic relationships, provide a voice for each group in the control of future developments in economic sustainability and to maximise the interests of the people represented by the treaty.

HISTORICAL IMPACTS OF COLONISATION

There are two important points here to understand in this section of the chapter. First, the **determinants of health**, which include political, environmental, economic and social factors, are an efficient way of understanding the impacts of colonisation on Māori society before and after the application of the Treaty of Waitangi; and second, that the effects of colonisation are ongoing and can still be seen in our current society.

Understanding the Treaty of Waitangi and the emergence of this country as a bicultural nation is fundamental to understanding how relationships can be built and our peoples can develop together. Understanding our history, including things that have and have not worked, can assist us to move forward. The history of Aotearoa, from both Māori and **Pākehā** perspectives, provides an account of what happened in the establishment of Aotearoa, and gives a context to how the social and economic position of Māori became what it is today. History gives us, as New Zealanders, an insight as to why health inequities and inequalities exist.

Since 1840 the Treaty has had an important impact, both in New Zealand society generally and on Māori in particular. The economic, health, education or social position of Māori within the wider society is based not on their **ethnicity** alone but influenced by many contributing factors. Therefore we can use the determinants of health to understand broader issues of equality within Aotearoa. In turn, we can appreciate our history and how the Treaty can be used for a platform for equality in Aotearoa, especially in relation to health and wellbeing.

One of the most significant effects of colonisation on today's society is that traditional Māori cultural knowledge systems and philosophy have been filtered and replaced with Western thinking systems and practice. Creation theories, knowledge of deities and their links to humankind have been categorised as myths and legends.

The role that the Treaty has played in Māori society has not been a positive one for the most part. However, over the last forty years, the Treaty has been reintegrated into Aotearoa society and has slowly made an impact on the resurgence of Māori knowledge. More importantly, the Treaty is being used to close the gaps in inequality across sectors in order to bring into existence the intention of the Treaty: a partnership for the development of two cultures.

TE TIRITI Ō WAITANGI

Ko Wikitoria te Kuini o Ingarani i tana mahara awatai ki nga Rangatira me nga Hapu o Nu Tirani i tana hiahia hoki kia tohungatia ki a ratou rangatiratanga me to ratou wenua, a kia mau tonu hoki te Rongo ki a ratou me te Atamoho kua wakaaro ia he mea tika kia tukua mai tetahi Rangatira—hei kai wakarite ki nga Tangata Māori o Nu Tirani—kia wakaaetia e nga Rangatira Māori te Kawanatanga o te Kuini ki nga wahikatoa o te wenua nei me nga motu—na te mea hoki te tokomaha ke nga tangata o tona Iwi Kua noho ki tenei wenua, a e haere mai nei.

Na ko te Kuini e hiahia ana kia wakaritea te Kawanatanga kia kaua ai nga kino e puta mai ki te tangata maori ki te Pakeha e noho ture kore ana.

Na kua pai te Kuini kia tukua e hau a Wiremu Hopihona he Kapitana i te Roiara Nawi hei Kawana mo nga wahi katoa o Nu Tirani e tukua aianei amua atu kit e Kuini, a mea atu ana ki nga Rangatira o te wakaminenga o nga hapu o Nu Tirani me era Rangatira atu enei ture ka korerotia nei.

Ko te tuatahi

Ko nga Rangatira o te wakaminenga me nga Rangatira katoa hoki ki hai i taua wakaminenga ka tuku rawa atu kit e Kuini o Ingarani ake tonu atu—te Kawanatanga katoa o o ratou wenua.

Ko te tuarua

Ko te Kuini o Ingarani ka wakarite ka wakaae ki nga Rangatira ki nga hapu—ki nga tangata katoa o Nu Tirani te tino rangatiratanga o o ratou wenua o ratou kainga me o ratou taonga katoa. Otiia ko nga Rangatira o te wakaminenga me nga Rangatira katoa atu ka tuku ki te Kuini te hokonga o era wahi wenua e pai ai te tangata nona te wenua—ki te ritenga o te utu e wakaritea ai e ratou ko te kai hoko e meatia nei e te Kuini hei kai hoko mona.

Ko te tuatoru

Hei wakaritenga mai hoki tenei mo te wakaaetanga ki te Kawanatanga o te Kuini—kia tiakina e te Kuini o Ingarnai nga tangata maori katoa o Nu Tirani ka tukua ki a ratou nga tikanga katoa rite tahi ki ana mea ki nga tangata o Ingarani.

Na ko matou ko nga Rangatia o te Wakaminetanga o nga hapu o nu Tirani ka huihui nei ki Waitangi ko matou hoki ko nga Rangatiratanga o Nu Tirani ka rite nei i te ritenga o enei kupu. Ka tangohia ka wakaaetia katoatia e matou, koia ka tohungia ai o matou ingoa o matou tohu.

Ka meatia tenei ki Waitangi i te ono o nga ra o Pepueri I te tau kotahi mano, e waru rau e wa te kau o to tatou Ariki.

Ko nga Rangatira o te Wakaminenga

Her Majesty Victoria Queen of the United Kingdom of Great Britain and Ireland regarding with her Royal Favor the Native Chiefs and Tribes of New Zealand and anxious to protect their just Rights and Property and to secure to them the enjoyment of Peace and Good Order has deemed it necessary in consequence of the great number of Her Majesty's Subjects who have already settled in New Zealand and the rapid extension of Emigration both from Europe and Australia which is still in progress to constitute and appoint a functionary properly authorized to treat with the Aborigines of New Zealand for the recognition of Her Majesty's sovereignty authority over the whole or any part of those islands—Her Majesty therefore being desirous to establish a settled form of Civil Government with a view to avert the evil consequences which must result from the necessary Laws and Institutions alike to the native population and to Her subjects has been graciously pleased to empower and to authorize me William Hobson a Captain in Her Majesty's Royal Navy Consul and Lieutenant Governor of such parts of New Zealand as may be or hereafter shall be ceded to

Her Majesty to invite the confederated and independent Chiefs of New Zealand to concur in the following Articles and Conditions.

Article the first

The Chiefs of the Confederation of the United Tribes of New Zealand and the separate and independent Chiefs who have not become members of the Confederation cede to Her Majesty the Queen of England absolutely and without reservation all the rights and powers of Sovereignty which the said Confederation or Individual Chiefs respectively exercise or possess, or may be supposed to exercise or to possess over their respective Territories as the sole sovereigns thereof.

Article the second

Her Majesty the Queen of England confirms and guarantees to the Chiefs and Tribes of New Zealand and to the respective families and individuals thereof the full exclusive and undisturbed possession of their Lands and Estates Forests Fisheries and other properties which they may collectively or individually possess so long as it is their wish and desire to retain the same in their possession; but the Chiefs of the United Tribes and individual Chiefs yield to her Majesty the exclusive right of Preemption over such lands as the proprietors thereof may be disposed to alienate at such prices as may be agreed upon between the respective Proprietors and persons appointed by Her Majesty to treat with them in that behalf.

Article the third

In consideration thereof Her Majesty the Queen of England extends to the Natives of New Zealand royal protection and imparts to them all the Rights and Privileges of British Subjects.

Now therefore the Chiefs of the Confederation of the United Tribes of New Zealand being assembled in Congress at Victoria in Waitangi and We the Separate and Independent Chiefs of New Zealand claiming authority over the Tribes and Territories which are specified after our respective names, having been made fully to understand the Provisions of the foregoing Treaty, accept and enter into the same in the full spirit and meaning thereof in witness of which we have attached our signatures or marks at the paces and the dates respectively specified.

Done at Waitangi this Sixth day of February in the year of Our Lord one thousand eight hundred and forty.

The Chiefs of the Confederation
(Orange, 2004)

PRE AND POST TREATY: SETTING THE CONTEXT

Māori were quick to see the advantages of establishing and maintaining relationships with the new settlers in Aotearoa New Zealand. Items imported by the Pākehā became sought after, and the Pakeha required assistance with acquiring land and resources for establishing themselves here. Rangatira forged relationships with missionaries and settlers to gain access to their knowledge and resources. Relationships between Māori and the new Pākehā settlers extended as far as marriages with Māori women of good social standing to solidify trade relationships and gain land as gifts for the new couple. In pre-Treaty times, Māori were the largest population, at an estimated 150 000. Māori, in the far north area around Kororāreka (Russell), had the population advantage and an established economic base. The Northern region was the site of most initial British settlements and had the economic monopoly in terms of trade relationships. William Busby, the representative of the British Crown, acknowledged this established trade economy and the need to gain recognition as a sovereign nation in order to trade internationally under a recognised flag. To this end the Confederation of Chiefs was established and in 1835 a Declaration of Independence was drafted and signed by the Chiefs under this Confederate. Under this Declaration, Aotearoa was recognised as a sovereign nation, and more importantly, it recognised the mana of the Chiefs, their role in a growing and changing economic and social society and the authority and governorship they had over their lands, resources and knowledge systems.

In 1835, British colonists acknowledged Māori **sovereignty** and independence by signing the Declaration of Independence, which was superseded by the signing of Te Tiriti o Waitangi on 6 February 1840. There, **kāwanatanga** (governance) was surrendered by Māori, while **rangatiratanga** (chieftainship) over lands, estates, forests, fisheries and **taonga** (treasured possessions) was guaranteed. Māori assumed that an equal balance would be gained between tāngata whenua and new settlers. The Treaty was intended as recognition of equal partnership and as a foundation for future relationships between Māori and the Crown (Orange, 1989).

The drafting of and the differences between the Māori and English versions of the Treaty have driven debate about the use of the Treaty by the government, and in turn, across society. Interpretation of the Māori version and English translation of the three articles of the Tiriti has given rise to considerable conflict, although the internationally recognised principle of Contraproferendum holds that when conflict arises between Tiriti versions, the version in the language of the non-drafting signatory (in this case Māori) should stand. The Waitangi Tribunal, however, must consider both versions, as directed by Section 5(2) of the *Treaty of Waitangi Act* 1975 (Reid, 1999).

Regardless of such conflicts, the Tiriti has significant relevance to health. Some would say that Normanby's instructions to Hobson, noting that he wanted to protect the rights and property of Māori, eager to ensure that they enjoyed peace and good order, implied protections of good health (Reid, 1999). Significant implications that emerge directly from various Tiriti articles with relevance to health (taonga) are participation and equity, processes of good governance, self-determination and development of iwi resources.

The constitutional guarantee of equity between Māori and other citizens of Aotearoa New Zealand is stipulated in Article 3 of the Treaty. This promises that Māori should experience equal enjoyment of all the benefits of New Zealand citizenship. Good health is clearly one of these benefits, which implies the inclusion of good health. In relevance to health outcomes for all New Zealanders, including Māori, one of the reasons the Treaty was entered into was to protect the interests of Māori and to address the rapid population decline due to disease and musket warfare.

CASE STUDY 12.1

PERSPECTIVES ON HEALTH AND WELLNESS

There are various currently accepted health paradigms that have been created with respect to a Māori health perspective. One such is **Te Whare Tapa Whā**, developed by Mason Durie (1984). Te Whare Tapa Whā is often referred to as the traditional approach to Māori health although it was developed in accordance with contemporary Māori thought. Te Whare Tapa Wha was conceptualised from a Hui Taumata held in 1984 between Māori leaders and active participants in Māori communities gathered to talk about what the priorities for Māori were to improve the status and position of Māori populations overall. This was the opportunity for Māori to again participate in determining better outcomes. Through consultation with Māori elders, Durie identified four dimensions that interact to maintain strength, symmetry and balance thereby ensuring good health. He models them upon the walls of the whare; the four dimensions are **taha wairua** (spiritual), **taha hinengaro** (thoughts and feelings), **taha tinana** (physical) and **taha whānau** (family) (Durie, 1994). With the development of a model of health that included Māori knowledge in both traditional and contemporary ways, this was a stepping stone for Māori to be able to address and be included in the improvement and development of Māori people at the top end of government and at the community level.

Medicalisation of childbirth in New Zealand appears to have had effects upon women parallel to those that colonisation had upon Māori as a whole. Guilliland and Pairman (1995) identified a loss of power and dispossession of motherhood knowledge as the descriptors of the alienation of the childbirth experience for women. Out of this realisation a model for practice within midwifery was offered. This model has become known as the 'partnership model'. The model has gained regulatory and professional recognition and is widely acknowledged as an important and unique contribution to the field.

POST-TREATY LEGISLATION

The signing of the Treaty of Waitangi basically yielded rights to the British Crown to establish a government and institutions congruent with British society. This was agreed upon in the Treaty by both Māori and the Crown; however, some legislation that followed that was extended to Māori society was both detrimental to Māori development, health and the economy and in conflict with the understandings of the Treaty articles.

Historically, legislation in Aotearoa New Zealand has been detrimental to Māori, and therefore has served to entrench the establishment of a 'New Zealand' colony based on British law post Treaty signing. The acquisition of land and the assimilation of the 'Natives' were the means by which this plan was to be achieved. The analysis of the determinants of health, in the context of Aotearoa New Zealand, presents an effective backdrop to understanding the effects of colonisation on Māori. Exploring these concepts provides an insight into why Māori health and socioeconomic status, on average, have been poorer than for other ethnic populations in Aotearoa New Zealand, and offers a rationale as to why movements have been made to close these gaps.

The health and wellbeing of Māori declined with the rapid sales, gifting (hoko whenua) and confiscation of lands. Economic stability was evident pre Treaty, as Māori undertook the majority of trading in food and natural resources (Durie, 1998). Land control allows production growth to provide economic wealth and the sustenance of the people. Land also provides an unseen wealth source that is linked to identity (both tribal and individual), social cohesion and sustainability. The Māori worldview, like that of many cultures worldwide, cannot differentiate between land, identity and health of their people. The *Native Lands Act* 1865, and amended 1873, included the individualisation of land title. Tribal ownership was no longer acceptable in the new society. Durie states that 'the law was not designed to develop Māori land, but to speed up its sale by overcoming collective Māori resistance' (Durie, 1998, p. 36). The breaking of ties with the land and the destruction of a social unity under tribal affiliations weakened Māori society. Land, economic stability, identity, social cohesion and unity are important factors for health. Māori have come to resist legislative changes that have had an impact on these factors, leading to inequalities in social, economic and general wellbeing.

Disease, dispossession of land, inequitable legislation, trade relationships and other changes in and around Māori society have contributed to Māori becoming the minority population with little or no power to control events over their own lives, including their health. These **disparities** in economic position, health status, educational attainment and social stability exist today. Over the last thirty years Aotearoa has seen changes in legislation to specifically address Māori wellbeing and health outcomes, but huge gaps are still evident. A history of attitudes, actions and legislation has seen the near extinction of the Māori language and knowledge systems. There is little evidence of the economy in which Māori fully participated, owned and managed resources. Māori society has been forced to adapt, adopting foreign belief systems and values along with social structures. Recent literature now shows that a person's culture and identity are as important to their health and wellbeing outcomes as a sound economic base, education and social structures (National Health Committee, 1998). Language, and the capacity and capability to participate equally and fully in society and to access good health and educational outcomes, are necessary to the good health of individuals, communities and societies (Baum, 2008; **Health Promotion** Forum of New Zealand, 2002).

CASE STUDY 12.2

HEALTH STATUS OF MĀORI

Up to the early 1980s the life expectancy gap between Māori and non-Māori was closing. The inaccuracy of statistical information collected during the 1980s and 90s meant that Māori mortality rates were seriously undercounted (Ajwani et al., 2003), nevertheless the findings show a steady decline in mortality rates for both genders at all ages for non-Māori ethnic groups (excluding Pacific ethnic groups) while in contrast there was little change in the rate for Māori. Results found a progressive widening of disparity in survival chances between ethnic groups in this period. For example, the life expectancy gap for Māori males at birth increased from 6.3 years to 9.9 years when compared to non-Māori.

Chronic disease is identified as the major cause for this increase in inequality. Māori are more likely to experience cardiovascular and cancer mortality, diabetes and chronic lung disease. The rates of unintentional injury and suicide mortality are also significantly evident (Ajwani et al., 2003). Māori have increased rates of preterm and low birth weight infants; these babies are then at higher risk of ongoing health issues, and a Māori baby is more likely to die within seven days of birth than non-Māori (excluding Pacific babies). Infant mortality rates are one and a half times higher than non-Māori.

THE TREATY IN LEGISLATION AND HEALTHCARE

Significant implications that emerge directly from various Treaty articles with relevance to health (*taonga*) are: participation and equity; processes of good governance; self-determination; and development of iwi resources. The constitutional guarantee of equity between Māori and other citizens of New Zealand is stipulated in Article 3 (TOW, 1840). This promises that Māori should experience equal enjoyment of all of the benefits of New Zealand citizenship, which implies the inclusion of good health. The *Treaty of Waitangi Act* 1975 was instrumental in the establishment of the Waitangi Tribunal. One of the primary purposes of the Waitangi Tribunal was to interpret the Treaty and render 'principles' that established a common understanding; these principles have since gained inclusion in healthcare legislation and facilitated a pathway to addressing the inequalities between Māori and non-Māori.

CASE STUDY 12.3

MĀORI HEALTH AND DISABILITY WORKFORCE DEVELOPMENT

One of the main threads within He Korowai Oranga is to increase participation of Māori at all levels within the health sector. The aim is to build the capacity of Māori to determine their health outcomes and participate in the services that are provided to and by mainstream and Māori organisations. In order to build the capacity of Māori communities and to improve the health of Māori patients, whānau and community members, one of the strategies is to increase the number of Māori in the health and disability workforce at all levels, especially in professions requiring higher education qualifications. This is consistent with international literature stating that ethnic concordance increases the likelihood of a person attending clinical visits and adhering to medical advice. To increase the number of Māori in the health and disability workforce at higher qualified health professions, a number of initiatives have been established over the last two decades.

Māori and Pacific Admissions Scheme (MAPAS)

This is a support program, through the Faculty of Health Sciences and the Department of Māori Health, University of Auckland, to recruit, retain and redirect Māori and Pacific Island students into medical careers. Target areas are medicine, pharmacy and nursing. This program has had success in creating the whānau support systems, Māori and Pacific Island student support liaisons and an environment where the students are supported throughout their studies (Ratima et al., 2008).

MĀORI HEALTH POLICY: INCLUSION AND PRACTICE

Effective public health policy includes goals that reflect a larger picture: a broader public policy framework. When implementing policy, strategic direction guides the action plan to achieve these overall goals. Public policy can be seen as an overarching aim, with subgoals that determine the direction of the strategy and action plan. Good practice requires asking what the most appropriate course of action would be for the population affected by specific health issues in order to attain the overall goal.

The New Zealand Government outlines policy and practice in publications such as the *New Zealand Health Strategy* (MOH, 2000). The need to focus on reducing race-based disparities in health status in Aotearoa New Zealand is widely acknowledged in these statements. For example, *He Korowai Oranga* (*Māori Health Strategy*) (MOH, 2002) advocates the need for an intersectoral approach, with the focus being on the achievement of whānau ora. Documents such as these provide the policy framework. However, such policy direction is yet to address Māori health issues comprehensively.

The *Public Health and Disability Act* 2000 was revolutionary in including the principles of the *Treaty of Waitangi*. This caused a shift in **health policy** and practice. District Health Boards (DHBs) comprise of (at least) two Māori members representing the area being served. Government strategies that acknowledge the status and needs of Māori include:

- *New Zealand Health Strategy* (2000)
- *New Zealand Disability Strategy* (2001)
- *Primary Health Care Strategy* (2001)
- *He Korowai Oranga Māori Health Strategy* (2002).

He Korowai Oranga (*Māori Health Strategy*) (2002) was developed to include Māori models of practice and Māori health priorities. The *New Zealand Health Strategy* identified thirteen health priority areas; some of these included Māori health priorities, such as reducing the incidence of obesity. *He Korowai Oranga*, along with the *New Zealand Health Strategy*, in essence work in partnership with each other to achieve good health outcomes. All other health strategies, including documents such as the *New Zealand Diabetes Toolkit*, the *Physical Activity and Nutrition Toolkit* and the *New Zealand Cancer Strategy*, must include Māori health priorities within their strategic implementation plans to reduce the health inequalities between Māori and non-Māori.

Figure 12.1: Depiction of the Treaty of Waitangi and overarching health policy and strategy and how they work in partnership with each other

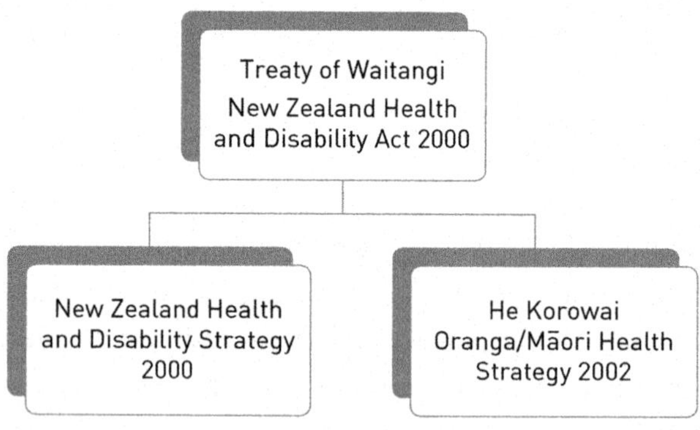

TREATY PRINCIPLES IN POLICY

CASE STUDY 12.4

The three main principles incorporated into recent public health policy are:

Partnership

Partnership refers to two parties of equal status working to achieve common goals, not necessarily in the same way, but enabling the achievement of both parties to benefit all. The significance of this principle within modern interpretations of the Treaty is its emphasis on how Māori and government can work together to achieve equitable outcomes within Aotearoa. Within the health sector, the emphasis is on improving Māori health outcomes, based on the overall goal of reducing the inequality gaps between Māori and non-Māori. Therefore, partnership interwoven in policy, strategy and practice ensures a way of improving Māori health outcomes and addressing community needs (Durie, 1998; 2011).

Participation

Participation at all levels in the health sector and health workforce is imperative to improving Māori health status. This includes community and primary healthcare, secondary and **tertiary healthcare**, and DHB and other agencies. This principle is interlinked with partnership, including the notion of tino rangatiratanga: the right of Māori to determine their own health outcomes and how those health outcomes will be achieved. It will require the participation of Māori at all levels within the health sector of Aotearoa to continue to build the capacity of the Māori health workforce so that Māori have equal and effective partnerships.

Protection

Protection as a principle is derived from Article 2 of the Treaty, which encapsulates the notion of tino rangatiratanga over nga taonga katoa; this being inclusive of health and wellbeing. Protection denotes the right of Māori to monitor government actions to ensure that policy, strategy and practice reflect partnership, and that Māori are participating in decisions affecting Māori communities and New Zealand overall.

Therefore the notions of partnership, participation and protection are intrinsically linked to ensure the realisation of the overall aims of improving Māori health and reducing inequities and inequalities.

CASE STUDY 12.5

TREATY PRINCIPLES: MIDWIFERY PARTNERSHIP MODEL

Guilliand and Pairman (1995) developed the 'partnership model', which has been adopted by the midwifery profession of Aotearoa. The backdrop of this model came from the demand of women realising the loss of autonomy over their childbirth experiences. This experience was almost a replica for the effects colonisation had on the Māori population and therefore Māori whānau embraced this model that facilitated recognition of these factors. The partnership model has been broadly established and professionally acknowledged by the regulatory bodies of the maternity sector.

The social environment and legislative structures providing the springboard for the partnership model in midwifery came from the constitutional base of the *Treaty of Waitangi*. Principles that emerged from the Cartwright enquiry (1987–1989) also fuelled the growing disillusionment with the medical model that had up to then shaped midwifery practice. Women had realised they were entitled to accountability, women-centred care, self-determination and cultural sensitivity (Guilliland & Pairman, 1994; Pairman, 1999).

The partnership model recognises pregnancy and birth as a normal physiological and biological process. It also places the total childbirth experience within its social and cultural framework (Guilliland & Pairman, 1994). The ideology of partnership evokes feelings of equality, which was the intention of the Treaty.

For Māori, loss of identity, dependency and loss of self-confidence had become a common reality. Māori women had been experiencing the alienating effects of healthcare twofold, and although the midwifery partnership model has now created a platform to challenge the earlier maternity services model, Māori women remain at a disadvantage.

A maternity sector that utilises a framework of partnership, recognised at a legislative level, must be effective in improving health outcomes for Māori birthing whānau. As discussed previously, this will only be realised when Māori are included at all levels of the maternity sector and there is an acknowledgment of the interdependence of the Treaty principals on improving health outcomes for Māori.

SUMMARY

Māori and the Crown are responsible for ensuring that the essence, intentions and principles of the Treaty of Waitangi are adhered to. Social and economic outcomes for a population are not based on ethnicity or the accepted status of one population by another, therefore language, identity, sound economic foundations, positive social connections and access to resources, including education, capacity building, self-determination and active participation in their communities, are vital ingredients for positive development. Historically, post-Treaty legislation has eroded these factors away from Māori, which in turn has contributed to the health and wellbeing outcomes and disparities we see in our society today. Therefore, as a society that was founded on a partnership agreement, legislation that includes the resurgence of Māori knowledge, language and practices, participation in society and economic development, improved educational outcomes and access to fair and equitable services, will contribute to the overall positive development of society in Aotearoa. The Treaty principles act as guides to ensure that the articles of the Treaty are alive and functional, from government to community level, including health policy and practice.

CRITICAL QUESTIONS

Cultural lens

- **How** can the obligation of partnership between Māori and the Crown address Māori health status?
- **How** can Māori be supported to actively participate in ways that contribute to health and wellbeing?

Social lens

- **What** is the overall aim of Whānau ora and Māori Health and Disability Workforce Development?

Gender lens

- **What** specific roles to kaumātua and **kuia** have in community wellbeing?

Political lens

- **How** can health policy and strategic planning address the broader determinants of health and wellbeing and include populations in high need?

Moral lens

- **How** can partnership be genuinely understood and enabled?

Media lens

- **How** can the media support policy developments and strategic initiatives?

FURTHER READING

Durie, M. (1998). *Whaiora: Māori Health Development* (2nd edn) (pp. 197–213). Auckland: Oxford University Press.

Durie, M. (2011). *Nga Tini Whetu: Navigating Māori Futures.* Wellington: Huia Publishers.

REFERENCES

Ajwani, S., Blakely, T., Robson, B., Tobias, M. & Bonne, M. (2003). *Decades of Disparity: Ethnic Mortality Trends in New Zealand 1980–1990* (pp. 45–54). Wellington: Ministry of Health and University of Otago.

Arato, J. (2010). Subsequent practice and evolutive interpretation: techniques of treaty interpretation over time and their diverse consequences. *Law and Practice International Courts and Tribunals, 9*, 443–494.

Baum, F. (2008). *The New Public Health* (3rd edn). Melbourne: Oxford University Press.

Durie, M. (1984). 'Te Taha Hinengaro': An integrated approach to mental health. *Community Mental Health in New Zealand, 1*(1), 4–11.

Durie, M. (1994). *Whaiora: Māori Health Development* (1st edn). Auckland: Oxford University Press.

Durie, M. (1998). *Whaiora: Māori Health Development* (2nd edn) (pp. 197–213). Auckland: Oxford University Press.

Durie, M. (2011). *Nga Tini Whetu: Navigating Māori Futures.* Wellington: Huia Publishers.

Guilliland, K. & Pairman, S. (1994). The midwifery partnership: a model for practice. *New*

Guilliland, K. & Pairman, S. (1995). *The Midwifery Partnership: A Model for Practice.* Wellington: Victoria University Press.

Health Promotion Forum of New Zealand (2002). *TUHA-NZ: A Treaty Understanding of Hauora in Aotearoa-New Zealand.* Auckland: Health Promotion Forum of New Zealand (Whakapiki Ake i te Hauora o Aotearoa).

Ministry of Health (2000). *The New Zealand Health Strategy.* Wellington: Ministry of Health.

Ministry of Health (2002). *He Korowai Oranga: Māori Health Strategy.* Wellington: Ministry of Health.

National Health Committee (1998). *The Social, Cultural, and Economic Determinants of Health in New Zealand.* Wellington: National Health Committee.

Orange, C. (1989). *The Story of a Treaty.* Wellington: Bridget Williams.

Orange, C. (2004). *An Illustrated History of the Treaty of Waitangi.* Wellington: Bridget Williams.

Pairman, S. (1999). Partnership revisited: towards midwifery theory. *New Zealand College of Midwives Journal, 21,* 6–12.

Ratima, M., Brown, R., Garrett, N., Wikaire, E., Ngawati, R., Aspin, C. & Potaka, U. (2008). *Rauringa Raupa: Recruitment and Retention of Māori in the Health and Disability Workforce. A Report Prepared for the Ministry of Health and the Health Research Council of New Zealand.* Auckland: Taupua Waiora Centre, Faculty of Health and Environmental Sciences, AUT University.

Reid, P. (1999). *Te pupuri I te Ao o te Tangata Whenua. Health and Society in Aotearoa-New Zealand.* Auckland: Oxford University Press, 38–47.

WEBSITES

<http://www.hauora.maori.nz/>

Māori standards of health.

<http://www.maorihealth.govt.nz/moh.nsf/menuma/About+Maori+Health>

Māori health information.

<http://www.msd.govt.nz>

Ministry of Social Development.

<www.nzhistory.net.nz/category/tid/133>

New Zealand history online.

<http://www.nzhistory.net.nz/politics/read-the-treaty/maori-text>

The text of Te Tiriti o Waitangi (the Treaty of Waitangi).

<http://www.ots.govt.nz/>

Office of Treaty settlements.

<http://www.waipareira.co.nz>

Te Whanau o Waipareira Trust.

<http://www.waitangi-tribunal.govt.nz/>

The Waitangi Tribunal.

<http://www.whariki.ac.nz/>

Social outcomes research and evaluation.

Media and Technology

AILSA HAXELL

CHAPTER OVERVIEW

This chapter covers the following topics:

- Defining media
- Marketing
- Technology
- Telemedicine
- Telesurgery
- Simulation
- Nanotechnology
- Genetic information technology
- Tissue engineering

KEY TERMS

Apps
Communication and computer technologies
Digital footprint
Direct-to-consumer advertising
E-health
Genetic information technology
Media
M-health
Nanotechnology
Simulation
Social networking
Stem cell research
Technology
Telemedicine
Telesurgery
Tissue engineering

Media is a word directly from the Latin: medium (the singular) indicates being in the middle, between people speaking to each other. At their most basic, media take the position between people as information is conveyed. They are carriers of ideas between people. This is the meaning we make when we think of media, such as newspapers and television, as they take information from one situation and provide the means of sharing it.

DEFINING MEDIA

Thinking about media as carriers of information suggests information is located somewhere, and it needs to get to someone else, separated most commonly by distance, but also by time. Media provide the means whereby information can traverse distances, plus they can stay intact despite being stored during the intervening days, weeks or years. In this way books are also a form of media. The capturing of information, whether in digital or other forms, provides an efficient means for both storing information and disseminating it widely.

CASE STUDY 14.1

ESCALATION OF AN EPIDEMIC IN THE NEWS MEDIA

During October 2011 a number of media articles sought to bring the notion of a 'measles epidemic' to the attention of the New Zealand public. These may be found by searching the *New Zealand Herald* website. They were characterised by titles such as:

- Auckland's measles outbreak continues to spread (4 October 2011) <http://www.nzherald.co.nz/nz/news/article.cfm?c_id=1&objectid=10756514>
- Thousands exposed to measles (14 October 2011) <http://www.nzherald.co.nz/nz/news/article.cfm?c_id=1&objectid=10759094>
- Doctors urge mass measles vaccination to beat outbreak (24 October 2011) <http://www.nzherald.co.nz/health/news/article.cfm?c_id=204&objectid=10761211>

The language used in the media quickly escalates from encouraging people to check their immunisation status to messages about 'outbreaks' of disease and 'epidemics'.

There are deeper concerns that are not fully apparent in such reporting. The information is not provided with the intent of providing an informed decision; it is provided as part of media sensationalism, as the core business of a newspaper is to sell papers. For dedicated health information, a source such as <http://www.ncirs.edu.au/immunisation/education/mmr-decision/index.php> is recommended rather than relying on information from the mass media about immunisation.

A complicating feature of mass media is that they do not easily engage in dialogue. The stories tend to stay small enough to provoke interest without being able to address detail. Addressing who is most at risk of measles, which could lead to death or lifelong complications, is left out of these stories. The level of detail doesn't allow an explanation that those most at risk are those with vulnerable immune systems, such as infants, or those whose immune systems are compromised, and therefore a mass immunisation approach is particularly benefiting those who cannot be immunised. Unfortunately, and particularly in the case of the measles, mumps and rubella (MMR) immunisation programme, dissemination of superficial information is not the biggest problem.

The bias towards publishing particularly sensationalist news implicated the MMR vaccinations in causing autism. The initial research (Wakefield et al., 1998) published in *The Lancet* (and which has since been retracted) conceded no definitive link had been found, but the lead researcher Andrew Wakefield, in a press conference, told the world he believed the measles, mumps and rubella vaccines in the form of the MMR vaccine should not be given (BBC News, 1998). This was front page news in *The Guardian*, and was repeated in a further 122 news items in the United Kingdom (Goldacre, 2008). A media frenzy was compounded by the then Prime Minister's wife conceding that she had not had their baby vaccinated.

In the United Kingdom relentless negative media coverage of vaccination is credited with having reduced immunisation rates by 30 per cent (Murch, 2003). A subsequent increase in measles cases can be mapped against this, with a 36 per cent increase in children contracting measles in 2008. Despite the research that had associated MMR with autism being discredited following discovery of fraudulent data, where none of the information of the twelve children studied could be verified (Deer, 2010, 2011) and a retraction of the research by ten out of twelve associated medical researchers (Murch et al., 2004), as well as widespread reporting of the unethical and irresponsible practices involved (see for example Boseley, 2010) and where the initiator of that research, Dr Andrew Wakefield, has since been removed from the medical register (General Medical Council, 2010), confidence in the MMR immunisation has yet to be restored, and many weblinks continue to repeat the claim.

The effects were not localised to the United Kingdom. The loss of confidence was felt worldwide, and the fear of vaccinations was generalised to other vaccines and immunisations, the fear still exerting an influence a decade later, with as many as one in four USA parents believing vaccines can cause autism (Freed et al., 2010). That the initial research paper received such a high level of media coverage and created significant damage to public health, as well as to confidence in health services more generally, has been described as unparalleled in the history of medical science (Godlee, 2011).

The message in the New Zealand media that a "mop-up" [was] required in poor vaccine delivery' illustrates how poor research can be compounded by poor media coverage. But this pales into insignificance when compared to the unnecessary suffering and deaths attributable to preventable childhood illnesses.

Until recent times mass media have been dominated by a one-way stream of information. This has led to a lack of detail and inability to relate to individual experiences in much material issued by various media. Problems associated include the bias towards reporting sensationalist news (as in the preceding case study). A further bias becomes evident when we look at the increasing concentration of news ownership in fewer hands. The interconnectedness of newspapers of the world with television broadcasting and channel ownership is evident in a list of assets owned by Rupert Murdoch's News Corporation. Another source of media control is the influence of advertisers, whose contribution to the financial viability of news is huge. Only recently has it become easy for publishing to move outside of this field of influence, such that anyone can publish most anything. The World Wide Web allows for publishing faster, further, by more people, and more cheaply than by any previous means. At the time that I write this, the web is credited as being twenty years old, Wikipedia is ten years old and Facebook is just seven years old.

These latter forms are referred to as social media, or alternately as **social networking** sites. The defining feature of such sites is that they are social; they are about coming together rather than being a recipient of information as supplied. While initial use of the internet tended to reflect earlier modes of communication where information was posted so that others could read it, a second generation of World Wide Web use (Web 2.0) has evolved. O'Reilly (2005) distinguishes this from earlier models because it is participatory. Rather than posting information targeting readers as consumers, Web 2.0 reflects a producer-driven environment where information can be added, edited and shared by anyone with the inclination and ability to follow instructions. Developments in social software have deconstructed the technical requirements of writing, editing and adding to web pages, enabling people to make use of what was previously controlled by those with specific technical skills.

Having information readily available presents challenges in terms of quality, contradictory information, bias and privacy. The extent of the database available can be overwhelming. As I write this, a search using the Google search engine on the MMR vaccine results in 14 600 000 'hits'. Some of this material, as has been discussed, is no longer credible; however, it demonstrates that digital information never really goes away. We are still learning about how to manage information that is so readily available, and which seems indifferent to international borders and to legislative control. Retracting information doesn't destroy it. As stated in a now famous quip, 'You can't take something off the Internet—it's like taking pee out of a pool' (author unknown, 1995; see <http://www.quotegarden.com/internet.html>). What a lot of people do not realise is that when they post something online, even if they delete that information, it may still be retrievable.

The control of personal information is increasingly a concern, and particularly where there is limited understanding of how the medium works. Placing information online provides for both storage and retrieval of information. The important aspect to consider is how it is archived so that it remains accessible, and how it is protected so only those with legitimate cause have access. How to ensure privacy and confidentiality, as information that is personal is increasingly being put into digital formats, is therefore a concern for all of us. This is not a new concern, but the newness of the medium requires that new strategies for ensuring security and privacy are maintained.

Media literacy is about understanding media as being more than a carrier of information. In putting information into a digital world, new understandings of how we relate to information is required. Who hasn't regretted pressing Send on a text message or an email that would have been better not sent, or posting something on Facebook that took on a life of its own never anticipated? When a paper record is passed from one person to another, the actual piece of paper moves—it moves from point A to point B—and so no longer exists at Point A. In contrast, a digital trace replicates at each point. The message coexists at the point of origin as well as where it is received, and this may also include leaving a digital trace at transit points. Once it leaves your hands you have little control over its replication, and very limited ability to control what the recipients will do with what was sent. Even if you delete the original message, this does not delete the message from where it has travelled to, or through.

A **digital footprint** accrues information posted both intentionally and unintentionally, and this information can be collected passively or actively by others. Passive collection includes the recording of 'hits' on a site and making a record of that IP address. Active collection involves data collection on entry to a site, such as requiring a password to have been logged. The digital footprint becomes big business in a competitive market where advertising might then be targeted; also, this type of knowledge is of interest to companies with a vested interest in knowing about people. Knowledge of the digital footprint highlights how concerns of openness and privacy may come into conflict, and these issues are of particular concern in relation to health information.

CASE STUDY 14.2

HEALTH AND NEW TECHNOLOGY

Despite the concerns identified, use of the World Wide Web for healthcare is generally considered favourably, particularly with regard to the empowerment of clients (Fox et al., 2000). The US-based Pew Internet Research Centre has identified that:

- 55 per cent of American adults with internet access have used the web to get health or medical information
- 92 per cent described the information they found as useful
- 48 per cent of web-based health seekers said the advice they found on the web improved the way they take care of themselves (Fox et al., 2000).

In 2011, further changes become evident:

- 80 per cent of internet users have looked online for health or medical information
- 34 per cent of internet users, which roughly translates to 25 per cent of all American adults, have read someone else's commentary or experience about health or medical issues on an online news group, website or blog
- 25 per cent of internet users, or 19 per cent of adults, have watched an online video about health or medical issues
- 24 per cent of internet users, or 18 per cent of adults, have consulted online reviews of particular drugs or medical treatments
- 18 per cent of internet users, or 13 per cent of adults, have gone online to find others who might have health concerns similar to theirs
- 16 per cent of internet users, or 12 per cent of adults, have consulted online rankings or reviews of doctors or other providers
- 15 per cent of internet users, or 11 per cent of adults, have consulted online rankings or reviews of hospitals or other medical facilities (Fox, 2011).

The changing trend is towards participatory use of health-related sites. Patients are no longer just finding out about their conditions; they are also posting their experiences online. While rating your hotel stay or experience of a restaurant has been around for a while, rating your health professional, and using such information to make choices about treatment providers, is a newer phenomenon. Validity regarding such ratings is highly problematic. Internet-based rating sites, such as Rate My Medical Doctor or Dentist <http://www.ratemds.com> or Rate My Midwife <http://ratemymidwife.com>, allow one disaffected person to post multiple times, or for the provider to be self-promoting without this being acknowledged. With globalisation, any ability to redress slander is small, as the server may well reside in a different country to the health practitioner.

MARKETING

Leverage and concerns of power through the media are nowhere stronger than in the use of **direct-to-consumer advertising (DTCA)** practised by pharmaceutical companies. Aotearoa New Zealand and the USA are the only two industrialised countries that allow direct-to-consumer advertisements for prescription-only medicines (Frosch et al., 2007). Rather than targeting healthcare professionals, this type of advertising is directed towards the general population, and specific patients.

The goal of direct-to-consumer advertising, as with all advertising, is to increase market share and to encourage switching to the advertised brand. This matters for healthcare professionals, as there are important consequences for public health. Such consequences include increased costs. Paying for the production of advertisements is hidden in the product cost, but there is also the pharmaceutical company's intended outcome of increasing prescriptions through the general public asking for specific products to be prescribed, and to prescribe the newer and often more expensive product.

Advocates of DTCA point to the potential benefits of increased health awareness, open communications between patients and healthcare providers, freedom of choice, greater compliance and better health outcomes (Gilbody et al., 2005). To these reasons Auton (2009) adds the potential of DTCA to address undertreatment and undiagnosed disease. The concern is that these interventions may not be clinically or fiscally supported. DTCA encourages uptake of newer pharmaceuticals before their safety, efficacy and cost effectiveness may be known (Hollon, 2005; Women's Health Action Trust, 2006). In addition, DTCA draws attention away from the social and economic determinants of health and sustains a focus on the individual (Moynahan, 2005; Women's Health Action Trust, 2006).

TECHNOLOGY

Future gazing is always an imprecise art. Predicting what will change, the direction and extent of this can never be known fully in advance. It is, however, possible to look at trends.

Ursula Franklin (1999) suggests the following approach to understanding the concept of **technology**:

> Technology is not the sum of the artefacts, of the wheels and gears, of the rails and electronic transmitters. Technology is a system. It entails far more than its individual material components. Technology involves organization, procedures, symbols, new words, equations, and, most of all, a mindset (Franklin, 1999, p. 12).

In other words, technology is less about tools and is more about our ways of doing things.

Webster (2007) suggests it is possible to see where things might be going by looking at what receives funding and media attention. Particular trends can then be explored. Taking this as a lead, the areas currently receiving significant interest are:

- **communication and computer technologies** (CCTs): extending the preceding discussion of health information data storage and retrieval, are applications of CCTs that allow for new treatment options within a digitally enhanced world
- **genetic information technology**: with the complete mapping of the human DNA sequence, diagnosis based on genetic screening of DNA becomes a very real possibility, as does the potential to treat disease before it eventuates through genetic modification
- tissue generation: currently there are combinations of biological tissue and synthetic materials being used to repair or regenerate damaged tissue.

TELEMEDICINE

The most direct applications for healthcare made possible by advances in CCTs are in the area of **telemedicine**. The rapid development of CCTs and the internet has completely transformed how health information is stored, retrieved and shared in healthcare services. Further transformation occurs with treatment options being provided electronically. The hope for any change in healthcare is that it addresses concerns of accessibility, affordability and appropriateness, directions that are supported by the Alma Ata Declaration (World Health Organization, 1978), *Health for All by the Year 2000* (World Health Organization, 1981), the *Ottawa Charter* (World Health Organization, 1986) and *Working Together for Health* (World Health Organization, 2006).

With advances being made in the telecommunications industry, the capacity to do more with less readily lends itself to efficiency in health services, both for learning about health and for healthcare delivery. The ability to work at a distance reduces cost barriers associated with travel, or with access issues related to disability, and also reduces barriers that may exist related to concerns of embarrassment or privacy. The genre of health applications available online is loosely referred to as **e-health** when provided via a computer, or **m-health** when accessed by mobile phone.

Smartphones are increasingly being used for self-managing of health. The majority of phones being sold in New Zealand today are smartphones (Commerce Commission New Zealand, 2011). This description relates to a mobile phone that is internet capable. Current costs of broadband access have been prohibitive for many, though costs are decreasing and are anticipated to keep decreasing following government regulation of the telecommunications industry (Commerce Commission New Zealand, 2011).

A recent study by Pew Internet identified that, of the 85 per cent of adults in the USA who own a cell phone (mobile phone), 9 per cent say they have software applications or '**apps**' on their phones that help them manage their health (Fox, 2011). There are apps for tracking dietary intake and exercise, weight, blood sugar levels, menstrual cycles as indicators for fertility and managing addictions; even apps that track and inform on smog, through to apps that will assist you with yoga and meditation. If you are worried about the appearance of a rash, there are also apps that will attempt diagnostic advice based on pattern recognition of a photographed image of the rash. Similarly, there are apps that will attempt pattern recognition based on the sound of a cough. More recently, apps are becoming more personalised and more interactive. An app for tracking asthma has been shown to significantly increase people's abilities to manage their own symptoms by taking into account the history of a person and making suggestions for when medications should be increased (Asthma control? We've got an app for that, 2010). In-home equipment monitoring devices are also being developed and connected to apps; for example, the Withings Blood Pressure Monitor cuff that connects directly to the iPhone (a branded smartphone), keeping a graphed record of blood pressure that can also be sent directly from the iPhone to your health professional (Corney, 2011).

Apps are rapidly increasing as adjuncts to timely healthcare. Whether you are well, unwell or just curious, there is probably an app for that. Over 300 000 apps have been developed in the last three years, especially since the advent of smartphones and iPhones. Usefulness and effectiveness are, however, difficult to assess. Anecdotal evidence suggests people wouldn't buy them if they were not useful, but actual effectiveness studies remain sparse. As reported in Live Science <http://www.livescience.com>, it can take six months to build an app, then a further six to fifteen months to run a study, and a further year, involving editing and peer reviews, prior to publication. Independent studies, those not funded by the developers, are only just beginning to come out now, and by the time they are published, new apps will have replaced them (Pappas, 2011).

TELESURGERY

Many procedures that can now be performed laparoscopically with robots used to be performed as open surgery. With laparoscopic interventions, rather than a large wound being required to access internal parts of the body, a puncture or keyhole is opened, enabling the use of video and extended reach tools surgery. More recently, **telesurgery** has become possible. With telesurgery, computer-mediated procedures make it possible for procedures to occur remotely. The tools used in the surgery are manipulated at a distance through a computer. The first reported surgery occurring at a distance involved surgeons in the United States removing a gall bladder from a patient in eastern France by remotely operating a surgical robot arm (BBC News, 2001, 19 September). Two healthcare surgical teams were involved, linked by video and high-speed fibre optics, making the surgery feasible despite the 14 000-kilometre distance. Surgical expertise mediated by CCTs and available globally is possible, but the costs involved, as with any new technologies, render it prohibitive in all but exceptional cases.

SIMULATION

Students and practitioners in the field of healthcare often learn tasks through **simulation** entities such as SimMan (Laerdal, 2008). Simluation is valuable, in that it reduces the burden of access to clinical areas to teach simple and technical skills. There are challenges, however, including the need to ensure that people can engage appropriately with the people they meet and work with. The development of these human skills requires interaction with real people in real environments, suggesting that the teaching of clinical and technical skills cannot be completely repositioned as a simulated process.

CASE STUDY 14.3

TECHNOLOGY AS COMPANION AND CARER

Paro is a robotic fur seal developed in 2003 as a companion for the elderly. More than 6000 have been sold worldwide (Paro Therapeutic Robot, 2011). Being with Paro apparently makes people happier, reducing stress and depression, and is advertised as improving quality of life <http://www.parorobots.com/whitepapers.asp>.

Paro could be considered a 'soft toy'. He or she might have been a doll, except that he or she costs considerably more at US$6000 and is marketed as a medical device (Paro Therapeutic Robot, 2011). Sherry Turkle, a psychologist and professor at the Massachusetts Institute of Technology, finds Paro deeply disturbing (Turkle, 2007). How can a soft toy disturb so deeply? Because Paro is marketed as companionship for people who are lonely, confused and/or needing social stimulation.

Paro has been described as the solution in a distressing phone call between a mother in the early stages of dementia, and her daughter who is unable to be there for her (Harmon, 2010).

Aliz-e, a robot, is described on the manufacturer's website as being able to have robust conversations that include analysis and synthesis of emotions (Aliz-e, 2010). This robot is still in the experimental stages, with research being conducted in hospitals to see if it can make children's experience of hospital more pleasant and to take over some tasks, including patient education (Hornyak, 2010).

In a seminal text, *Computer Power and Human Reason*, Joseph Weizenbaum (1976) asked that we consider the limits of what we delegate to computers. These examples of robots for healthcare provoke questions as to what are desirable and undesirable applications. The boundaries may well be blurred, but for most of us, the needs we have for understanding and for love may be better met by involvement with people than with things.

NANOTECHNOLOGIES

'Smaller is better' is a theme in technological advances. Multidisciplinary researchers are developing technologies so small, we can't see them. The science of **nanotechnology** is focused at the level of this smallest building unit, a nanometre (nm). To understand the size of what is being talked of, one nano is one-billionth of a metre. Most atoms are 0.1 to 0.2 nm wide, strands of DNA around 2 nm wide, red blood cells are around 7000 nm in diameter, while human hair has the width of approximately 80000 nm ('Nanotechnology', n.d.).

CASE STUDY 14.4

NANOTECHNOLOGY: NANO-SILVER AND THE RISK OF NANOTOXICITY

Silver has long been identified as having curative properties. It has been applied to wounds in the form of silversulpherdiazide for its antibacterial properties for more than fifty years. More recently it has been developed as nano-silver, and embedded in woven fabric, which prevents bacterial infections from occurring. 'Silver socks' are one such product. These would lessen the likelihood not only of bacteria-causing foot odour, but also reduce the incidence, particularly for people with diabetes, of developing bacterial infections on their feet that could lead to amputations. However, little is known about the potential risks of nanotechnology.

Benn and Westerhoff (2008) identify some brands of silver socks as losing as much as 100 per cent of their silver content within four washes, while alternate brands lost just under 1 per cent over the same number of washes. The ease with which silver nanoparticles can enter into wastewater during washing is disturbing, not only because of the huge loss incurred financially to make a product that quickly loses effectiveness, but because the effects of nanoparticles on the wider environment are simply unknown. Given that wastewater treatment is dependent on helpful bacteria, this poses a huge threat to the ecological system of wastewater.

The Swedish Environmental Protection Agency has protested against this application because wastewater may be contaminated with nano-silver (Wijnhoven et al., 2009). Recently, the United States Environmental Protection Agency has similarly moved to regulate this specific form of nanotechnology (Wijnhoven et al., 2009). Silver-ion generating devices for washing machines, which have the declared aim of killing bacteria, will no longer be listed as simple washing devices, but are now listed as pesticides. This ruling was not an action to regulate nanotechnology; it is the silver's bactericidal effect rather than the molecular size that led to the decision.

In view of potential effects in aquatic ecosystems, new purification methods need to be developed to remove the nano-silver, increasing costs to the government and therefore to taxpayers (Wijnhoven et al., 2009). Farmers are concerned that the antimicrobial activity of nano-silver will affect the beneficial bacteria in soil, essential particularly to organic farming (Murata et al., 2005). For healthcare professionals the concern is a reminder of what occurred when antibiotics were used unwisely and 'super bugs' evolved. The potential development of widespread antibiotic resistant organisms is worrying.

While there is a rapidly growing market of nano-enhanced products, gaps in knowledge are not being addressed at a pace in keeping with the market or the products themselves.

GENETIC INFORMATION TECHNOLOGY

There is rapid development of technologies associated with genetics; these include the areas of genetic screening for diagnostic purposes through to gene therapies, which modify human DNA so as to prevent disease development. The hereditary nature of some diseases has been known for centuries; however, it is only with the completion of the Human Genome Project in 2004 that the long chains of DNA that make up the human genetic structure have been mapped. The potential is a major shift in healthcare away from disease management to disease prevention as the deliberate manipulation of genes, known as genetic engineering, would allow individual genetic structure to be modified to correct for mutations before they eventuate.

Genetic engineering is a highly controversial area of research that has disturbing implications for our understandings of what is, and is not, desirable in the human condition. If diseases with a hereditary component could be avoided, should they be? At what point do we decide that altering human DNA should be restricted? The eugenics movement that was associated with Hitler's Aryan race theories was widely condemned, as have been other practices of 'ethnic cleansing'. In what ways will human genetic engineering differ from these widely condemned practices?

TISSUE ENGINEERING

Tissue engineering, also known as regenerative medicine, is an emerging multidisciplinary field involving biology, medicine and engineering that aims to improve the health and quality of life for millions of people worldwide by restoring, maintaining or enhancing tissue and organ function. In addition to the therapeutic application where the tissue is grown in a patient, or outside a patient and transplanted, tissue engineering also involves applications of tissue grown in vitro to test medicines for harmful effects. With transplants from donors there is substantial risk that the recipient's immune system will reject the transplant; in contrast, tissues engineered from stem cells have not yet differentiated and so are less likely to be rejected. Stem cells develop early in embryonic development, providing a template for the differentiation and growth of all other cells in the body.

Stem cell research has the potential to change dramatically the treatment of human disease. A number of treatments already exist, such as bone marrow transplants for treating leukaemia. Anticipated future applications include treatment for neurological disorders such as strokes, Parkinson's disease and multiple sclerosis. However, there still exists a great deal of social and scientific uncertainty surrounding stem cell research. Significant controversy surrounds stem cell research, as most current stem cell technology requires the destruction of the human embryo to obtain these embryonic cells. In response Coles (2010), writing on the ethics of stem cell research, suggests the controversy hinges on how human life is defined. If the cells harvested are from the pre-implanted blastocyst that has the potential to be a person but is not yet a person, then a different biological, philosophical, legal and moral argument is being proposed. There are obvious ethical challenges involved in this. Nonetheless the interest in reversing cellular damage makes it possible to imagine that healthcare in the future could be radically transformed. Life expectancy could be prolonged, as organs at risk of failure could be replaced, changing patterns of morbidity and mortality. Given the costs currently involved, there is risk that patterns of inequality between rich and poor would widen.

SUMMARY

Changing technologies have implications for the context of health, both worldwide and within Aotearoa New Zealand. The media have obvious applications in disseminating information, which might also involve bias; nonetheless, media can also contribute towards a more participatory healthcare system, democratising processes through greater knowledge sharing and improving access.

The effects of technological innovations are never fully known in advance. The best future gazing we can muster tends to look at effects that are immediate, in the short term rather than the long term, and are closely associated with our intentions rather than consideration for a wider context. In addition, technological innovations are increasingly oriented towards the prevention of disease rather than its treatment. This may create a shift in healthcare away from the sick towards the well, away from the old towards the young, and away from the poor towards the rich. This has the potential to increase rather than reduce current social inequalities. Nonetheless, this is not an argument against innovation, but a plea for thoughtfulness.

CRITICAL QUESTIONS

Cultural lens

- **What** are cultural barriers to accessing and engaging in e-health?

Social lens

- **What** are the potential social control risks in relation to e-health?
- **Who** are likely to be the winners and losers in relation to the increasing use of technology?

Gender lens

- **How** do men and women engage differently with technology, and what impact is this likely to have on health?

Political lens

- **What** are the risks in relation to healthcare if technology is seen as having political advantage?

Moral lens

- **How** should risks of access to and security of health information be managed?

Media lens

- **How** does science fiction extrapolate from current technological developments?
- **How** do the media handle bias in relation to new technology?

FURTHER READING

Bushko, R.G. (ed.) (2002). *Future of Health Technology*. Amsterdam: IOS Press.

Koppel, A., Kahur, K., Habicht, T., Saar, P., Habicht, J. & van Ginneken, E. (2008). Estonia: health system review. *Health Systems in Transition*, *10*(1), 1–230.

Norris, A.C. (2002). *Essentials of Telemedicine and Telecare*. Chichester: John Wiley & Sons.

Rodrigues, A. (2008). Data security lapses in developed societies: public and private sector cases. In J. Aisbett, G. Gibbon, A. Rodrigues, K. Joseph, R. Nath & G. Renardel (eds), *Strengthening the Role of ICT in Development* (pp. 203–214). East Lansing, MI: Michigan State University Press.

Webster, A. (2007). *Health, Technology and Society: A Sociological Critique*. New York: Palgrave Macmillan.

Whetton, S. (2005). *Health Informatics: A Socio-technical Perspective*. Melbourne: Oxford University Press.

REFERENCES

Aliz-e (2010). *Welcome to the Aliz-e Project* <http://www.aliz-e.org/>.

Asthma control? We've got an app for that (2010). 9 June <http://www.sciencedaily.com/releases/2010/06/100609201302.htm>.

Auton, F. (2009). The case for advertising pharmaceuticals direct to consumers. *Future Science*, *1*(4), 587–592.

BBC News (1998). *UK Child Vaccine Linked to Autism*. 27 February <http://news.bbc.co.uk/2/hi/uk_news/60510.stm>.

BBC News (2001). *Doctors Claim World First in Telesurgery*. 19 September <http://news.bbc.co.uk/2/hi/science/nature/1552211.stm>.

Benn, T.M. & Westerhoff, P. (2008). Nanoparticle silver released into water from commercially available sock fabrics. *Environmental Science and Technology*, *42*(11), 4133–4139.

Boseley, S. (2010). Andrew Wakefield found irresponsible by GMC over MMR vaccine scare. *Guardian*, 28 January <http://www.guardian.co.uk/society/2010/jan/28/andrew-wakefield-mmr-vaccine>.

Coles, L.S. (2010). The ethical basis for using human embryo stem treatment for aging. In G.M. Fahy, M.D. West & L.S. Coles (eds), *The Future of Aging. Pathways to Human Life Extension* (pp. 63–86). New York: Springer.

Commerce Commission New Zealand (2011). *First Mobile Monitoring Report Shows Encouraging Early Trends*. Retrieved 28 October 2011 from <http://www.comcom.govt.nz/telecommunications-media-releases/detail/2011/first-mobile-monitoring-report-shows-encouraging-early-trends>.

Corney, D. (2011). *Withings Releases iPhone Blood Pressure Monitor*. 20 June. Retrieved 11 November 2011 from <http://news.cnet.com/8301-17938_105-20072505-1/withings-releases-iphone-blood-pressure-monitor/>.

Deer, B. (2010). Wakefield's 'autistic enterocolitis' under the microscope. *British Medical Journal, 340*(1127).

Deer, B. (2011). How the case against the MMR vaccine was fixed. *British Medical Journal, 342*(5347).

Fox, S. (2011). *The Social Life of Health Information, 2011* <http://pewinternet.org/Reports/2011/Social-Life-of-Health-Info.aspx>.

Fox, S., Rainee, L., Horrigan, J., Lenhart, A., Spooner, T., Burke, M., et al. (2000). *The Online Health Care Revolution: How the Web Helps Americans Take Better Care of Themselves* <http://www.pewinternet.org/PPF/r/26/report_display.asp>.

Franklin, U. (1999). *The Real World of Technology* (rev. edn). Toronto: House of Anansi Press.

Freed, G.L., Clark, S.J., Butchart, A.T., Singer, D.C. & Davis, M.M. (2010). Parental vaccine safety concerns. *Pediatrics, 125*, 654–659.

Frosch, D., Kruegar, P., Hornick, R., Cronholm, P. & Barg, F. (2007). Creating demand for prescription drugs: a content anlaysis of television direct-to-consumer advertising. *Annals of Family Medicine, 5*(1), 6–13.

General Medical Council (2010). *Dr Andrew Jeremy Wakefield: Determination on Serious Professional Misconduct (SPM) and Sanction* <http://www.gmc-uk.org/news/306.asp>.

Gilbody, S., Wilson, P. & Watt, I. (2005). Benefits and harms of direct to consumer advertising: a systematic review. *Quality and Safety in Health Care, 14*, 246–250.

Godlee, F. (2011). The fraud behind the MMR scare. *British Medical Journal, 342*(1), 22.

Goldacre, B. (2008). *Bad Science*. London: Harper Perennial.

Harmon, A. (2010). A soft spot for circuitry. *New York Times*, 4 July <http://www.nytimes.com/2010/07/05/science/05robot.html?pagewanted=all>.

Hollon, M.F. (2005). Direct-to-consumer advertising: a haphazard approach to health promotion. *Journal of the American Medical Association, 293*, 2030–2033.

Hornyak, T. (2010). *Robot companions to befriend sick kids at European hospital*. 1 September <http://spectrum.ieee.org/automaton/robotics/artificial-intelligence/robot-companions-to-befriend-sick-kids-at-european-hospital>.

Laerdal (2008). *Training Products: Patient Simulators* <http://www.laerdal.com/document.asp?docID=1022609>.

Moynahan, R. (2005). The marketing of a disease: female sexual dysfunction. *British Medical Journal, 330*, 192–194.

Murata, T., Kanao-Koshikawa, M. & Takamatsu, T. (2005). Effects of Pb, Cu, Sb, In and Ag contamination on the proliferation of soil bacterial colonies, soil dehydrogenase activity, and phospholipid fatty acid profiles of soil microbial communities. *Water Air Soil Pollution, 164*, 103–118.

Murch, S.H. (2003). Separating inflammation from speculation in autism. *Lancet, 362*(9394), 1498–1499.

Murch, S.H., Anthony, A., Casson, D.H., Malik, M., Berelowitz, M., Dhillon, A.P., Tomson, M.A., Valentine, A., Davies, S.E. & Walker-Smith, J.A. (2004). Retraction of an interpretation. *Lancet, 363*(9411), 750.

Nanotechnology (n.d.). *NewScientist.* Retrieved November 2011 from <http://www.newscientist.com/topic/nanotechnology>.

O'Reilly, T. (2005). *What is Web 2.0?* <http://oreilly.com/web2/archive/what-is-web-20.html>.

Pappas, S. (2011). *Health App Downloads Soar, But Do They Work?* <http://www.livescience.com/13328-health-smartphone-apps-weight-loss-quit-smoking.html>.

Paro Therapeutic Robot (2011). *Paro Therapeutic Robot* <http://www.parorobots.com/index.asp>.

Turkle, S. (2007). Can you hear me now? *Forbes.* 5 July <http://www.forbes.com/forbes/2007/0507/176.html>.

Wakefield, A.J., Murch, S.H., Anthony, A., Linnell, J., Casson, D.J., Malik, M. & Walker-Smith. J.A. (1998). Ileal-lymphoid-nodular hyperplasia, non-specific colitis, and pervasive developmental disorder in children. *Lancet, 637–41*, 351.

Webster, A. (2007). *Health, Technology and Society: A Sociological Critique.* New York: Palgrave Macmillan.

Weizenbaum, J. (1976). *Computer Power and Human Reason.* San Francisco: W.H. Freeman.

Wijnhoven, S.W.P., Peijnenburg, W.J.G.M., Herberts, C.A., Hagens, W.I., Oomen, A.G., Heugens, E.H.W., Roszek, B., Bisschops, J., Gosens, I., Van De Meent, D. et al. (2009). Nano-silver: a review of available data and knowledge gaps in human and environmental risk assessment. *Nanotoxicology, 3*(2), 109–138.

Women's Health Action Trust (2006). *Direct-to-consumer Advertising of Prescription Medications in New Zealand.* Auckland: Women's Health Action Trust.

World Health Organization (1978). Declaration of Alma-Ata. Paper presented at the International Conference on Primary Health Care, Alma-Ata, USSR.

World Health Organization (1981). *Global Strategy for Health For All by the Year 2000.* Geneva: World Health Organization.

World Health Organization (1986). The Ottawa Charter for Health Promotion. Paper presented at the First International Conference on Health Promotion, Ottawa, Canada.

World Health Organization (2006). *Working Together for Health* <http://www.who.int/whr/2006/en/>.

WEBSITES

<www.biotechlearn.org.nz/>

Biotechnology Learning Hub NZ.

<www.cdc.gov/vaccines>

The Centers for Disease Control and Prevention (CDC).

<http://fhti.org/>

The Future of Health Technology Institute, focusing on key technologies and challenges to the future of global healthcare to enhance health and lives.

<http://www.ncirs.edu.au/immunisation/education/mmr-decision/index.php>

National Centre for Immunisation Research and Surveillance.

<http://ocw.mit.edu/OcwWeb/Health-Sciences-and-Technology/HST-921Spring-2007/CourseHome/index.htm>

Massachusetts Institute of Technology.

<http://videolectures.net/i2010conf_smits_eheal/>

Topic on e-health on Vidoelectures.net website.

READING 30

Gender and Wellbeing

KIRK REED, CHRIS TAUA AND SUE WALKE

CHAPTER OVERVIEW

This chapter covers the following topics:

- Understanding differences between male and female
- Feminism and patriarchy
- Gender and identity in Aotearoa New Zealand
- Gender in relation to health and disability
- Gender-related issues

KEY TERMS

Discrimination
Fa'afafine
Feminist/feminism
Gay
Gender/gender identity
Homosexual
Lesbian
Male and female
Masculinity and femininity
Medicalised
Metrosexual
Morbidity
Patriarchy
Postmodernist
Sex
Sexism
Sexual orientation
Social construction
Socioeconomic status
Sociology

To begin any discussion on gender in relation to health, it is essential to establish the distinction between the terms **sex** and **gender** and realise they are not synonymous. Sex describes the genetic, physiological or biological characteristics of people, which indicates whether they are **male** or **female**. Sex refers to the biologically recognised differences between men and women, related to reproduction.

UNDERSTANDING DIFFERENCES BETWEEN MALE AND FEMALE

The term gender refers to the **social construction** of being feminine or masculine: our identity. Gender must then be understood 'as a structure of social relations, particularly power relations' (Connell, 2000, p. 8). Gender is a social category that defines the social and cultural construction of **femininity** and **masculinity** in society, justifying the differential allocation of resources and power (Ostlin, 2002).

Given that the word gender refers to the differences between men and women, masculinity or feminity, it is therefore often used to describe a sexual stereotype. In social sciences it often refers specifically to social differences between the genders, and is commonly referred to in relation to gender roles. **Gender identity** is about how people see themselves, an individual's own sense of being masculine or feminine. Those people whose gender identity feels incongruent with their physical bodies may describe themselves as transgender or genderqueer. **Feminist** thinking argues that many gender roles are socially constructed; that is, determined by society rather than the individual. In this chapter we will explore the differences between male and female, feminine and masculine, and how they are socially constructed in Aotearoa New Zealand.

FEMINISM AND PATRIARCHY

Feminism is the organised movement that began in the 1960s to promote equality for men and women in political, economic and social spheres. Throughout history men have had greater power in both the public and private spheres (the system known as **patriarchy**). To maintain this power, it is suggested that men created boundaries and obstacles for women, thus making it harder for women to hold power. It is important, though, to realise that this system does not only apply to women, but also wherever there is an unequal access to power; for example, the oppression of minority groups, such as people who identify as **homosexual**. Essentially, though, if there is one characteristic that defines patriarchy, it is not just biology or the actual male control of society, but rather a structure of a social organisation with a powerful dogma or a dominator at the top and less powerful individuals or groups underneath (White, 2002).

Feminist ideology has taken on many different forms. In the 1970s women began to propose a theory to explain their oppression and thereby challenge the concepts and constructs of patriarchy. By the 1980s feminists started disagreeing on particular issues linked to feminism. What was once one theory began to branch out into a diversity of theories focusing on feminist issues. Today, there are many definitions of feminism, and each one depends on a number of factors, including not only its purpose, but also beliefs, history and culture.

Socialist feminists believe that although women may be divided by class, ethnicity, race and religion, they all experience the same oppression simply because they are women. However, while socialist feminists challenge the patriarchal ideologies, rather than focusing primarily on women they concentrate on a broader context, and believe that the way to end oppression is to put an end to class and gender difference and to function side by side with men as opposed to excluding them (Welch, 2001). They promote collaboration and a consideration of each other as equals.

Cultural feminists express beliefs regarding primary biological differences between men and women, emphasising that women should celebrate these differences. Cultural feminists suggest that Western society values male thought and the ideas of independence, hierarchy, competition and domination. Cultural feminists are usually non-political, and focus instead on transforming society through individual change. The cultural feminist believes that females value ideas such as interdependence, relationships, cooperation and community, and argues that these ideas are not always valued in contemporary Western societies (Alcoff, 1994). They espouse that women are inherently more kind and gentle, advocating that if women ruled the world, it might be a better place. While not supporting a complete disconnection, cultural feminists generally advocate separate female countercultures as a way to change society.

FEMINISM AND HEALTH

In relation to health, feminists have explored how medicine itself is filled with tensions, contradictions, ambiguities and uncertainties, and feminist scholars have also uncovered ways in which medicine has also been beneficial to women (Barry & Yuill, 2002). Feminist scholars and activists examine ways in which medicine produces diagnoses and treatments that are harmful to women.

A common aspect of women's lives that has been **medicalised** is their reproductive capability. A medical textbook from the nineteenth century suggested:

> childbearing is essentially necessary to the physical health and long life, the mental happiness, the development of the affections and whole character of women. Woman exists for the sake of the womb (Holbrook, 1871, pp. 13–14, cited in Marks et al., 2005, p. 39).

Barry and Yuill (2002) argue that women have been depicted in textbooks and scholarly reports in negative clichéd ways that are neither objective nor value free. The fundamental feminist argument in relation to health is that 'medicine and patriarchy control women by enforcing passivity, dependence, and submission as appropriate feminist traits' (White, 2002, p. 130). The roots of this thinking from early medical teachings are premised on the idea that women were simply lesser versions of men, and that data on the male body was therefore acceptable for both sexes. When male norms influence health service delivery and health services provided to women, women's bodies will always be seen as flawed.

The history of medical beliefs regarding menopause also saw extremes of either dismissal of symptoms, treating it as an illness requiring a pharmacological response, or offering some psychological explanation. The problem then is that a normal developmental function of women becomes medicalised, seen as requiring a medical solution, and the normal aspects of a woman's life, such as fertility, sexuality, menopause and ageing, are pathologised.

MEN'S HEALTH FROM A GENDER PERSPECTIVE

Considering men's health from a gender perspective has been a challenge to some feminist sociological thinking. While early feminists were focused on acknowledging women as equal in health considerations, there is now recognition that for both theoretical and practical reasons, gender in relation to health must include both men and women. Indeed, to ignore men's health is to 'leave the dichotomy between men and women intact at a theoretical level and inhibit any political movement towards equity…' (White, 2002, p. 148). Ignoring the health of men might maintain the stance that men are well and women by contrast are sick. Returning also to the earlier assertion that men's bodies were the norm and women's were flawed, there is a paradoxical issue in that many men struggle to recognise, accept and respond to personal health concerns (White, 2002). Chronic illness is sometimes seen as a challenge to men's masculinity, as they are expected not to complain but to stay in control, and it is this issue that is played out frequently in studies around men's health. An obvious example of this is the late detection of prostate cancer.

HEALTH PROFESSIONAL RELATIONSHIPS AND GENDER ROLES

Traditional roles in health were the physician (doctor) and nurse relationship, where the physician was in a position of power and the nurse cast in a subservient role. Alongside this was a perceived social order between nurses and doctors in relation to gender, where men were predominantly doctors and women the nurses. Historically, nurses learnt early in their training that physicians were to be respected, and indeed feared, while physicians were trained to have an air of self-assurance. Nurses were thereby indoctrinated into their subservient role. Nurses sustained this in seeking praise and approval from the physicians. However, it seems this was not the actual intention of early nursing leaders, and that nurses were actually seen to have the skills of reflection and critical thinking. Schattschneider (2005) highlighted this in reviewing the Florence Nightingale era where

> the profession developed in a military context. Although nurses were expected to maintain their position of loyalty and obedience, they did question orders; since the nurses were expected to follow orders, they became adept at questioning in a way that allowed the physician to save face and to maintain ultimate authority (Schattschneider, 2005, p. 2).

Although medicine may continue to be seen as the dominant discourse in relation to health and disease, medical knowledge is now being challenged in **postmodernist** thinking as only one interpretation of reality. There are many more health professional roles in today's societies with diverse gender mixes. There is an ethic of liberation and a drive among health professionals to respect each other, share common goals and to work interprofessionally and in partnership with the client.

GENDER AND IDENTITY IN AOTEAROA NEW ZEALAND

The formation of gender identity is a complex process. As we discussed earlier, the notion of gender identity is a person's own sense of identification as masculine or feminine. The term gender identity is intended to distinguish between the psychological association with identity and the biological aspects of sex.

Sociology has reinforced a view of gender as 'something that we become; we are shaped into being feminine or masculine by powerful social structures' (Holmes, 2007, p. 40). These social structures that influence our understanding of gender include family, school, the media, politics and social interaction. The media particularly has a huge impact on our understanding and beliefs around gender. The prevalence of images in the mass media gives us an indication of who and what is valued in society. We see many more images of the tough guy rugby player than the softly spoken caring male. These expected roles of being tough or caring are reinforced by society's expectations of what being male means. However, the expectation that men are strong, tough, protect women and provide for their families is being disintegrated by women's own expectations of being capable of looking after themselves. It is now even more of a reality for many women, who either by choice or necessity, provide for themselves and their families. Images of women too are socially constructed. The media depicts women as being size 10 or smaller, glamorous and kindhearted.

In Aotearoa New Zealand we receive clear messages from an early age about the roles and occupations that are more masculine or feminine and how these define who we are. For example, working with or caring for people is considered more feminine, while those occupations that are more technical and require strength and dexterity, such as being a builder or farmer, are considered more masculine. These ideas also translate to our expectations of the sports and hobbies we engage in, which are passed down and across generations. As previously noted, the image of the tough guy rugby player is common in this country—rugby is considered to be a masculine sport. Not being interested in, or not having an understanding of, rugby has the potential to challenge a male's masculinity, just as being female and playing rugby leads to a female's femininity being challenged. Interestingly though, the rural–urban divide in Aotearoa New Zealand means that occupations in rural settings are undertaken by both men and women. A female farmer is just as likely to milk the cows or repair a fence. So if where we live determines what we do and how we perceive our gender identity, perhaps there is a perception that milking the cows and repairing a fence makes a female less feminine.

Not all people believe that their gender identity corresponds to their biological sex. The term genderqueer is used by people who identify as other than male or female. People who are genderqueer may think of themselves as falling outside the gender binary of male or female. This could be related to identity or could be biologically based. In some Pasifika societies **Fa'afafine** (a Samoan word meaning literally in the manner of woman) are considered to be a 'third gender' alongside male and female. Fa'afafine is accepted as a natural gender within many Pasifika societies, and is neither looked down upon nor discriminated against.

While the discussion so far has focused on gender, this should not be confused with **sexual orientation**. Homosexuality refers to sexual behaviour with, or an attraction to, people of the same sex. In general terms, **gay** commonly refers to male homosexuality and **lesbian** to female homosexuality, although the term gay is used by either gender. A person's sense of personal and social identity based on these attractions, behaviours and membership of a community is referred to as homosexuality. Therefore sexual orientation can be clearly distinguished from biological sex and gender identity, and as such should be considered separate.

Gender may also be considered on a continuum anywhere between the typical masculine and feminine roles. For example, individuals who identify as genderqueer may consider themselves at different places on the continuum. It is important to note that, as society changes, so do the ideas surrounding gender and identity. Since the 1990s the term **metrosexual** has come into use, and is seen by some as signifying the deconstruction of understandings of gender. The advent of the metrosexual, where it is more accepted for heterosexual men to take pride in their personal appearance, use skin care products and be aware of and express their feelings, is seen as a challenge to traditional ideas of masculinity.

These cultural changes in the environment and changing views on gender have been reinforced in the media through such television programmes as *Shortland Street*, *Happy Endings* and the talk show *Ellen* and in the increase in marketing material aimed at men to improve their appearance. In addition, traditional views on masculinity have been challenged in Aotearoa New Zealand by the *National Depression Initiative*, where ex-All Black John Kirwan features in a media campaign talking about his experiences of depression. The aim is to raise awareness and reduce the impact of depression, with a powerful message that it is acceptable for a tough rugby player to acknowledge vulnerability. This campaign not only gives a message about mental health issues but serves to break down the stereotypical views we have of what it means to be male and masculine in this country. These examples within the Aotearoa New Zealand media show understandings of gender are dynamic and are constantly being challenged.

GENDER IN RELATION TO HEALTH AND DISABILITY

We now know that gender is a social construction. This knowledge also relates to gender differences in health and disability. In relation to health, both sex and gender influence the differences in men's and women's health outcomes. In industrialised societies today, men die earlier than women (mortality) but women have poorer health (**morbidity**) than men. The main determinants of health are generally considered to be income, employment, housing, education, culture and ethnicity. It is within these areas that inequalities are revealed and women are often disproportionately represented at the lower end of the spectrum. Interestingly, where health services benefit women they often benefit the health of all, therefore gender may be considered a health determinant. Studies of health inequalities are a potentially useful gender-sensitive way of contributing to an understanding of the causes and effects of gender inequality.

When thinking about people with disabilities, the issues of both disability and gender need to be considered, and we argue that **discrimination** is a continuing issue for all people with disabilities. The New Zealand Disability Strategy describes disability as

> not something individuals have. What individuals have are impairments. They may be physical, sensory, neurological, psychiatric, intellectual or other impairments. Disability is the process which happens when one group of people create barriers by designing a world only for their way of living, taking no account of the impairments other people have (Ministry of Health, 2001, p. 1).

Men and women may experience disability differently. Disabled men may struggle with the cultural expectations that as males they should be strong, with a body that performs well. Similarly, women may struggle with expectations about reproducing and raising children (Sakellariou, 2006). Because New Zealand women live longer than men, they are more likely than men to have a disability. In the 1996–97 disability surveys, more than one-fifth (23.2 per cent) of all women aged 15 years or over reported at least one disability, and women represent 54.3 per cent of all adults with a disability in Aotearoa New Zealand (Statistics New Zealand, 2006).

Disabled people have often been assumed to be without gender or as asexual (not interested in sex) (Chance, 2002). For example, a disabled woman wanting to have a child may be seen by some in society as not being normal, as selfish or unable to care for a child. Not only is she discriminated against for being disabled but also for being a woman, so in a sense being a disabled woman may be seen as a double negative where the woman is subjected to **sexism** as well as disability bias. They are also less likely to be married or in a partnership, or are more likely to be left alone than disabled men. Disabled women may also be at greater risk of physical or sexual abuse. So you can see how gender stereotypes interact with disability stereotypes to create a deep set of complexities in society. Gender as a social construct can be even more oppressive for both men and women with disability.

WOMEN'S HEALTH STATISTICS AND ISSUES

Statistics show life expectancy outcomes for women in Aotearoa New Zealand have increased over time (Statistics New Zealand, 2004). However, the gap between males and females in terms of life expectancy is narrowing. Based on the mortality experiences of New Zealanders in the period 2007–09, life expectancy at birth for males was 78.4 years and for females 82.4 years. Since the mid 1980s gains in longevity have been greater for males than for females (Ministry of Social Development, 2010). There are also marked differences in life expectancy for Māori and non-Māori females. From 2005–07 the life expectancy for Māori females was 75.1 years compared with 83 years for non-Māori (Ministry of Social Development, 2010). Life expectancy at birth for Pacific Island females was estimated to be 6.5 years more than for Pacific Island males, and Asian females could expect to live about 5 years longer than Asian males.

The leading cause of death for women in Aotearoa New Zealand is cancer (Statistics New Zealand, 2004). There is scientific evidence that suggests breast cancer screening reduces deaths from breast cancer and that cervical screening reduces the risk of developing and dying from cervical cancer. This is why there are national screening programmes for these two cancers. Interestingly, while women typically fear breast cancer, the reality is that more die from lung cancer than from breast cancer. Cardiovascular disease is thought to be an additional concern for women, with more than half of female deaths over age 50 due to heart attacks, strokes and congestive heart failure, yet somehow these are still considered to be predominantly male conditions. Given the previous recognition that women live longer than men, we could expect that women might live longer with a disability, and may experience increased non-fatal chronic illnesses and more acute illnesses.

MEN'S HEALTH STATISTICS AND ISSUES

There are a number of health determinants that have an impact on the lower morbidity yet higher mortality rates for men. Lifestyle includes higher-risk sports pursuits, riskier employment activities and different coping mechanisms when unwell. Men are more at risk of accidents, injuries, suicide and some illnesses. The statistics for men of lower **socioeconomic status**, and men who live alone, are similar to the findings for women, in that they have more health problems, and Māori and Pacific men have been shown to have poorer health overall (Statistics New Zealand, 2004). Prostate cancer is an important health issue for men in Aotearoa New Zealand. It is the third most common cause of cancer mortality (13 per cent), following lung and colorectal cancer, and it is estimated that 500 men a year die of prostate cancer. Some health centres offer men-specific health checks. Males have a significantly higher rate of death by suicide than females, with an age-standardised rate of 17.4 deaths per 100 000 males in 2007, compared with 4.9 deaths per 100 000 females (Ministry of Social Development, 2010). Men are also less likely to visit a health professional, potentially missing out on opportunities for early detection and treatment for life-threatening illnesses. Men often find it difficult to talk to health professionals about their emotional worries or personal health concerns.

Both men's and women's health is affected by gender roles, and policies and programmes need to be sensitive to the impact of gender on exposure to health risks, health services utilisation and health outcomes. Risk factors such as exposure arising from labour segregation (both in the workplace and the home) and varied access to social and economic resources contribute to gender differences in health outcomes. We need to understand better how gender influences health inequalities in order to develop gender-sensitive policies and programmes that are more effective at reducing socioeconomic and ethnic inequalities in health between men and women, as well as among men and among women. The best sources of information to gain an understanding of gender-related health and disability issues is through data available through the Ministry of Health website <www.moh.govt.nz> and Statistics New Zealand <www.stats.govt.nz>.

A GENDER-RELATED ISSUE: FAMILY VIOLENCE

While there are many gender-related issues in contemporary Aotearoa New Zealand society, family violence is one that receives significant media attention. Family violence is a gender-related health issue that is so serious the government has created strategies, budget and advertising to raise awareness in an attempt to address it. Most family violence is perpetrated by males and most victims are females (Busch & Robertson, 2000).

Statistics New Zealand reported in 2006 that:

- one woman is killed by her partner or ex-partner every five weeks
- ten children are killed every year in acts of domestic violence

- half of all female homicides are the result of domestic violence
- domestic violence is the fifth leading cause of death in Aotearoa New Zealand.

Family (or domestic) violence is considered by the 1995 *Domestic Violence Act* (New Zealand) to be violence by one person against another with whom he or she has or has been in a domestic relationship. Family violence instils fear in order to control, coerce, manipulate or dominate others. Violence is a form of power and control that makes victims fearful and afraid.

Many people and groups of people may be affected by family violence. Violence crosses all boundaries of gender, age, race, culture and socioeconomic status. Members of marginalised groups, such as disabled people and migrants, may be particularly at risk. Family violence includes intimate partner or ex-partner abuse, sexual abuse, physical abuse, psychological–emotional abuse, homicide, child abuse and neglect, elder abuse and neglect, violence towards parents, sexual assault and rape, sibling violence and incest, financial exploitation, same-sex partner abuse, and neglect. Women are the victims in most of these situations.

The cost of family violence on health and wellbeing in Aotearoa New Zealand is immense. Conservative estimates indicate that the financial cost of family violence in this country is of the order of approximately $4–5 billion per annum. This cost is partially comprised of the following: greater use of health services; significant use of police and court time by perpetrators of family violence; greater use of mental health services by both victims and perpetrators; and loss of income and work for employees through family violence. The Domestic Purposes Benefit (DPB) was introduced in the 1970s to provide financial support to a sole parent caring for dependent children. This enabled women with violent partners to be financially independent if they chose to leave the relationship. The government funds family violence intervention coordinator positions in all District Health Boards (DHBs), and the Violence Intervention Programme (VIP) supports health sector family violence programmes throughout Aotearoa New Zealand. Advertising campaigns such as 'Are You OK?' are designed to raise awareness of family violence and to encourage people to come forward and seek help.

CASE STUDY 15.1

GENDER INEQUALITY IN DISABILITY HEALTHCARE

That people with intellectual disability (ID) have a much higher risk for developing mental illness is well known. What is less known are the specific risk factors women with ID face in regard to developing mental illness. It has been suggested that this group of women may have higher rates of mental illness compared with women without ID. In response to this, Taggart and colleagues (2010) undertook a study to dispel the myths that women with ID were 'a gendered' [sic] and 'a sexualised' [sic]. They explored perceptions of staff working with this population in relation to the possible risk factors facing women with ID, revealing several interrelated risk factors. First, having both an ID and being female led to experiences of 'exploitation, abuse, stigmatisation and made to feel different' (p. 93). Alongside this were negative feelings of not fitting the normal female roles of their mothers and sisters, not having a boyfriend or children and not having the freedom to live away from home. This notion of being different was found to lead to self-esteem issues and increased vulnerability to mental illnesses such as depression. Even more disturbing was the disempowerment that arose from abuse, emotional mistreatment and sexual abuse that occurred within their families and relationships. Hormonal issues were also particularly relevant for this group, in that many women with ID have very little understanding of their body and hormonal changes over the lifespan. Taggart and colleagues (2010) suggested that the use of hormone replacement therapy was almost nonexistent for this group of women.

It is acknowledged that these findings are not completely exclusive to women with ID; however, the evidence is that these women experience these issues to a much greater extent than the non-ID group, yet their needs as females are often ignored or not considered. Taggart and colleagues (2010) refer to gender-blind ID services, suggesting that staff need to use gender-sensitive assessment tools, and have knowledge of gender-specific agencies for referral to ensure best care and effective response to gender-particular needs.

SUMMARY

Coming to understand the differences between sex and gender requires delving into the historical context in which understandings about gender have emerged over time. Recognising that gender is a construct informed by social structures creates an opportunity to explore how gender is considered on a continuum, typically between masculine and feminine, but with many combinations in between. It is also important to recognise that traditional ideas about gender are challenged and reframed as society develops. The notion of how power relationships show themselves in relation to gender has been explored; in particular, how power contributes to understandings of health, health inequalities and the way in which health services are delivered. Issues related to gender and wellbeing are raised for consideration, along with how, as we come to new understandings of gender, these have the potential to influence the way in which health services are funded and delivered along with fundamentally changing the way in which we understand and view health and wellbeing.

CRITICAL QUESTIONS

Cultural lens

- **How** is gender viewed in Māori, Pacific and Pākehā traditions, and how is it related to wellbeing?

Social lens

- **What** are the community impacts of not appreciating or acknowledging gender differences and preferences?

Gender lens

- **Why** are the concepts of gender and sex confused, and what are the impacts of using the terms interchangeably?

Political lens

- **What** changes would need to occur to officially recognise the difference in health and disability outcomes for males and females in Aotearoa New Zealand?

Moral lens

- **How** should decisions about gender-related support services and resources be made and evaluated?

Media lens

- **What** gendered assumptions about health are regularly presented in the media?

FURTHER READING

Appignanesi, L. (2009). *Mad, Bad and Sad: A History of Women and the Mind Doctors from 1800 to the Present*. London: Virago.

REFERENCES

Alcoff, L. (1994). Cultural feminism versus post structuralism: the identity crisis in feminist theory. In N. Dirks, G. Eley, & S. Ortner (eds), *Culture, Power, History: A Reader in Contemporary Social Theory* (pp. 96–122). Princeton, NJ: Princeton University Press.

Barry, A.M. & Yuill, C. (2002). *Understanding Health: A Sociological Introduction*. London: Sage.

Busch, R. & Robertson, N. (2000). Innovative approaches to child custody and domestic violence in New Zealand: the effects of law reform on the discourses of battering. *Journal of Aggression, Maltreatment and Trauma*, *3*(1), 269–99.

Chance, S. (2002). To love and be loved: sexuality and people with physical disabilities. *Journal of Psychology and Theology*, *30*(3), 195–208.

Connell, R.W. (2000). *The Men and the Boys*. Cambridge: Polity.

Holmes, M. (2007). *What is Gender? Sociological Approaches*. Los Angeles: Sage.

Marks, D.F., Murray, M., Evans, B., Willig, C., Woodall, C. & Sykes, C. (2005). *Health Psychology: Theory, Research and Practice*. London: Sage.

Ministry of Health (2001). *The New Zealand Disability Strategy: Making a World of Difference: Whakanui Oranga*. Wellington: Ministry of Health.

Ministry of Social Development (2010). *2010 The Social Report: Te Purongo Oranga Tangata*. Wellington: Ministry of Social Development.

Ostlin, P. (2002). Gender perspective on socioeconomic inequalities in health. In J. Mackenbach & M. Bakker (eds), *Reducing Inequalities in Health: A European Perspective*. London: Routledge.

Sakellariou, D. (2006). If not the disability, then what? Barriers to reclaiming sexuality following spinal cord injury. *Sexuality and Disability*, *24*(2), 101–111.

Schattschneider, H. (2005). Power relationships between physician and nurse. *Journal of the Art and Science of Medicine*, *6*(3).

Statistics New Zealand (2004). *Women in New Zealand*. Wellington: Statistics New Zealand.

Statistics New Zealand (2006). *A History of Survival in New Zealand: Cohort Life Tables 1876–2004*. Wellington: Statistics New Zealand.

Taggart, L., McMilland, R. & Lawson, A. (2010). Staffs' knowledge and perceptions of working with women with intellectual disabilities and mental health problems. *Journal of Intellectual Disability Research*, *54*(1), 90–100.

Welch, P. (2001). *Strands of Feminist Theory* <http://pers-www.wlv.ac.uk/~le1810/femin.htm>.

White, K. (2002). *An Introduction to the Sociology of Health and Illness*. London: Sage.

WEBSITES

<www.hrc.co.nz>

Human Rights Commission.

<www.mwa.govt.nz>

Ministry of Women's Affairs.

<www.socialreport.msd.govt.nz>

The Social Report.

<http://www.who.int/topics/gender/en>

World Health Organization information on gender.

Interprofessional and Consumer Focus

DUNCAN REID AND BRENDA FLOOD

CHAPTER OVERVIEW

This chapter covers the following topics:

- Why interprofessional collaboration? An Aotearoa New Zealand perspective
- Interprofessional education (IPE) and collaborative practice (IPCP)
- Patient–client–family–community-centred care (consumer focus)
- Interprofessional communication
- Interprofessional teamwork
- Role clarification

KEY TERMS

Interprofessional collaboration
Interprofessional communication
Interprofessional teamwork
Patient–client-centred care
Primary healthcare
Role clarification
Secondary healthcare

Interprofessional working and thinking are among the most important current and future developments in healthcare and disability.

CASE STUDY 17.1

INTRODUCING MRS J.

Mrs J. is a seventy-eight-year-old woman who has lived alone for five years since her husband died. She has diabetes and an arthritic right knee. Two weeks ago she missed taking her medication for her diabetes and as a consequence had a reduction in her blood glucose levels (hypoglycaemia), which left her lightheaded. During this time she fell and scraped her leg badly against the coffee table in the lounge. Following the fall she was able to call her daughter who lives nearby, and she was admitted to hospital for one night's observation. She also received six stitches to the cut in her lower leg. Once she left hospital she was to have her leg dressed daily by a district nurse, and an occupational therapy home visit to review her home environment and ensure she was able to participate in those activities that she finds meaningful. She was also given a referral for the community physiotherapist to help with some leg-strengthening exercises, and she was supposed to have a review of her medications from her local general practitioner (GP). She is still a little confused since the fall, and has been anxious about leaving the house for fear of falling. Since being at home she has been visited by four different district nurses, two different physiotherapists and an occupational therapist. Her GP has been to visit and reviewed her diabetes medication, but he is a little concerned about her continued confusion and has referred her for a specialist geriatrician appointment. Mrs J. has commented to one of the district nurses that she is concerned. She has been telling her story of the fall and the subsequent treatment to all the health providers who have visited her this week and is getting confused as to whom she has told what.

What are your first thoughts?

- What do you think Mrs J.'s main goal for treatment might be? Has this been taken into consideration by the health professionals involved? Does she have a role in setting her own goals? Do you think this would be consistent with the health professional's goals?
- How can we be sure that all these health professionals have talked to each other and that the systems are in place to record this interaction?
- Which health professional should coordinate all this care?
- What are the consequences of this care not being coordinated?

Keeping this case study in mind, it is useful to reflect on these questions as you read the next sections of this chapter.

WHY INTERPROFESSIONAL COLLABORATION? AN AOTEAROA NEW ZEALAND PERSPECTIVE

Aotearoa New Zealand, along with many other developed countries in the world, has some significant challenges in the provision of healthcare presently and in the future. As a consequence of improved healthcare we have a population that is living longer, but is living with an increasing number of health conditions. Since the 1950s life expectancy for both men and women in New Zealand has increased by 8.8 and 9.6 years respectively (Zodgekar, 2005). The median age of the population is moving upwards in most developed countries, and the percentage of the population over 65 is increasing dramatically as Western societies reduce early age mortality and prolong life. New Zealand's population is ageing particularly rapidly, with the number of people over 65 predicted to increase from 18 per 100 today, to 45 per 100, within the working lifetime of today's new graduates, and by 2051 they will make up one-quarter or more of all New Zealand residents (Statistics New Zealand, 2007).

The changing demography of the population will have a profound effect on the provision of healthcare services over the next twenty years, with some suggesting a 40–69 per cent increase in demand by 2021 (New Zealand Institute for Economic Research, 2004). Quite clearly, the present healthcare systems, and their inherent workforce structures and design priorities, will need to undergo radical reform if the present working age populations are to expect adequate and ongoing care. Given the increasingly complex health issues that an ageing population produces, practitioners need to be prepared to work collaboratively.

Since 1978 the World Health Organization has promoted collaboration in primary care (see Declaration at Alma Ata <http://www.who.int/hpr/NPH/docs/declaration_almaata.pdf>). The general emphasis has been on promoting health for all. At that time, health professionals worked alongside each other in multidisciplinary teams, making decisions about client care separately. A second report (World Health Organization, 1988) emphasised the need for interprofessional learning and interdisciplinary teamwork. That report drew attention to the processes of collaboration. Health professionals who had been educated in isolation from each other had to learn how to collaborate and work together interprofessionally (McCallin, 2005). Collaboration has always been important for **primary healthcare** service delivery, as client needs have become increasingly complex and they need a larger number of health professionals with wide-ranging expertise to manage their care (Meads & Ashcroft, 2005; McCallin, 2005).

The New Zealand Primary Health Care strategy states, 'The world of primary health care is changing and old isolated ways of working must be replaced by new collaborative models' (Ministry of Health, 2001, p. 28). More recently, the latest international report, the *Framework for Action on Interprofessional Education and Collaborative Practice* (World Health Organization, 2010), suggests that **interprofessional collaboration** is essential to manage the global health workforce crisis. The worldwide shortage of 4.3 million health workers means that health workers (includes anyone involved in health service delivery) must be educated differently. 'The health workforce [needs to be] more flexible, and better prepared to maximise limited resources' (World Health Organization, 2010, p. 13). Clearly, the emphasis in collaborative practice has altered substantially. Given the lack of resources and increasing population demands placed on a smaller number of providers, the need to work more collaboratively with other health professionals is another concern for the future. One way of doing this is to engage in a greater level of interprofessional practice. This will require both new ways of education, but also new ways of practising collaboratively.

INTERPROFESSIONAL EDUCATION (IPE) AND COLLABORATIVE PRACTICE (IPCP)

The World Health Organization (2010) identifies some key messages in relation to interprofessional education and collaborative practice. These include:

> Interprofessional education occurs when students from two or more professions learn about, from and with each other, to enable effective collaboration and improve health outcomes. Interprofessional education is a necessary step in preparing a collaborative practice-ready health workforce that is better prepared to respond to local health needs.
>
> A collaborative practice-ready health worker is someone who has learned how to work in an interprofessional team and is competent to do so.
>
> Collaborative practice happens when multiple health workers from different professional backgrounds work together with patients, families, carers and communities to deliver the highest quality of care. It allows health workers to engage any individual whose skills can help achieve local health goals (World Health Organization, 2010, p. 7).

The World Health Organization recognises the need for a strong, flexible and collaborative global workforce to tackle positively the range of health challenges the world is currently facing. Collaboration when addressing maternal and child health; the detection, treatment and prevention of global diseases; the responses to humanitarian crisis; the management of epidemics and pandemics; the prevention and management of chronic conditions; and the contribution this makes to health systems, is an essential ingredient to improve health outcomes and strengthen health systems (WHO, 2010).

Providing an educational structure from which students and practitioners can develop an interprofessional worldview is important in order to ensure that optimal interprofessional learning occurs. One of the first challenges to working within an interprofessional and collaborative practice framework is that many tertiary education programmes continue to teach in silos, where each profession learns in isolation to others. This has a direct impact on the development of the student's professional worldview, as we are likely to assume the professional values, attitudes and knowledge modelled by those professionals we surround ourselves with. If, for example, a physiotherapy student spends all her or his time with other physiotherapists, she or he will increasingly see the world through the eyes of that profession, resulting in a limited ability to view the world from other perspectives, and may assume that her or his view is the correct one. Orchard (2010) summarises the findings from a number of authors, which suggests that myths and inaccuracies about other professions persist in the minds of students and are carried through into professional practice if they are not corrected early on in educational programmes. Other consequences of this narrowing of perspectives include **interprofessional communication** difficulties or misunderstandings (Charles et al., 2010).

In order for students to gain an understanding of interprofessional education and collaborative practice, an educational framework has been proposed (Charles et al., 2010). The first stage of the framework is Exposure, whereby students are exposed to the roles, contributions and differing perspectives of others and are introduced to the concept of interprofessional collaboration. The second stage is Immersion, where students begin to apply their knowledge and skills collaboratively with other students. Students at this stage have a greater confidence in their own professional identity and are considered to be more open to the views of others. The third and final stage is Integration, where students and/or practitioners are able to use and adapt their interprofessional knowledge and skills in the practice environment.

Figure 17.1: AUT interprofessional education model

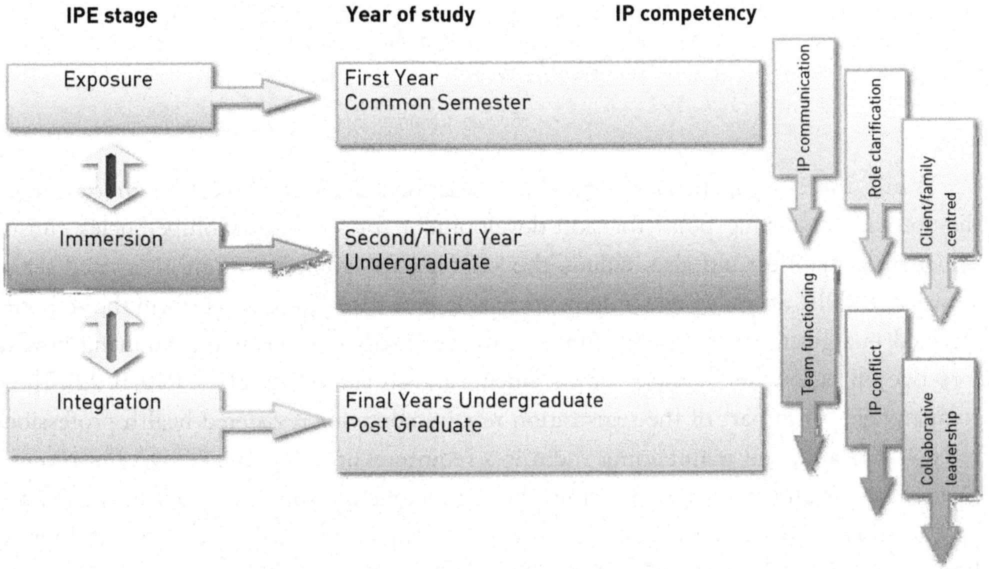

Source: adapted from University of British Columbia Model of Interprofessional Education (Charles et al., 2010).

Collaborative practice goes hand in hand with effective interprofessional education. The Canadian Interprofessional Health Collaborative (CIHC) has developed a competency framework that highlights the required skills, knowledge, attitudes and behaviours that aim to provide a practical guide for interprofessional education and collaborative practice (CIHC, 2010). There are six competency domains that have been described below; see Table 17.1.

Table 17.1: Summary of the Canadian Interprofessional Competencies

Competency	Description
Patient–client–family–community-centred care	'A partnership between the team of health providers and a patient where the patient retains control over his/her care and is provided access to the knowledge and skills of team members to arrive at a realistic team-shared plan of care and access to the resources to achieve the plan' (Orchard et al., 2010, p. 249)
Interprofessional communication	'Learners/practitioners from different professions communicate with each other in a collaborative, responsive and responsible manner' (CIHC, 2010, p. 16)
Team functioning	'Learners/practitioners understand the principles of teamwork dynamics and group/team processes to enable effective interprofessional collaboration' (CIHC, 2010, p. 14)
Role clarification	'Learners/practitioners understand their own role and the roles of those in other professions, and use this knowledge appropriately to establish and achieve patient/client/family and community goals' (CIHC, 2010, p. 12)
Collaborative leadership	'Learners/practitioners understand and can apply leadership principles that support a collaborative practice model' (CIHC, 2010, p. 15)
Dealing with interprofessional conflict	'Learners/practitioners actively engage self and others including the patient/client/family, in dealing effectively with interprofessional conflict' (CIHC, 2010, p. 17)

Source: Canadian Interprofessional Health Collaborative (2010)

While these competencies are being researched and are subject to modification, they provide a starting point for skill development for students. Competencies consist of personal qualities, and also include the 'ongoing development of an integrated set of knowledge, skills, attitudes, and judgments enabling one to effectively perform the activities required in a given occupation, or function to the standards expected in knowing how to [practice] in various and complex environments and situations' (CIHC, 2010, p. 22). These competencies form part of the registration requirements for registered health professions in New Zealand, and maintaining them is a requirement under the *Health Practitioners Competency Assurance Act* (2003). How the competencies are represented or articulated by the different registration bodies varies. For example, the NZ Occupational Therapy Board competency document, under Section 4.8, states under the overall communication competency that a therapist must develop effective and cooperative relationships within teams (including multidisciplinary teams) and with other workers and agencies <http://www.otboard.org.nz/Competence/CompetenceOverview.aspx>, whereas the NZ Physiotherapy Board competencies refer to 'contributing to relevant health professional teams' <http://www.physioboard.org.nz/docs/PHYSIO_Competencies_09_for_web.pdf>.

This means that undergraduate students who are exposed to interprofessional learning opportunities will not only need to be better prepared for future practice but also have the ability to ensure they retain these key competencies. Evidence shows that interprofessional education and collaborative practice result in improved health outcomes for communities and individuals in primary health and **secondary healthcare** settings (Reeves, 2001; Zwarenstein & Bryant, 2000). Curran and colleagues (2007) argue that interprofessional collaborative practice has the potential to increase efficiency and coordination of services, to enhance professional relationships and improve job satisfaction. More recently, Suter and Deutschlander (2010, p. 1) reported that 'there is sufficient evidence to suggest that interprofessional interventions improve workplace quality, provider satisfaction, student clinical placement and graduate employment choice, and strong evidence suggests that interprofessional interventions have cost benefits for patient care'. Overall, there is little doubt that health professionals need to be competent to deliver collaborative, patient-centred care.

To be an effective interprofessional practitioner it is essential to adopt the values that encourage and foster interprofessional collaboration. These are intrinsic within each of the competency domains, four of which will be discussed in more depth below.

PATIENT–CLIENT–FAMILY–COMMUNITY-CENTRED CARE (CONSUMER FOCUS)

This approach to delivering services firmly locates the client at the centre of interactions. It is achieved by actively engaging the patient, client, family and community in the process of care, through promoting participation, sharing and providing information in a way that is respectful and supports understanding, focusing on the person rather than solely on the disease or impairment, as well as learning about and listening to the needs of all parties involved in order to effectively shape services (Hammick et al., 2009, CIHC, 2010; Orchard, 2010; Reeves et al., 2010). Working in this way implies a shared vision, where the team and the patient, client, family and community work together to achieve goals.

In order to genuinely implement **patient–client–family–community-centred care**, practitioners need to have an understanding of the concept of power and the importance of enhancing power for their patient. Power is related to patients' ability to set their own goals, achieve objectives and effect outcomes, and gives control to individuals (Raatikainen, 1994; Swaffield, 1990). Sumsion and Law (2006) suggest that this balance of power needs to shift from the professional to the client in order to foster mutual interdependence and partnership.

A consumer focus can save time, enable time to be used more efficiently and enhance job satisfaction, but it is important that the appropriate organisational structures and attitudes are in place in order to effectively support patient–client–family–community-centred practice (Sumsion & Lencucha, 2009). This was also highlighted by Orchard and colleagues (2010, p. 254), who believe that 'The values within health organizations need to be underpinned by collaborative interprofessional patient-centred practice'. Some of the mechanisms, organisations and institutions put in place to achieve optimum collaborative practice include having clear protocols and policies that support teamwork; providing a culture where shared decision-making is the norm, and where regular team meetings and effective communication and information strategies are in place; and that a suitable shared physical environment is provided to enable practitioners to work in an interprofessional way (WHO, 2010).

INTERPROFESSIONAL COMMUNICATION

An essential part of working interprofessionally is the selection and effective use of different forms of communication. Communication within interprofessional teams can take many forms, from verbal and non-verbal to formal and informal, but the central focus or purpose of communication is to progress the patient's or client's care. Health professionals must develop skills for working with colleagues from other professions, so that they can communicate effectively with each other and work together to improve patient–client care. Some of these required skills include; being an active listener, ensuring that interactions are fully focused on the person; using questioning to clarify issues to ensure meanings are understood and shared; being aware of body language; and having the skills to provide effective feedback (Hammick et al., 2009).

Between 1995 and 2004, communication failures were identified as the leading root cause for medication errors, delays in treatment and wrong-site surgeries, as well as the second most frequently cited root cause for operative and postoperative events and fatal falls in Canada (Joint Commission on Accreditation of Healthcare Organizations, 2005). Formal communication can be facilitated through regular team meetings (Youngwerth & Twaddle, 2011), and can assist with breaking down professional barriers, assist with developing effective relationships and resolving conflicts. Informal communication can be as important, and is often reliant on members working within the same geographical area. Opportunities for informal communication can assist with the development of interpersonal relationships and the development of trust and respect within the team.

INTERPROFESSIONAL TEAMWORK

As highlighted by the World Health Organization (2010), working collaboratively in teams can make a positive contribution to some of the world's most urgent and significant health challenges. Working as a team member sits at the centre of interprofessional collaboration. Collaboration is a highly complex form of communication, and is a key element of **interprofessional teamwork,** which requires a significant degree of interaction. In order to understand interprofessional teamwork it is useful to consider the different types of collaboration evident within different types of teams represented in health and social care. A collaborative continuum is a useful way of conceptualising the levels of collaboration undertaken by different teams, although the amount of collaboration may change depending on the specific context and complexities in relation to the issues at hand. Therefore the teams may move up and down the continuum (see Figure 17.2).

A multidisciplinary team (MDT) is one where health professionals representing different health and social care professions may work closely with one another, but may not necessarily interact, collaborate or communicate effectively (Atwal & Caldwell, 2006). They are typically hierarchical in structure, where the professional identities of the members are placed above team membership (Youngwerth & Twaddle, 2011). They have described MDTs as working like 'wedges of a pie', where there is a clearly defined membership in the team but their contributions may be in relative isolation from each other. Orchard (2010) believes that most practice is multidisciplinary, where each discipline assesses and plans patient care independently, but will meet with other team members to discuss individual care plans primarily for information-sharing purposes.

An interdisciplinary team (IDT) is a term for which a consensus on the definition of which is not apparent from the literature; however, there are a number of perspectives that have been outlined below. Interdisciplinary collaboration was a term used in the 1970s, coming from evidence that suggested better coordination and collaboration in the health services saved lives (Yeager, 2005). It has also been described as an interpersonal process that leads to the achievement of specific goals that would not normally be achieved by a single team member (Wittenberg-Lyles et al., 2010). Reeves and colleagues (2010, p. xiii) describe it as 'the collaborative efforts undertaken by individuals from different disciplines such as psychology, anthropology, economics, geography, political science and computer science'. It would appear to involve a wider range of 'disciplines' than would traditionally be considered within health and social care arenas. The term 'interdisciplinary team' is often used synonymously with 'interprofessional teams', both in practice and in the literature. More recently it would appear that the literature supports the use of 'interprofessional', with little reference made to interdisciplinary teamwork.

An interprofessional team (IPT) has been described by Reeves and colleagues (2010) as occurring when two or more different health and/or social care professionals work in an interdependent and integrated way to problem-solve and provide services. It involves a high level of collaboration, which requires an active and ongoing partnership, between team members who come from diverse backgrounds (Freeth et al., 2005). Freeth and colleagues (2005) identified a number of key aspects underpinning interprofessional teamwork. These include having clear team goals, a shared commitment, role clarity, interdependence, open communication, teambuilding opportunities, mutual respect and regular team meetings. Orchard (2010) has identified a shift towards collaborative practice where all health professionals come together with the patient, developing and working towards a shared plan of care. Interprofessional teamwork involves continuous interaction and the sharing of knowledge to solve issues, while at the same time attempting to maximise patient–client participation.

A transdisciplinary team (TDT) occurs where 'team members share information among each other so that the boundaries of each discipline begin to be removed and professionals gain skills in other practice areas' (Batorowicz & Shepherd, 2008, p. 613). This collaboration enables members to utilise not only their own specialist skills and knowledge but also allows them to assimilate the knowledge and skills of other team members (Bell et al., 2009). Discussions are made rich through knowledge gained from working with other professionals (Batorowicz & Shepherd, 2008). Members develop trust and confidence in each other to overcome traditional boundaries and adopt a more holistic approach. The development of this type of team may require long-term commitment among professionals to build trust and establish mechanisms for regular and consistent communication.

In a review of research into the benefits of the different team approaches, Bell and colleagues (2009) identified that the more collaborative team models had advantages for both the teams and the patient–client–whānau–community that they served, as compared to the multidisciplinary team model. Some of these advantages included better team cohesion, cooperation, communication, integration, participation and satisfaction.

Figure 17.2: Suggested collaborative continuum

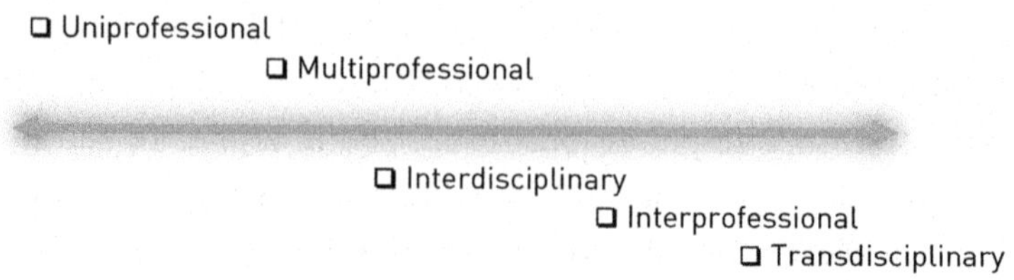

- ❑ Uniprofessional
- ❑ Multiprofessional
- ❑ Interdisciplinary
- ❑ Interprofessional
- ❑ Transdisciplinary

ROLE CLARIFICATION

Role clarification is the understanding health professionals have of their own professional role and the roles assumed by other disciplines within the team, which support the establishment and achievement of patient–client-centred goals (Orchard et al., 2005). The formation and maintenance of clear roles is considered important in maintaining effective team performance and relationships (Reeves et al., 2010).

Practitioners who understand what other health professionals do and their role in the care of patients have a better idea of how to provide a coordinated approach to the care. Often this requires a team leader or case manager to coordinate the processes, but other systems, such as access to and use of common patient records and generic assessment templates that capture relevant demographic and critical health information that all practitioners can access, are vital to effective care. Most of the critical incidents in the health area relate to a lack of information sharing and knowing what the key goals of treatment are.

CASE STUDY 17.2

WHEN THINGS GO WRONG

Mrs A. was a fifty-three-year-old woman who was referred by her GP to a specialist in his private practice following a ten-day history of acute abdominal pain. Following the specialist's examination he operated on her in a private hospital for a bowel obstruction. This appeared to resolve the issue but one month later the abdominal pain returned. Initially this was thought to be an infection and she was treated with antibiotics. The pain did not settle and five days later she was admitted to the private hospital again. On this occasion Mrs A. had her gall bladder and appendix removed. After the operation Mrs A. still complained of significant abdominal pain. She was treated with strong pain relief (pethidine) but deteriorated further, and nursing staff contacted the anaesthetist. He suggested not using this medication as it has strong sedative properties and an alternative pain relief was prescribed. With no further reduction in pain the on-call doctor was contacted. He did not contact the anaesthetist, and although he discussed the case with a nurse he prescribed pethidine for the pain. Over the next few days Mrs A. became increasingly unwell, and was seen on two more occasions by the original surgeon, who did not seem overly concerned and felt the pain was still mostly postoperative discomfort. The nursing staff continued to express their concern about the lack of progress, but received little feedback from the surgeon as to how to progress. There was also little information from the surgeon in Mrs A.'s notes as to how to proceed. Six days after the operation, as the pain continued to increase, Mrs A. was seen by yet another on-call doctor. He did a very brief assessment but did not change the management plan and indicated he would not be available for further consultations that day as he would be in surgery. He did not contact the original surgeon. By the end of day seven, despite the nurses requesting an urgent assessment from the surgeon, Mrs A. went into cardiac arrest, she was resuscitated and taken to theatre for emergency surgery. It was discovered she had a perforated bowel and significant internal infection. Following surgery she was admitted to the intensive care unit of the private hospital but did not improve and was transferred to the intensive care of a public hospital. She did not recover and died the next day.

Questions

- Was Mrs A. at the centre of the care here, and did she or her family have a say in the management plan?
- What aspects of effective team functioning were missing in this case?
- Was there a clear clarification of roles?
- Was the communication clear?
- Was there collaborative leadership?
- How was the interprofessional conflict around the lack of key decisions at key times managed?

In this case, the Health and Disability commissioner in his report concluded that the doctor should have recognised her postoperative complications at an earlier stage, and acted sooner. The commissioner concluded that the doctor had failed to provide Mrs A. services with reasonable care and skill, and failed to cooperate with other clinical staff to ensure quality and continuity of services. Accordingly, he breached Rights 4(1) and 4(5) of the *Code of Health and Disability Services Consumers' Rights* (the Code) (HDC Surgeon, Dr B, private hospital 06hdc13334 (2006), www.hdc.org.nz).

CASE STUDY 17.3

EXAMPLES OF INTERPROFESSIONAL EDUCATION AND COLLABORATIVE PRACTICE AT WORK

Akoranga Integrated Health (AIH)

AUT University has a teaching clinic on the Akoranga campus for undergraduate and postgraduate health students called Akoranga Integrated Health (AIH). This clinic has developed a project that promotes interprofessional collaboration. The project is centred on people with a chronic health condition, arthritis. AUT has developed a relationship with Arthritis NZ (a nongovernmental support group for those with arthritis who needed help and education). These people enter the project via a referral from Arthritis NZ or their general practitioner, or they can self-refer. Two or more students assess and work with these arthritis patients throughout their time in the clinic.

Interprofessional collaborative placement

Students from a number of different professions participate in an interprofessional placement with the Waitemata Primary Health Organisation (Waitemata PHO). The placement is based within a rural community, and provides students from different disciplines the opportunity to learn from, with and about each other. The placement aims to provide an environment where students are able to develop and modify attitudes and perceptions of interprofessional collaboration and teamwork; acquire some of the knowledge and skills required for interprofessional collaboration; as well as contribute to improvements in the health and wellbeing of individuals and groups within the local community. Students are provided with opportunities to better understand how interprofessional learning fosters interprofessional collaboration and improves health and social outcomes for clients, and they gain a greater understanding of the community and the people living in it. Their understanding of the models of primary health care (PHC) and community-centred care, with particular emphasis on the interprofessional model of care, are developed, as well as skills required for effective interprofessional teamwork.

Students are supported in their interprofessional learning through engagement in a range of activities. They live in shared accommodation from 4 to 12 weeks; they meet weekly for interprofessional education sessions that draw on their practice learning and experiences; they spend time with a wide range of other disciplines in the local community; and they work together on an interprofessional project that is relevant to the local community and individual students' learning needs.

The outcomes of this project have demonstrated that students leave the project with a greater understanding of the community health environment, greater understanding of their own profession and its interaction with other health providers and a desire to work in this area.

SUMMARY

The future provision of healthcare services in Aotearoa New Zealand faces significant challenges because an ageing population is living longer with an increasing number of illhealth conditions. It will not be possible to equip enough health professional to meet the needs of these people in the way that services are currently designed and delivered. One way to address this challenge is to improve the way in which future health professionals work together. There is a growing body of evidence that interprofessional education and collaborative practice is an appropriate strategy to ensure that services are effective and safe. In order to work this way, education of emerging health professionals must ensure they are competent in the areas of patient–client–family–community-centred care, interprofessional communication, have the skills to work as part of highly functioning teams, and understand their own and others' roles. The process to achieve this will involve exposure and theoretical education about the concepts, followed by immersion in areas of clinical practice, and developing integrated approaches to working with clients.

CRITICAL QUESTIONS

Cultural lens

- **Discuss** how culture has an impact on interactions among practitioners and with patients.

Social lens

- **What** level of collaboration is most likely to occur in any particular environment?

Gender lens

- **Are** teams of practitioners more likely to be led by men or women, and what would the differences be?

Political lens

- **What** organisational structures could be put into place to promote a patient–client-centred approach to care?

Moral lens

- **Do** you think health professionals always work from a patient–client–family-centred perspective? Why? Why not?

Media lens

- **How** could the public become better informed about interprofessional collaboration, learning and practice?

FURTHER READING

Humphris, D. (2007). Multiprofessional working, interprofessional learning and primary care: a way forward? *Advances in Contemporary General Practice Nursing Role of the Practice Nurse.* Special issue of *Contemporary Nurse, 26*(1), 48–55.

Humphris, D. (2008). Changing clinical care and workforce development. In A. Gray, P. Degeling & H. Colebatch (eds), *Changing Clinical Care: Experiences and Lessons of Systematisation* (pp. 211–223). Oxford: Radcliffe Publishing.

Humphris, D. & Macleod Clark, J. (2007). Embedding interprofessional learning in Hampshire and the Isle of Wight: the New Generation Project. In *Piloting Interprofessional Education: Four English Case Studies, Occasional Paper 8*. London: Higher Education Academy: Health Science and Practice.

REFERENCES

Atwal, A. & Caldwell, K. (2006). Nurses' perceptions of multidisciplinary team work in acute health-care. *International Journal of Nursing Practice, 12*, 359–365.

Bainbridge, L., Nasmith, L., Orchard, C. & Wood, V. (2010). Competencies for interprofessional collaboration. *Journal of Physical Therapy Education, 24*(1), 6–11.

Batorowicz, B. & Shepherd, T. A. (2008). Measuring the quality of transdisciplinary teams. *Journal of Interprofessional Care*, *22*(6), 612–620.

Bell, A., Corfield, M., Davies, J. & Richardson, N. (2009). Collaborative transdisciplinary intervention in early years: putting theory into practice. *Child: Care, Health and Development*, *36*(1), 142–148. doi:10.1111/j.1365-2214.2009.01027.x_1027 142.

Canadian Interprofessional Health Collaborative (CIHC) (2010). *A National Interprofessional Competency Framework*. Vancouver: Canadian Interprofessional Health Collaborative, University of British Columbia.

Charles, G., Bainbridge, L. & Gilbert, J. (2010). The University of British Columbia model of interprofessional education. *Journal of Interprofessional Care*, *24*(1), 9–18.

Curran, V.R., Sharpe, D. & Forristall, J. (2007). Attitudes of health sciences faculty members towards interprofessional teamwork and education. *Medical Education*, *41*(9), 892–896.

Freeth D., Hammick, M., Reeves, S., Koppel, I. & Barr, H. (2005). *Effective Interprofessional Education*. Oxford: Blackwell Publishing.

Hammick, M., Freeth, D., Copperman, J., Goodsman, D. (2009). *Being Interprofessional*. Cambridge: Polity Press.

Joint Commission on Accreditation of Healthcare Organizations (2005). *The Joint Commission Guide to Improving Staff Communication*. Oakbrook Terrace, IL: Joint Commission Resources.

McCallin, A.M. (2005). Interprofessional practice: learning how to collaborate. *Contemporary Nurse*, *20*(1), 28–37.

Meads, G. & Ashcroft, J. (eds) (2005). *The Case for Interprofessional Collaboration in Health and Social Care*. Oxford: Blackwell.

Ministry of Health (2001). *The Primary Health Care Strategy*. Wellington: Ministry of Health.

New Zealand Institute for Economic Research (2004). *Ageing New Zealand and Health and Disability Services: Demand Projections and Workforce Implications, 2001–2021: A Discussion Document*. Wellington: New Zealand Institute for Economic Research.

Orchard, C. (2010). Persistent isolationist or collaborator? The nurse's role in interprofessional collaborative practice. *Journal of Nursing Management*, *18*(3), 248–257.

Orchard, C., Curran, V. & Kabene, S. (2005). Creating a culture for interdisciplinary collaborative professional practice. *Medical Education Online*, *10*(11), 1–13 <http://www.med-ed-online.org>.

Orchard, C., King, G., Pallaveshi, L. & Bezzina, M.B. (2010). Assessing interprofessional health teams for their collaboration: a new instrument. Presentation. Sydney: All Together Better Health Conference. 7 April.

Raatikainen, R. (1994). Power or lack of it in nursing care. *Journal of Advanced Nursing*, *19*, 424–432.

Reeves, S. (2001). Community-based interprofessional education for medical, nursing and dental students. *Health and Social Care in the Community*, *8*(4), 269–276.

Reeves, S., Lewin, S., Espin, S. & Zwarenstein, M. (2010). *Interprofessional Teamwork for Health and Social Care*. Oxford: Blackwell Publishing.

Sladden, N. (2001). Ethics and professional responsibility. Presentation. Auckland: Medicine in the New Millennium: Fringe or Frontier? Aotea Conference Centre.

Statistics New Zealand (2007). *New Zealand's 65+ Population: A Statistical Volume*. Wellington: Statistics New Zealand.

Sumsion, T. & Law, M. (2006). A review of evidence of the conceptual elements informing client-centred practice. *Canadian Journal of Occupational Therapy*, *73*(3), 143–150.

Sumsion, T. & Lencucha, R. (2009). Therapists' perceptions of how teamwork influences client centred-practice. *British Journal of Occupational Therapy*, *72*(2), 48–54.

Suter, E. & Deutschlander, S. (2010). *Can Interprofessional Collaboration provide Health Human Resources Solutions?* <http://www.usask.ca/ipe/Documents/Suter%20Deutschlander%20et%20al%20IPC%20and%20HHR%20outcomes%20Final%20Report%20March%2023%202010%20%282%29.pdf>.

Swaffield, L. (1990). Patient power. *Nursing Times*, *86*(48), 26–28.

Wittenberg-Lyles, E., Oliver, D.P., Demiris, G. & Regehr, K. (2010). Interdisciplinary collaboration in hospice team meetings. *Journal of Interprofessional Care*, *24*(3), 264–73.

World Health Organization (1988). Learning together to work together for health. Report of a WHO study group on multiprofessional education for health personnel: The team approach. Technical Report Series, 769, 1–72. Geneva: World Health Organization.

World Health Organization (2010). *Interprofessional Education and Collaborative Practice.* Technical Report. Geneva: World Health Organization.

Yeager, S. (2005). Interdisciplinary collaboration: the heart and soul of health care. *Critical Care Nursing Clinics of North America*, *17*(2), 143–148.

Youngwerth, J. & Twaddle, M. (2011). Cultures of interdisciplinary teams: how to foster good dynamics. *Journal of Palliative Medicine*, *14*(5), 650–654.

Zodgekar, A.V. (2005). The 'greying' of Aotearoa New Zealand: policy implications of demographic change and structural ageing. In K. Dew & P. Davis (eds), *Health and Society in Aotearoa New Zealand.* Auckland: Oxford University Press.

Zwarenstein, M. & Bryant, W. (2000). Interventions to promote collaboration between nurses and doctors. *Cochrane Database* CD000072.

WEBSITES

<http://www.otboard.org.nz/Competence/CompetenceOverview.aspx>

Competencies for Occupational Therapists in Aotearoa New Zealand.

<http://www.physioboard.org.nz/docs/PHYSIO_Competencies_09_for_web.pdf>

Competencies for Physiotherapists in Aotearoa New Zealand.